THE BIRTH OF A GENETICS POLICY

T0271865

The Birth of a Genetics Policy
Social Issues of Newborn Screening

JOËLLE VAILLY

National Institute for Health and Medical Research,
Interdisciplinary Research Institute on Social Issues, France

Translated by Lucy Garnier

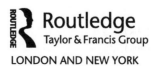

Routledge
Taylor & Francis Group

LONDON AND NEW YORK

First published 2013 by Ashgate Publishing

Published 2016 by Routledge
2 Park Square, Milton Park, Abingdon, Oxfordshire OX14 4RN
711 Third Avenue, New York, NY 10017, USA

First issued in paperback 2016

Routledge is an imprint of the Taylor & Francis Group, an informa business

British Library Cataloguing in Publication Data
A catalogue record for this book is available from the British Library

The Library of Congress has cataloged the printed edition as follows:
Vailly, Joëlle.
   [Naissance d'une politique de la génétique. English]
   The birth of a genetics policy : social issues of newborn screening / by Joëlle Vailly.
      pages cm
   Text in English, translated from French.
   Includes bibliographical references and index.
   ISBN 978-1-4724-2272-9 (hardback)
   1. Cystic fibrosis in children--Diagnosis--France.
   2. Newborn infants--Diseases--Diagnosis--France. 3. Medical screening--France.
   4. Medical genetics--Government policy--France. I. Title.

   RJ456.C9V3513 2014
   618.9237200944--dc23

                                            2013023949

ISBN 13: 978-1-138-27950-6 (pbk)
ISBN 13: 978-1-4724-2272-9 (hbk)

Contents

List of Abbreviations		*vii*
Preface		*ix*

Introduction   1
> The Importance of Health Issues and How Those Issues
> Are Evolving   5
> An Analytical Framework   7
> Screening Newborns   9
> Presentation of the Study   13

1   The Birth of a Screening Policy (Brittany-France)   21
> A Breton Tale   23
> History of a National Debate   44

2   On Scientific Grounds   57
> When Conviction Prevails   61
> Looking for Evidence   68

3   Governing   87
> Power Relations   91
> Governing in Time and Space   99

4   Extending Abnormality   119
> Techniques and Biological Abnormality   122
> Managing Uncertainty   129

5   Living with the Disease   143
> Paediatric Semantic Networks   146
> Social Life and Biological Life   154

6   Maintaining a Quality Life   169
> Gaining Time and Passing Time   170
> The Impact of Newborn Screening on Prenatal Diagnosis   182

Conclusion   197

References   *207*
Index   *223*

List of Abbreviations

AFDPHE	*Association française pour le dépistage et la prévention des handicaps de l'enfant* [French Association for Screening for and Preventing of Handicaps in Children]
AFLM	*Association française de lutte contre la mucoviscidose* [French Association against Cystic Fibrosis]
AFM	*Association française contre les myopathies* [French Association against Muscular Dystrophy]
CAF	*Caisse d'allocations familiales* [National Family Allowance Fund]
CCNE	*Comité consultatif national d'éthique pour les sciences de la vie et de la santé* [The National Consultative Ethics Committee for Health and Life Sciences]
CF	Cystic Fibrosis
CFTR	Cystic Fibrosis Transmembrane Conductance Regulator
Cnamts	*Caisse nationale d'assurance maladie des travailleurs salariés* [French National Health Insurance Fund for Employees]
CRCM	*Centre de ressource et de compétence de la mucoviscidose* [Centre of Resources and Competence in Cystic Fibrosis]
DGS	*Direction générale de la santé* [Department of Health]
DHOS	*Direction de l'hospitalisation et de l'organisation des soins* [Department of Hospitalization and Health Care Organization]
DRASS	*Direction régionale des affaires sanitaires et sociales* [Regional Department for Health and Social Affairs]
EBM	Evidence-Based Medicine
ERCF	European Epidemiologic Registry for Cystic Fibrosis
NSCF	Newborn Screening for Cystic Fibrosis
ONM	*Observatoire national de la mucoviscidose* [National Cystic Fibrosis Observatory]
RCT	Randomized Controlled Trial
VLM	*Vaincre la mucoviscidose* [Beating Cystic Fibrosis]
WHO	World Health Organization

List of Abbreviations

Preface

Fifty years ago this year Robert Guthrie, an American doctor, invented a technique for collecting blood samples from newborns on filter paper in order to carry out tests, thus allowing thousands of children to be protected from the harmful side effects of phenylketonuria, a rare genetic disease. In 2013, more than 50 conditions are now screened for at birth in the United States, most of which are genetic. An important stage in this rapid development was the 2005 report by the American College of Medical Genetics recommending screening for a panel of 29 core conditions and 25 secondary conditions. Today, certain States in the United States screen for diseases that affect people during their adult life as well as for little known conditions or those in which early screening presents limited benefits. Moreover, recent developments in rapid DNA sequencing, and the so-called 'chip' method, mean that genome sequencing of newborns is not such a distant possibility. In a context where screening meets with substantial public approval, particularly from parents of sick children, several national debates are now beginning to consider these genome-related technologies in terms of adapting them to newborn screening. At the same time, observers raise questions about the kind of information that should then be provided to parents, given the large quantity and considerable complexity of the data collected. As we shall see in this book, questions that arose due to changes in newborn screening find a new source in these genome-related techniques, and may even increase as a result. This book focuses specifically on newborn screening for cystic fibrosis (NSCF)[1] in France and many of the arguments that were successful in the debate about this screening programme are now called upon by those advocating an increase in newborn screening more widely. This screening programme for cystic fibrosis (CF) called directly upon DNA analysis in the case of an initial positive test, showing that genetic testing has already entered into the routine of clinical practices and public health.

Therefore, rather than focusing on spectacular medical practices such as new techniques of assisted reproductive technology or so-called synthetic biology, this book looks at seemingly ordinary practices linked to the medical genetics of today; practices that are advancing and yet remain outside of the limelight. However, despite the fact that newborn screening has increased considerably in both the United States and Europe, relatively few social science studies have looked at this question so far. The present study approaches this topic in an entirely new

---

1   When abbreviations involve French institutions or organizations, the French title is given along with the English translation.

fashion. It analyzes all at once the scientific knowledge, political dimensions and moral questions related to newborn screening, while also examining the interplay between these elements. The methodological framework for the study also takes an original form. It brings together ethnographic observation and sociological analysis, as well as questions from broader spheres. In doing so, this book creates a dialogue between biomedical anthropology, science and technology studies, sociology, and political and moral anthropology, while also fostering exchanges between the Anglo-Saxon and French social sciences.

Of course, certain aspects vary according to social and political contexts, and understanding how these practices are instituted in France may shed some light on certain differences between countries, such as how care provision is organized and the legal framework in place. That being said, there are striking similarities between countries in the field of biomedicine, where knowledge and arguments circulate quickly. Three examples among those outlined in this book can testify to this. First, a study carried out in the United States had a significant impact on the French decision to screen for CF. Second, on a European level, a consensus conference took the same position as the French paediatricians regarding so-called borderline forms of cystic fibrosis. Finally, the decrease in incidence of cystic fibrosis related to newborn screening that has been observed in France has also been noted in certain regions of the United Kingdom and Australia. Above and beyond newborn screening itself, this book looks to offer an account of what screening can tell us about broader societal changes. Indeed, the key issues analyzed in the context of France – evidence, government, norms, the links between the social and the biological, etc. – are also of much wider relevance.

Finally, this book is likely to be of interest to those who find that Michel Foucault's work provides fertile ground upon which to develop their own analyses. His work is used here as something of a 'tool box', as he himself recommended, while taking care to remain rooted within the social dynamics of the early twenty-first century – in other words, taking care to avoid fixing any form of Foucauldian dogma (which would be a somewhat inappropriate homage to a philosopher who displayed such concern for dynamics). Moreover, as we will see, this flexible approach makes it possible to develop a critical perspective that remains respectful of the actors involved, who often find themselves perplexed in the face of their own practices.

I would like to end these preliminary remarks with a few words of thanks. I would particularly like to express my deepest gratitude to Didier Fassin for his consistently sound advice and his constant attention, which both testify to his great academic and personal qualities. My thanks also go (in alphabetical order) to Jean-Paul Gaudillière, Thomas Lemke, Vololona Rabeharisoa and Didier Sicard for having agreed to read and comment on the study that led to this book, despite their extremely busy timetables. I am also very grateful to Vincent Boissonnat, Hélène Bretin, Cécile Ensellem, Boris Hauray and Carine Vassy for our many discussions. Thanks also to Anne-Claire Baratault for her invaluable help with documentary resources and to Lucy Garnier for her care and attention in translating this book. I would also like to thank the health professionals who gave generously of their time to answer my questions and enable my observations with a view to enlightening my research. I am also indebted to the different people, whether family members with sick children or not, who kindly agreed to talk to me about their lives and allowed me to be present during medical consultations. I would also like to express my gratitude to the members of the jury for the 'Le Monde' Prize for university research, who gave visibility to my work and to Marion Colas from the Presses Universitaires de France (PUF) who assisted me in the process of publishing this English version of my book *Naissance d'une politique de la génétique. Dépistage, biomédicine, enjeux sociaux*, published in French in 2011. Finally, I would like to dedicate this work to the people close to me who have given me strength, and who continue to do so, particularly the strength to change direction when necessary.

Joëlle Vailly, Paris, 20 February 2013.

Acknowledgements

This research received funding from the Gis-Institut des Maladies Rares. The translation was funded by the Institut de Recherche en Santé Publique, the MiRe-DREES, the Fondation Perharidy, and the Institut de recherche interdisciplinaire sur les enjeux sociaux (Iris).

Introduction

We are in a modern maternity hospital; uniformed staff move busily about. We can hear a voice saying, 'Now, only seconds old, the exact time and cause of my death was already known'. A drop of blood is taken from a newborn. A nurse in green hospital scrubs reads printed sheets emerging from a computer: 'Neurological condition, 60% probability; manic-depression, 42% probability; attention deficit disorder, 89% probability; heart disorder'... She looks over at the father... '99% probability. Early fatal potential. Life expectancy: 30.2 years'. 'Thirty years', the father murmurs.//

We see a little boy running in a garden. His mother calls to him; he falls. A voice says: 'From an early age, I came to think of myself as others thought of me: chronically ill. Every skinned knee and runny nose was treated as if it were life-threatening'.//

The parents and the little boy are in a very clean, extremely modern hospital. From the back we see a man behind a desk, explaining: 'Your extracted eggs, Marie, have been fertilized with Antonio's sperm. After screening, we are left, as you see, with two healthy boys and two very healthy girls. Naturally, no critical predispositions to any of the major inheritable diseases. All that remains is to select the most compatible candidate. First we may as well decide on gender'. The man rises: 'Have you given it any thought?' He sits down facing the parents. The mother: 'We would want Vincent to have a brother, you know, to play with'. The man smiles at the little boy sitting on the floor playing with the molecule models. ... The man: 'You have specified: hazel eyes, dark hair and fair skin. I have taken the liberty of eradicating any potentially prejudicial conditions: premature baldness, myopia, alcoholism and addictive susceptibility'. The father moves his head; the mother looks at him. The man continues: 'Propensity for violence, obesity, etc.'. The woman intervenes: 'We didn't want... I mean diseases, yes, but...' The father: 'We are just wondering if it's good to just leave a few things to chance'. The man: 'You want to give your child the best possible start. Believe me; we have enough imperfection built in already. Your child doesn't need any additional burdens'.

This is how the future of genetic screening was imagined in the North American film *Gattaca*, which came out in the late 1990s to considerable box-office success. The near-future depicted in the film was characterized by several notions: screening for a series of traits at birth, personalized life expectancy estimates, embryo choice and prenatal selection of genetic traits. This crude entertainment-industry vision of the issue sought to highlight the dangers of scientistic totalitarianism in a fantasy vision of the future. Let us see how recent history and developments in medical genetics gave a foothold to the film's projections.

In the second half of the twentieth century, biologists considered the genome – that is, the sum of an individual's genetic material – to be a programme that controlled the cellular events and characteristics of living beings. Although some geneticists were cautious in their statements, genetics was nonetheless supposed to influence how we conceived of a wide range of questions: abilities, handicaps, social problems, family relationships and the quality of life (Conrad and Gabe 1999). When the human genome sequence was established at the turn of the millennium, geneticists, particularly in North America, used rhetoric infused with a sense of the sacred, referring to the 'Holy Grail' and the 'Bible', thereby bringing social science researchers to speak of the 'DNA mystique' (Nelkin and Lindee 1994). However, it was precisely this sequencing that shook their certainties, for it did not provide the keys to the secrets of life that most of them had naively hoped for. The very concept of 'gene' became fragmented (Fox Keller 2000). It became necessary to develop more complex and less deterministic models based on the general notion that genetic and non-genetic factors mutually affect one another (Atkinson, Glasner and Lock 2009, Lock and Nguyen 2010). This shift towards greater complexity has given rise today to projects involving large banks of samples in order to understand the respective and combined roles of DNA and the environment in the etiology of multifactorial diseases. Research on 'epigenetics' is now developing, focusing on the effects of the environment on how DNA is used by cells and the inheritability of these changes in the absence of modified genetic sequences (Niewöhner 2011). Moreover, the range of psychiatric and psychological conditions considered to have a genetic component is widening. The molecularization of the living being is thus pursuing its path, integrating greater levels of complexity along the way, and the attention paid to DNA continues.

More broadly, the constituted knowledge called genetics spreads – albeit only in part – throughout societies. Even without taking into account new practices such as paternity tests, choosing embryo sex on the Internet, police identification methods and genetic information on people's origins, which are beyond the scope of this book, the dissemination of genetics knowledge manifests itself in several ways. Patient organizations and the media have their own ways of propagating knowledge about genetics, and the related hopes. In France, the *Association Française contre les Myopathies* (AFM – French Association against Myopathies), among others, actively contributes to 'concern about genes' in the population at large (Rabeharisoa and Callon 1999), thanks to the famous Téléthon, a television fund-raising event calling on viewers to show solidarity and compassion to patients with rare genetic diseases. The Téléthon mobilizes tens of thousands of volunteer workers and collects nearly 100 million euros every year. Anthropologist Paul Rabinow (1999: 39) has described the period during which, for the president of this patient organization, 'the "gene" became the key symbol, the embodiment of fate, the evil locus from which arose death and ruination of innocent life, and, simultaneously, the site of hope.' Obviously, the co-production of genetic culture within societies also affects decision-makers and political leaders. In this regard, it is of interest to recall the controversy triggered among biologists and sociologists alike by remarks made by presidential candidate Nicolas Sarkozy during his 2007 election campaign.[1] Sarkozy's words, which are consistent with a current of thought that is usually better represented in the United States than in France, expressed belief in the idea of a genetic predisposition to paedophilia and suicide. In sum, people are born paedophiles or suicidal, a representation that de-socializes those behaviours or acts. Private companies have joined in to defend and take advantage of that general understanding. In a context of internationally circulating ideas, knowledge, methods and biological materials, company investments in biotechnology have made great leaps in wealthy countries and the so-called developing countries alike (Rose 2008). In 2011, forty or so companies were selling genetic tests on the Internet (Ducournau and Beaudevin 2011). For a few hundred dollars (the average fee), they analyze their customers' genomes and inform them – so they claim – about predispositions to a great variety of diseases and traits: cystic fibrosis, Tay-Sachs disease, but also breast cancer, susceptibility to heart attack, obesity, in some cases manic-depressive tendencies, hyperactivity, alcohol-dependence, having an above-average IQ, etc. Meanwhile the press takes up stories of customers who have been reassured on certain points – 'I'm not at higher-than-average risk for cancer' – and made to worry about others: 'I'm likely to develop a degenerative eye disease.'[2] There is also a market for pre-pregnancy genetic tests: for $350 a company in the United States called Counsyl will screen would-be parents for a set of 100 diseases but in doing so neglect the question of the diversity of possible conditions. These various tests, openly for sale on the Internet, elicit opposition from some geneticists, who contest their scientific validity and express concern about their psychological and social effects. As early as 2007, the Council of Europe, France's *Agence de la Biomédecine* and the French health ministry, likewise alarmed, organized a conference to analyze the implications of this development and determine what to do about it. Such tests are not permitted in France as they do not comply with French 'bioethics' laws, which, as we shall see, strictly regulate the principles on which genetic testing may be done and genetic tests used.[3] Of course the fact that they can be purchased today

---

1 Candidate Sarkozy's remarks were as follows: 'For my part, I would be inclined to think that one is born a paedophile – and the fact that we don't know how to treat that pathology is a problem. There are 1,200 to 1,300 young people who commit suicide every year in France, and not because their parents didn't take good care of them! But because, genetically, they had a vulnerability, a pre-existing distress' (see 'Dialogue entre Nicolas Sarkozy et Michel Onfray' in *Philosophie Magazine*, March 2007).

2 Cf. 'Ton génome pour 1 000 dollars,' *Le Monde*, June 7, 2008, and 'Hints of future health from a drop of saliva', *The New York Times*, Dec. 8, 2007.

3 Various French national authorities for regulating biomedical practice have recently put forward proposals for how to frame these practices legislatively.

on the Internet does not say anything about their future. We cannot know what will happen when their limitations as predictors and their potential negative effects on individuals are better known or, conversely, when they start getting greater publicity and the price goes down (in the case of a company called 23andMe, the cost fell quickly from $1000 to $400). Still, this example of the way genetics is developing illustrates that there are strong social dynamics at work. In sum, biologists, those who fund them, patient advocacy groups, biotechnology firm economics, the media, political officials and many other actors are fully implicated in a way of thinking where the inclination is to find explanatory causes for diseases and to orient social questions in the direction of genetics, yet the situation appears relatively complex due to fears of scientist manipulation on the one hand and hope for cures on the other (Vailly 2013). This duality should be understood in relation to the fact that these new practices are situated at the intersection of science, health and life (Vailly, Niewhöner and Kehr 2011).

Precisely because these developments give rise to fantasies, it is useful to analyze not only what science and medicine *might be able to do* but what they are actually doing in this area today. In this spirit, my book makes use of anthropological and sociological approaches and is therefore rooted in practice. Taking up an idea defended by Michel Foucault, I have sought to view the present up close without falling into a 'theatrical declaration that this moment in which we exist is one of total perdition, in the abyss of darkness, or a triumphant daybreak', but understanding it instead to be 'a time like any other, or rather, a time which is never quite like any other' (Dean 1999: 43). Genetics has a certain propensity to elicit studies that are either extremely alarmist or excessively enthusiastic about current or contemplated practices, or that focus on questions that have already sparked widespread public debate. The investigation on which my study is based is distinguished both by its approach and its type of research focus. It concerns a rapidly developing type of practice applied to entire populations: newborn screening. First of all, let me specify that screening by definition involves identifying individuals within a given population who are at risk for a certain disease or disorder (in which case the screening is followed by a conclusive diagnostic test) or who already have the disease or disorder without knowing it (Armstrong and Eborall 2012). Newborn screening has not drawn much attention outside professional circles, despite the fact that it is the most widely used means of detecting genetic conditions. Specifically, I studied newborn screening for cystic fibrosis, and we shall see why this is an emblematic example of the way norms and techniques in this area are changing. In other words, while seeking to steer clear of false assumptions, my book aims to account for ordinary practices and discourses in medical genetics at the start of the twenty-first century – although the questions it asks are much less ordinary – and to show what screening can tell us about the ways that medicine and our societies are currently changing. But before moving to the heart of the matter, it is important to present the set of analytical tools that will enable us to identify clearly what is at stake.

The Importance of Health Issues and How Those Issues Are Evolving

Questions related to the body, health and well-being are a central preoccupation of contemporary Western societies. This is illustrated by recent fears of epidemics – such as H1N1 flu – as well as increases in screening practices, and the numbers of treatment and well-being centres. This general trend is related to a still more general process of medicalization, by which all sorts of questions become medical ones, including those that used to be located outside medicine's area of intervention (Foucault 2001b: 48-49). As anthropologist Didier Fassin has explained (1996), the medicalization process is manifest in the current expansion of the health field in three directions. The first concerns the targets of health policy – that is, its aims and the people or groups of people it is geared towards. Clinical medicine, which used to handle patients' complaints and involve a direct relationship with a doctor, is combined today with preventive medicine focused on risk and the screening of populations, even though certain screening programmes have given rise to debate due to the anxiety that they can create and due to problems of over-diagnosis (Armstrong 2012). More specifically, screening, anticipation and disease prevention practices are simultaneously addressed to populations as a whole and to individuals. Each person within a given population is urged to get screened whenever possible and to behave in ways that will protect them from the risk of disease. Encouraging individuals to take care of themselves and to exercise vigilance over their own behaviour can work to transfer responsibilities in highly significant ways. Problematizing the issue of lung cancer by emphasizing an approach in terms of genetic predisposition will not target the same people as emphasizing the responsibility of the smoker or occupational exposure to carcinogenic substances. In the first case, the 'target' is the family; in the second, the individual; and in the third, employers. And it does not imply the same research campaigns or health policies: the first approach leads to investigating DNA; the second to prohibiting tobacco use; the third to implementing workplace safety measures. In sum, the first point to be made about newborn screening is that it is consistent with, and part of, a general concern about health and the general expansion of screening practices. The second direction in which the medicalization process is moving concerns the people who intervene. This general category of actors is becoming much more diverse and the relationships between the various components more complex. An example can be seen in patient advocacy groups, increasingly likely to intervene in the public arena to make decision-makers and the population at large aware of their problems. With regard to the history of health and patient organizations in France, the case of AIDS has given salience to a model that involves criticizing delegation and what was termed medical 'paternalism' (Pinell 2004a). It is in this context that we must situate users' increasing demand for information on health. Moreover, patients are now increasingly able to obtain that information through their own efforts, particularly through the media and the Internet. The third direction, less directly related to my study, concerns the diversification of the areas in which health policy is applied. This can be illustrated by 'conduct disorder' in children, today considered a medical problem after long being thought of as mere agitation. Regarding the primary focus of this study, we can say that given the fact that health has become a precious good and individuals are increasingly considered responsible for their own health, it has become morally reprehensible not to take care of oneself and not to prevent a loved one's suffering. Likewise, for anthropologist Margaret Lock (2000), well-being and steering clear of disease have become a sort of virtue – especially, she adds, among the middle classes. For make no mistake, taking care of one's health requires skills and resources that are not equally available to all, and the technicizing of medicine in rich countries is obviously no threat to stratification based on socio-economic inequalities. The observed collective sensitivity to health and life-related issues does not mean we can assume that health care is a priority in all circumstances. What are we to think of a prison population exposed to serious health risks and going untreated, or employees who remained exposed for decades to asbestos in France when the danger had already become clear, or groups of Roma living in unhealthy conditions, and similar problems? This study will partially mirror this last observation, for it analyzes a health policy and programme that concern very few sick people and handle them in a particularly concentrated, active way. It remains to be seen what the conditions of possibility were for implementing this policy. Another apparent contradiction is that although bodies exposed to suffering elicit compassion, this does not mean that people with handicaps have their full place in society. There is indeed a general concern for health but, on the one hand, not all health problems are taken into account the same way, and, on the other, while there is compassion for suffering bodies, the other's physical otherness is not fully accommodated. All of this means that different, and in some instances clashing, elements come into play, which need to be analyzed. Because Michel Foucault's analytical framework enables us to attend at once to knowledge, policies, norms and morality, it will enable us to move forward in this direction. First, however, it is important to specify certain changes that have taken place in the field of health.

The medicalization of people's existences is accompanied today by a movement that sociologists call 'biomedicalization', which affects primarily, but not exclusively, Western countries. This term designates the process by which the techno-scientific approaches associated with the life sciences are being hybridized with those used in clinical practice. This process, which developed during the second half of the twentieth century (Gaudillière 2006), has been greatly accelerating since the 1980s (Clarke et al. 2010). It obviously does not imply that all earlier approaches to medicine have disappeared, but rather that new practices, changes and replacements will gradually be added. One characteristic of biomedicalization, then, is related to the emergence of new knowledge and the effect it has of obscuring the boundaries between sciences, techniques and medicine. Because biomedicine means to be both scientific and medical, it raises issues related to the status and productions of science, and these are of interest to anthropologists of biomedicine as well as sociologists of science and epistemologists. The question of what role should be granted to social processes versus intrinsic characteristics of nature is debated at length by these thinkers and researchers. Many social science researchers today agree that instead of analyzing science's finished products, the priority is to study science in action, meaning ethnographic studies and studies of science's material forms (Cambrosio, Young and Lock 2000). The point is to investigate the dynamics of science, the social conditions in which it develops, and the way it legitimizes actors and is itself legitimized by those actors' social position. However, precisely because biomedicine intersects with clinical work and implicates people as living beings and their lives, it has its own issues and values that are not necessarily to be found in the sciences *per se*. In other words, because biomedicine applies at once to people, organs, and molecules, it brings into play both 'living beings' (*les vivants*) and life itself (*le vivant*).

An Analytical Framework

Michel Foucault's theories provide keys for analyzing health care questions and the larger issues they raise precisely because they highlight how life and health care have made their way into political strategies. Foucault's notion of biopower refers to the emergence in the seventeenth century of a 'power over life' that was deployed at an individual level and somewhat later at a collective level as well (Foucault 1998). At an individual level, because this power focused on the body for the purpose of training it and increasing its strength by ridding it of bodily, sexual and social habits that might hurt its health; at a collective level in that it aimed to control the species, which then became a stake in political strategies for ensuring proliferation and longevity, strategies grounded in demography and epidemiology. These two elements, which Foucault referred to respectively as 'anatomopolitics' of the human body and 'biopolitics of population', constituted two poles that could also intersect with each other. From the early twentieth century, the desire for health no longer consisted solely in avoiding diseases or premature death but also in seeking to optimize the body so as to attain a sort of general well-being (Rose 2001). The World Health Organization (WHO) went even further, defining health as 'a state of complete physical, mental and social well-being and not merely the absence of disease or infirmity'.[4]

This already enables us to better grasp this process of the biomedicalization of human lives. However, if we were to leave things there, the historical movement I have just briefly retraced would seem somewhat linear. First, it seems oblivious to disparities between the goal of good health and the means available and actually used in societies to reach that goal. In Western countries, this presentation of things would have to be clarified and refined by studying various social worlds;

---

4   Cf. 'Preamble' to the World Health Organization Constitution adopted by the International Health Conference, New York, June 19-July 22, 1946, http://www.who.int/suggestions/faq/en/.

specifically, worlds marked by social inequalities and unfavourable living conditions, where having enough to eat and a roof over one's head is more urgent than taking care of one's health. Moreover, established as it has been on the basis of various European countries, the process seems to ignore the countries where health is not really taken into account in political or policy strategies. Anthropological studies in South Africa (Fassin 2007) and Brazil (Biehl 2005) are working to expose and illuminate this rather large blind spot. By showing how the political is inscribed in human bodies, Foucault's analytical framework enables us to integrate situations such as social inequalities, divergent interests, etc., that may counterbalance the very real general progression of medicalization. Second, this presentation would have to take into account historical periods in which promotion of health and biological life comes up against other strategies, such as those for waging war. While this question would take us too far afield, this possibility of integration was suggested by the philosopher himself (Foucault 1988). It should also be noted that some authors think that life became a focus of political strategies much earlier than the seventeenth century (Agamben 1998), while others have suggested that the development was triggered by general mechanisms that can be found in other historical periods and places, such as ancient Rome (Fassin 1996). Lastly, it should be stressed that using Michel Foucault's analytical framework implies following the modulations of thought that changed over time.

Indeed, the philosopher later introduced the notion of 'government' and this shifted the focus of his theories of power. He did so at least in part in response to critics who had faulted him for not acknowledging potential resistances to the seemingly omnipotent power he had defined (Gros 1996). With its notions of control, surveillance and the production of docile, submissive bodies, the first version of his biopower theory did indeed leave itself open to this critique. What Foucault added more clearly later was a dimension of freedom. This term immediately calls for two remarks. First, in a crucial way, Foucault's freedom is internal to power, for not only does that power encompass freedom in its own techniques but it can only endure by relying on that same freedom. What bolsters the stability of that power is that it neither represses nor forbids – this explains the metaphor of the bumblebee ruling without using its stinger – but rather urges and produces. Second, the philosopher is not analyzing one or several powers so much as power *relations*, understood to be exercised over a recognized 'other' who is to be maintained as an acting subject. Foucault thus defined government as the set of more or less conscious, calculated modes of action aimed at affecting other individuals' possibilities of acting. In this sense 'government' refers not only to political structures and state management but to a way of structuring others' potential fields of action ('*conduire les conduites*' or 'leading conduct'). Consistent with the fact that power in this conception is not located exclusively 'at the top', the analytical framework includes a 'microphysics' of power, composed of all the apparently minor power processes that get diffused within society. It is therefore important not only to perceive and seek to understand the strategies and instruments of government previously defined but also power at its extremities, where it comes to resemble capillaries. The question of propagating genetic knowledge in society must therefore be related to Foucault's concept of diffuse, diffused power.

Toward the end of his life, Michel Foucault turned back to his past work, taking as his theoretical focus 'the field of experience', a concept that provided a new foundation for the body of his previous work. Although he did not develop this idea as fully as his theory of government, he did write of it in the following terms: 'In these three areas – madness, delinquency, and sexuality – I emphasized a particular aspect each time: the establishment of a certain objectivity, the development of a politics and a government of the self, and the elaboration of an ethics and a practice in regard to oneself. But each time I also tried to point out the place occupied here by the other two components necessary for constituting a field of experience' (Rabinow 1984: 387). In other words, the field of experience was conceived as a fold situated between a question of truth linked to knowledge, a question of power, and a question of the subject's relationship to the self (Gros 1996). It should be emphasized that because the subject's relationship to the self is conceived as an 'experience' it is not at all metaphysical but necessarily anchored in practices and discourses.

Foucault thus moved from biopower and biopolitics to government, the subject and ethics by reshaping his concepts. My argument here is that these concepts provide a particularly suitable framework within which to study newborn screening and biomedicine. This might be linked to the fact that Michel Foucault was a student of the philosopher and historian of biology and medicine Georges Canguilhem. The fact is that these tools allow several notions to be both reconciled and linked together, which I will of course have occasion to discuss at several points further on. The question of 'forms of knowledge' will be taken up in connection with the role of genetics and statistics in the history and practice of newborn screening for cystic fibrosis; the role of the body and health in policies such as screening will be resituated in the framework of 'biopolitics'; and 'subjectification' – that is, the constitution of choice-making subjects and their dialectical relationship to passive 'objects' – will be analyzed in connection with the notion of 'informed consent', a notion increasingly present in medical law, as we shall see. Equipped with this highly relevant analytical framework, we are now ready to move to the heart of the subject of newborn screening.

Screening Newborns

The screening of newborns, usually carried out to detect genetic conditions, is consistent with the changes described above both in terms of politics and policies of life and the living being, medicalization and disease prevention, and in terms of the development of biomedicine and the genetic approach. It also involves the question of how public policy handles issues involving young children. During the twentieth century, children were the target par excellence of screening-based medicine, through vaccination and health education campaigns, as well as the study of children's physical and mental development (Armstrong 1995). The practice of keeping track of how newborns are developing reflects an even more longstanding concern about the health of children in their first months and years of life. Although this concern obviously does not explain everything, it should nonetheless be seen as related to the substantial quantitative development of newborn screening in wealthy countries. As early as 2001, an article published in the prestigious biomedical journal *Science* made the following announcement: 'The ability to scan one sample for some two dozen inherited disorders is about to cause an explosion in neonatal screening; few health systems are prepared for the consequences' (Marshall 2001: 2272). In the United States, more than four million newborns are screened every year. Today no fewer than 50 conditions are screened for on average in the country's various states – rare diseases, as most affect between one child in several thousand and one child in several hundred thousand.[5] In Europe as I write, Germany screens for 14 diseases at birth, while Great Britain screens for five and France for six.[6] This has brought about two developments. First, the standardization and routine use of new techniques mentioned in connection with the rise of biomedicine has made it possible to use those techniques on large populations and to analyze a greater variety of conditions. Spectrometry, chromatography and direct study of certain sections of the DNA chain have led to the practice of analyzing a great number of proteins and genetic anomalies using a few drops of a newborn baby's blood. Second, these new screening practices are modifying some of the legitimacy criteria for newborn screening that had hitherto been in effect. Until about 15 years ago, newborn screening had to meet a set of criteria known as Wilson-Jungner (Wilson and Jungner 1968), established by the WHO in 1968 and reapproved by a North American consensus conference in 1988. Among other things, these criteria defined disease or disorder characteristics (the disease has to be known, serious, etc.), the way diseases might be identified (signs and markers have to be reliable, etc.), public health care requirements (screening cost should not be too high nor exceed the cost of treating the sick identified, etc.) and the information provided to screened populations (they have to be clearly informed about the test and cannot be tested without their consent). Among the criteria relating to the characteristics of the disease, the existence of a cure was considered to be a prerequisite. Gradually, however, this has been replaced by the idea that there must be benefits to treating the disease or the condition early, even in cases where, at the existing state of medical knowledge, there can be no return to normal health. Obviously the decisive point here is what is meant by 'benefits' and 'treatment'. Moreover, the fact that it was in parents' interest to be informed of any disease

---

5   For further information on newborn screening in the United States, see the site of the National Newborn Screening and Genetics Resource Center, http://genes-r-us.uthscsa.edu/.

6   Newborns in France are screened for the following diseases: phenylketonuria, hypothyroidism, congenital adrenal hyperplasia and cystic fibrosis (CF). In France's overseas *départements* and territories, screening for sickle cell disease has been generalized while in mainland France it is restricted to populations of African origin or from the Mediterranean basin. Screening for deafness was added to this list in 2012.

their newborn might have began to be taken into account, independently of the benefits the children themselves might draw. Despite these changes, until recently there has been little social science study of newborn screening compared to the attention given to genetic diagnoses of the foetus and what are known as 'genetic counselling' practices aimed at informing people about the origins of a disease, the risk of transmission, and the possibilities of detecting a potential genetic disorder in the foetus.

My research examined newborn screening for cystic fibrosis (NSCF). This genetic disease, which can vary greatly in severity, is primarily characterized by usually serious respiratory disorders, due to the accumulation of a viscous mucus that causes infections, as well as digestive disorders. A salient feature of the disease is that it is both rare and the most frequently occurring monogenic disease in populations of European origin.[7] It is estimated that in France one out of 4,400 people is born with CF; in France today there are approximately 6,000 people with the disease. Some of these aspects – severity, relative frequency – amount to factors that work to mobilize social actors around the disease. Above all, CF fits into the fundamental socio-historical developments by which chronic diseases became a priority concern in Western countries (whereas up until the Second World War, these countries were primarily affected by acute diseases). Biologists and geneticists have devoted and continue to devote much research to CF at the international and national levels; there has been much hope among both researchers and patients and their families that a form of gene therapy will be found for this disease; that is, a therapy that will correct the defective gene in the sick person. It is in this context that in 2002 France launched nation-wide NSCF. Two points should be made in this regard. First, France occupies an important position in that it was the first country to have adopted this practice, along with much of Australia and New Zealand. Second, NSCF is emblematic of newborn screening and how it is evolving, first of all due to the fact that there is no known cure for the disease. While patients' life expectancy has risen by 15 years in the last approximately 15 years, it is no higher than 40 years in Europe. The absence of curative treatment was (and to some extent continues to be) an issue in the debate in biomedical and health administration circles on whether NSCF was a good idea and whether and how it could be justified, given that the benefits for children who screen positive had not been clearly established (MMWR Recommendations and Reports 1997, 2004). An exploration of biomedical literature shows that this debate has been medical – Does NSCF offer enough patient benefits given its drawbacks? – and/or scientific – Is there scientific proof of those benefits? – and/or moral – Is it ethical to take into account possible benefits to parents? I will of course be returning to these questions. Today the cursor seems to be shifting in favour of NSCF, and other countries, including the United States and Britain, have begun the practice. There is also a

---

7 A monogenic disease involves one major gene, although other genetic factors as well as social and environmental ones can affect how serious the disease is.

techno-scientific indication of NSCF's position at the transition point between already established and new newborn screening tests. The technical aspects of the practice will be specified below, but here it is important to know that NSCF involves direct study of the DNA of people who have tested positive once – and this is the first time that such study has occurred on this scale in France. Direct DNA study may induce various effects that would not occur with other biomedical practices. It may work to diffuse particular representations related to the image of DNA (Nelkin and Lindee 1994); it may focus family ties on biology rather than emotional relations. And in France it is subject to stricter legal regulations than traditional biological tests: it requires written consent of the concerned party – in this case, the newborn baby's parents.

At a time when genetics is undergoing the important developments indicated above, it is worth analyzing the social issues raised in connection with an actual policy and real practices. The point is to study what that policy and those practices can tell us about the fact that the issue of the living being and life has become part of political strategies and about wider societal changes. What are the defining characteristics of a policy of the living being (*le vivant*) or living beings (*les vivants*), that uses the form and content of the knowledge called genetics? Under what scientific and social conditions is such a policy possible? What does it tell us about the politics and government of people-as-living-beings? How is it involved in producing norms and values? In the present study, the point is to analyze *as a field of experience* (in the sense defined above) a *policy that developed out of medical genetics*; that is, to analyze it three-dimensionally: *in scientific, political and moral terms*. The aim, then, is less to assess the benefits of the policy and point out its limitations than to analyze the conditions under which it is possible to implement such a policy, the varieties of political logic underpinning it, and its effects on norms and values. In doing so, I will show in particular that *newborn screening outlines a new political and moral space of genetics*. My study encompasses an apparently heterogeneous set of discourses and practices, decisions, laws, administrative measures, scientific statements and moral propositions, all organized around a field of experience whose three dimensions – scientific, political and moral – may be interrelated. From the outset we can hypothesize that each of these dimensions helps constitute the other two: knowledge affects moral understanding and political practices, etc. This hypothesis will lead us to consider questions that, although certainly not meant as universal, may well reach beyond the frame of biomedicine, questions that may be described as sociological or anthropological knots. Borrowing that term from psychiatry, Ian Hacking (2005) defined a knot as an issue produced by contradictory tendencies. Here those issues are truth (versus seeming), choice (versus being forced), the norm (versus deviance) and a quality life (versus a poor quality life). In other words, we will also be studying a policy of the living being and living beings in the framework of a historically situated social dynamic, determining and defining what it tells us about the more general issues it both reflects and fuels.

Presentation of the Study

To answer the questions formulated above, a qualitative study was schematically conducted over two periods. In the first period, 2002-2004, I analyzed the history and issues involved in the decision-making process that led to implementing NSCF in France, especially the history of NSCF in Brittany, one of the two pilot screening regions, which set up the practice in the late 1980s.[8] The first study in Brittany was carried out through interviews with the main actors (biomedical personnel in charge of the regional programme, patient organization board members, journalists, elected officials, etc.) and supplemented by analysis of scientific articles and documents. Also during the first period, I studied the history of NSCF at the national level. In terms of organization, it is important to know that the responsibility for proposing and performing newborn screening in France belongs to a professional association made up of paediatricians and, to a lesser extent, geneticists called the *Association Française pour le Dépistage et la Prévention des Handicaps de l'Enfant* (AFDPHE – the French Association for Screening for and Preventing of Handicaps in Children). The AFDPHE is overseen by the *Caisse Nationale d'Assurance Maladie des Travailleurs Salariés* (Cnamts – French National Health Insurance Fund for Employees), the public authority that funds France's universal health insurance programme, including newborn screening, and the *Direction Générale de la Santé* (DGS – Department of Health), a department within the Ministry of Health. I interviewed officials from the AFDPHE, the Cnamts, the DGS and a patient support organization called '*Vaincre la mucoviscidose*' (VLM – Beating Cystic Fibrosis).[9] I also analyzed biomedical articles and in-house specialized material, namely from the national AFDPHE headquarters. This gave me a better understanding of how newborn screening is organized and the relationships between the various organizations involved.

In the second period, 2003-2005, I studied the practices used once NSCF had been put in place. My methods here were observation and interviews. The work carried out during the first period had brought two particular issues to light at several points: on the one hand, the question of borderline (very mild) cases of the disease; on the other, and more indirectly, the relationship between a policy that might give rise to debate in terms of validity, but remained fairly consensual on the moral count, because its focus was suffering children (newborn screening) and a more controversial policy, focused on foetus selection (prenatal diagnosis). Hypothesizing that birth was a particularly revealing moment at which to study how these two approaches did or did not come together, I decided to investigate the question within the framework of a field study. The research method was therefore

---

8   The other region was Normandy. I chose Brittany over Normandy in part because of the scientific scale of the programme there, as attested by biomedical publications on CF; second because of local doctors' involvement in the patient organization and an initial hypothesis regarding the role played by this organization in deciding to implement NSCF.

9   Formerly called AFLM (see abbreviations).

chosen as a function of these two questions – borderline varieties of CF and how two approaches, newborn screening and prenatal diagnosis, did or did not come together. Other aspects of the practice were therefore left aside. The field study comprised two components. First, I observed meetings on newborn screening (collective study days, scientific meetings, etc.), including all major national-level meetings on the matter. Second, I conducted a seven-month qualitative study in a major Paris hospital chosen for being one of the top paediatrics and genetics hospitals in France on both medical and scientific grounds. The study was conducted simultaneously in a paediatrics unit that has won national recognition for its special work on CF and monitors a large cohort of people with the disease, and the highly renowned genetics unit in the same hospital, collaborating with the afore-mentioned paediatrics unit in the framework of NSCF, though not specialized in CF (the disease accounts for approximately 5% of its activity). These units are in turn linked to the centre in charge of organizing newborn screening in the Ile-de-France region. The centre receives newborn blood samples and transfers them to biology laboratories; it is also in charge of all correspondence with parents, laboratories and clinicians. This is a major screening centre, managing almost a quarter of babies born in France. The originality of my method lay in observing consultations in both paediatrics and genetics, consultations likely to provide answers to the questions above. This part of the inquiry also involved interviews with the relevant professionals (primarily paediatricians and geneticists) and parents (often mothers) of children who had tested either positive or negative for the disease, supplemented by reading of biomedical journals and in-house written documentation. Lastly, I conducted observations and interviews in two maternity hospitals in the Paris area regarding mothers' consent to NSCF for their newborns.[10] Altogether, the study was conducted at three different levels: regional (Brittany), national (France) and local (a Paris area hospital and two maternity hospitals). In addition to my reading of biomedical articles and in-house literature, I conducted nearly 80 interviews (as well as approximately 40 short interviews in the maternity hospitals) and over 160 observation sessions (as well as 30 briefer sessions in the maternity hospitals). All interviews were recorded and all observation carried out with the explicit consent of the individuals concerned: clinicians, meeting organizers, parents and children (except very young children). All individuals remain anonymous or have been given false names (this explains why in some cases no names are given at all).

As has already been mentioned, in my research I call upon work in anthropology, sociology and occasionally philosophy (when historicized and contextualized). In practical terms, the idea was to use all relevant tools that could help understand and analyze. From a more theoretical perspective, the point was to integrate my thinking into a current of thought the purpose of which is to 'do social science'; in other words, to bring together the various social sciences in a synthetic approach. That

---

10   The study in the maternity units was conducted in collaboration with Cécile Ensellem.

approach relies in particular on a type of anthropology that includes power relations and social relations in its scope – phenomena traditionally emphasized more in sociology. The aim of this interdisciplinary approach is to combine explanations in terms of political and social context, social dynamics and historically situated processes with attention to what can be learned from observation and with a world of more general investigations and questioning. The approach is founded on the wager that not only can it remain coherent – despite disciplinary differences – it can also bring its own analytical and methodological advantages. It aims to get beyond the classic antagonism between individual actions and structures; neither an 'individualist' approach nor a 'holistic' (all-encompassing) one can account for everything that has been in play, at stake and in process in NSCF. The point, then, is to connect the level of social micro-processes and strategic actions by actors in a position to influence their environment to the level of structural constraints, which exert a counter influence on these processes and actions within a 'society of individuals' (Elias 1991).

Lastly, it is important as part of this presentation to examine my own position as a researcher. As Daniel Bizeul (2007: 75) has pointed out,

> it is with what he or she *is* – the gaps or deficiencies in his or her knowledge, his or her difficulties, physical nature, social history – that the researcher studies the world of others. ... Not speaking of those things and not imagining their possible effects on research study results puts the reader in a difficult position as it requires him or her to make a blind judgment.

My understanding here is that it is methodologically fairer to lay out any issues that may be implicated in the researcher's social position rather than insisting on some self-declared neutrality, which is often an illusion. Let me therefore lay these out to the reader. I initially trained in biology. After completing a PhD in the life sciences, I joined the *Institut National de la Santé et de la Recherche Médicale* (National Institute for Health and Medical Research, Inserm) as a biologist, where I worked as a molecular biology and genetics researcher for approximately ten years. A number of critical questions (to which I will return) and my diminishing enthusiasm for the discipline, combined with a keen (if at the time somewhat vague) interest in the social sciences, led to me to choose to retrain in that discipline. This itinerary offers obvious advantages when it comes to conducting social science research on the issues involved in screening for a genetic disease. It does, however, raise its own issues, because it also had an impact upon that research. On the one hand, my accumulated knowledge of biology made the technical aspects and the reading of biomedical texts easier. My scientific background has also given me some critical habits when it comes to analyzing scientific articles: as Dominique Vinck put it (1995: 108), the scientist learns to be sceptical, to disbelieve and mistrust what colleagues present and to question and debate data and information with peers. On the other hand, and in addition to the retraining in social sciences implied by my itinerary, I had to engage in a particular form of reflexive work, considering my own results critically. Norbert Elias (1987) emphasizes the need for social science researchers to free themselves from 'emotional involvement'; that is, the 'involvement' they are likely to feel toward their research subject. As he understood it, involvement and detachment are not two distinct sets of phenomena but rather the two ends of a continuum on which researchers are situated. How is one to find a balance between involvement (the involvement that fuelled my criticism of biology here) and detachment (the detachment necessary for conducting the inquiry and analyzing the results)?

This means working first on the 'involvement' aspect, which I shall look at here in two ways: explaining the issues at stake, and thinking critically about them. First, let me therefore outline the reservations I had with regard to my original scientific discipline that could potentially affect my study (and I shall only mention those specific reservations). The questions I asked myself as a biology researcher, which are linked to the research presented here, concern the following things: the *a priori* of action (the idea that if something can be done, it should be done); scientific evidence (how researchers establish scientific 'facts' without verifying them); and biology researchers' low level of reflexivity (they are unlikely to reflect on the social effects of their practices and to contest the fiction that science is neutral). On these three points, I had to be careful not to apply past questions that were not raised by my field studies to the research in progress. However, prior experience can also be used to raise research questions. To paraphrase Max Weber, what defines the researcher's involvement, at least in part, is how their research object is constructed. The point is also to specify the nature of the issues at stake in order to ensure that one's criticisms, if there are to be criticisms, are balanced. In this case, the questions I have raised (which will appear more clearly in the course of the study) concern how knowledge is used, competition among public issues, modes of governmentality and views of disease or abnormality.

The second concern is to further develop the notion of critique, distinguishing 'critical anthropology' from the type of 'critique' inspired by Michel Foucault. Critical medical anthropology looks to detach the discipline from its emphasis on face-to-face relationships between patient and doctor by showing the role that macro-social levels, class and political structures play in health care issues (Singer 1995). Its great strength – which should be emphasized – is that it introduces questions of class, gender relations and ethnic origin into studies of the tensions that may exist in clinical situations, rather than focusing on cultural or cognitive misunderstandings between health care providers and patients. However, as I see it, critical medical anthropology has a tendency to rigidify oppositions between the two groups, namely when it states that 'doctor-patient and other relationships in the health field [are] unavoidably conflictual meeting points between parties with fundamentally different and objectively opposed sociopolitical and political-economic interests' (Singer 1995: 84). While study of a hospital may show that people have divergent interests, for example, the hospital is not only a battlefield but also a locus of negotiation and values (some of which may be shared by health care providers and patients alike, such as sensitivity to the suffering of children) that exists within a wider socio-political context. From a different perspective, Michel Foucault et al. (2001: 456) explained: 'A critique ... consists in seeing on what type of assumptions, of familiar notions, of established unexamined ways of thinking the accepted practices are based. ... Criticism consists in uncovering that thought and trying to change it: showing that things are not as obvious as people believe.' In other words, bringing to the fore the conditions that make a given politics or policy possible and acceptable enables us to adopt a 'critical attitude' towards it, the understanding being that those conditions are not self-evident. I have given priority to this attitude.

The second issue is detachment. Distancing oneself from a familiar milieu entails both an initial technical aspect (one needs to remain capable of being surprised by familiar practices) and a second deeper aspect, related to interpretation (one needs to remain free of presuppositions). Regarding the technical aspect, I chose to study an area that did not correspond to practices I was particularly familiar with. This is not a study of biology laboratories but of hospitals; it involves not scientific research but biomedical policies and not biologists but paediatricians and geneticists. This shift enabled me to connect with the wellsprings of surprise and to escape familiarities (though I may add that those familiarities are fading with time in any case). Regarding the second aspect, the study actually seemed to generate its own detachment, for reasons I shall now attempt to explain. Because I remained in touch with and followed the movements of a certain number of actors for several years (paediatricians, geneticists, etc.), I was able to observe that these people were devoid of cynicism. In general they put a great deal of effort into their work, making the best of decisions that in some cases they had not made themselves and often showing a considerable degree of commitment and conviction. While these surely went hand-in-hand with professional interests, this was probably no more or less the case than in any other professional category. This illustrates the extent to which '[the anthropologist] takes on embarrassing aspects of the existence [of the people they study] and attests in return to their ordinary humanity' (Bizeul 2007: 76). And that in turn means that working to rid ourselves of false assumptions does not necessarily lead to attributing a conscious will to manipulate to the different actors involved (some of whom may be roughly qualified as 'pleasant dominators'). The detachment engendered by the study itself should also be related to the particular level of knowledge and conceptualization operative here, which influences the way one experiences 'whatever affects [one's] senses' and the 'meaning' one gives to perceptions, as suggested by Norbert Elias (1987: 4 and 11): a circular movement gets established between understanding events and 'inner control'. In short, the researcher ends up attempting to show usages and practices and to call into question (in the sense of wonder about) rather than 'criticize' (in the common sense of that word).

With these clarifications in mind, we can move on to the outline of the book, which is organized into six chapters. Chapter 1 gives a historical account of how newborn screening for CF was set up in France, emphasizing and explaining the relations between a set of actors, decisions, power relations, laws and moral questions. I identify and define the conditions that made it possible to launch this policy and programme, which was quite controversial in biomedical circles, and to keep it going for a decade in Brittany before extending it to France as a whole, bringing to light the major phases, the main actors and the key issues raised by the policy.

In Chapter 2, I consider the scientific side to the policy programme by looking at the evidence it provides about its benefits and the process through which what is considered to be 'true' in biomedicine today is constituted. The focus here is not only on the epistemic frameworks of actors implementing a public policy but also on the way these frameworks are made and come apart – in short, the dynamics of evidence. This allows for analyzing production and dissemination of evidence as well as for grasping the relative place of 'evidence-based medicine' in a process where knowledge, rumour, and emotion all operate together.

Chapter 3 examines the political side of screening and the meaning of governmentality in connection with a genetic disease. Here I examine how different actors either do or do not assume the position of choice-making subjects, the design of the policy from the perspective of individuals and/or populations, and the means and tools used to implement it. I show the subtle power relations operating between professionals and patient organization members, and the way screening was partially designed as a political technique for orienting patients in time and space. Lastly, the policy is analyzed at the capillary level, far from the centres of power and decision-making; that is, among mothers in maternity hospitals.

Using the example of this policy, I attempt to show in Chapter 4 how biomedicine's approach to abnormality and the norm has evolved. I show the technical limitations of screening, which has the effect of extending the application of the notion of biological abnormality, and the professional approaches and practices involved in paediatric follow-up care of patients, which have extended clinical abnormality. Lastly, on the basis of my hospital field studies, I analyze the consequences of these practices, located as they are at the interface between newborn screening and prenatal diagnosis, showing how the norm can be modified, this time with regard to foetuses.

At this point it will have become quite clear that the issues at stake in screening practices encompass the living being, life and ultimately existence itself. That is why I propose in this chapter reversing the concept of 'quality of life' (*qualité de vie*) widely used by professionals and replacing it with 'a quality life' (*une vie de qualité*).

Chapter 5 uses the field study to explore the efforts being made to treat sick children in a way that will enable them to lead better lives, and what this objective covers. Here I focus particularly on the semantic networks of the disease, how life prospects are envisaged and the way social life (going out, going to school, having fun, etc.) and biological life (taking care of oneself, avoiding infection, etc.) are linked or co-produced. Far from any genetic essentialism, I show the process through which CF patients are stigmatized in the hospital setting and the core issue of social inequalities in the area of health, a problem related to living conditions.

In Chapter 6, I explore how the aim of maintaining a quality life is pursued by analyzing how newborn screening and foetal screening interfere with one another. Above and beyond the various professional practices involved, I show how the two approaches – screening after birth and screening before birth – are linked, as well as the tension between them. I also examine how the idea of taking action early and more generally the question of time, operate to create this tie. If moral safeguards are in place, the goal of attaining good health (treatment) and the goal of eliminating poor health (foetal testing) may converge.

In the conclusion, I identify certain boundary areas of the biomedicalization process and the political and moral space that has been opened up by screening, a space that needs to be considered within the new politics of the living being. I show how this health policy informs us about social processes that extend beyond newborn screening and genetics, and may even seem far removed from them: the confrontation between different medical approaches; regimes of evidence; techniques of governmentality; tensions between moral values; the value of lived life or life yet to be lived. All these questions remain open ones of course, but this work does purport to shed some light on them.

Chapter 1

The Birth of a Screening Policy (Brittany-France)

For a number of reasons, the time is particularly ripe for analyzing the inception of a policy grounded in the recent developments of biomedicine and genetics. Indeed, genetics is permeating both discourse and practice in a variety of fashions: new newborn screening policies for genetic conditions are increasingly announced or feared (Goldenberg and Sharp 2012), the question of the alleged genetic origin of paedophilia or suicides caused controversy during a recent French presidential election campaign, DNA fingerprinting is used more and more extensively within police procedures (Hindmarsh and Prainsack 2010) and DNA tests for immigrants asking for family reunification are developing in certain countries (Heinemann and Lemke 2013). Of course, these different examples should not be considered on the same level – they have very different aims, and clearly some are consensual while others spark controversy. However, in all cases, the key issue remains the emergence of a debated scientific discipline in the field of politics and public action. Newborn screening for cystic fibrosis offers a choice medium through which to approach this question.

First, however, we should consider what exactly is meant by 'public policy'. For Yves Mény and Jean-Claude Thoenig (1989), a public policy is a programme of government action in a societal sector or geographical space. The term therefore refers to a view focused on government institutions and the State, unlike 'public action'. Indeed, the latter refers to the actions of State institutions but also to those of multiple actors, both private and public, working together and with various interdependencies, at national, but also local and sometimes supranational, levels (Commaille 2006). Given that a variety of social actors were involved in setting up NSCF, the term 'public action' will be used most often here.

When screening was decided upon in France in the early 2000s, it generated lively debate in the international medical sphere. France therefore offers a prime field of inquiry to study the conditions in which such a health policy was able to develop. The key issue in this chapter will be to try and understand *the conditions that made public action for a genetic disease possible*, in a situation where its benefits remained uncertain.[1] A number of questions will be addressed. How is a health policy based on recent data from genetics developed on a regional and national level, and what are the possible limitations of this development? How,

---

1 The question of the uncertainty of its benefits will be examined in more detail in Chapter 2.

in this particular case, can the roles of local actors be linked with a structural and global dimension that reaches far beyond them? In comparison with other health or screening policies, what are the specificities of policies that call upon genetics? In order to answer these questions, the history of the implementation of NSCF in Brittany and in France will be traced, tracking the process from inception to generalization. Analyzing both regional and national policies presents the advantage of revealing the specificities and stakes of both, and allows the intersections between different levels of decision making to be studied.

This first chapter will therefore retrace and analyze the history of this screening policy, initially on a regional level, identifying the conditions that allowed the policy to be launched and then stabilized over a decade in Brittany. I will first show how a policy's scientific dimension is one of the means through which global concerns are taken into account within public action. We will then see how the production of this regional health policy depended upon material and human resources afforded by coalitions of actors. The study of the intersections between the local, regional and national levels will show multi-level public action, driven by local actors making their voices heard and negotiating regulations on a national level. I will go on to focus on the national level, showing how screening practices were able to be generalized on the basis of legitimate professional links with institutions, certain technical conditions and the shift towards a new form of scientific rationale intersecting with organizational stakes. We will also see how hospital structures and large health care centres were consolidated during this period. And in conclusion, I will identify the specificities of public action involving genetics.

On a theoretical level, as I examine the regional level I will call in particular upon constructionist sociology, which focuses on the processes that structure collective attention in the public arena. In the widest possible variety of fields, constructionist sociologists analyze and illustrate the processes that transform a given situation into a 'problem', through the work of social actors (Becker 1966, Berger and Luckmann 1966, Hilgartner and Bosk 1988, Kunitz 1974, Spector and Kitsuse 1977). The inflation of studies on 'social construction' led Ian Hacking (1999) to highlight the tendency to overuse this expression. Regarding these different studies, two concerns inform more particularly the present work. The first stems from the fact that this book is connected with a domain – that is, health – where the reality of bodily suffering collides with the construction of social problems. Describing public health as a 'constructed reality', Didier Fassin (1998: 15) explains:

> Of course no one would dream of denying that public health has a very real epidemiological foundation, with its pathologies and instruments to measure how frequent and serious they are. Nonetheless, the entire history of public health shows that we cannot content ourselves with such a substantialist view, according to which health problems exist independently of the social intervention that defines them as such, or with such a positivist view, according

to which scientific knowledge affords objective and ahistorical criteria allowing them to be identified.[2]

Rather than the strictly constructionist approach (according to which social actors construct a problem), I shall therefore take up this approach combining realism and constructionism (according to which a clinical reality becomes social by being constructed by individual and collective actors). The work of these actors appears clearly in the study by sociologists Vololona Rabeharisoa and Michel Callon (1999) concerning the role of the patient organization AFM, even though it is not analyzed as such in the text. The president of the organization describes the nature of these efforts for recognition in strategic terms: 'It is necessary to create a trend in favour of genetics so that the whole medical system can be mobilized under the pressure of public opinion, so that medicine ... can commit firmly to the fight against all genetic diseases, which would inevitably benefit the AFM' (Rabeharisoa and Callon 1999: 37). There seems to be a wilful resolution to foreground genetic diseases through the mobilization of the relevant actors. And the second concern informing this study is related to the fact that, in the case in hand, it is not simply a question of health, but of genetic diseases. During the 1980s and 1990s, at a time when genetics seemed to seek increasingly to reveal the essence of the individual, the way in which people's idea of a genetic disease such as CF was constructed became particularly salient. There was just as much a tendency towards an essentialist view of the person as there was a tendency towards a substantialist view of health, particularly through the genetics of behaviour (with the genetic approach claiming to explain human behaviour, such as violence or alcoholism, through genes). This shows to what extent genetics was considered as the opposite of any form of social construction: it was a reality, or even *the* reality of the individual. Of course, this conception was above all defended by geneticists, although not all. However, it was also largely taken up in people's common understanding. The approach that could be described as 'real-constructionist' should be considered within this perspective, where it takes on even stronger meaning than with other issues. After these clarifications, let us now enter the heart of the subject and look at the history of the screening programme in Brittany.

A Breton Tale

The NSCF programme developed rapidly in the 1990s in Brittany. And yet a few years prior, not only was there no question of screening but the illness itself was little known in the region. This section will show how this screening policy formed and what issues were at stake.[3] First, we must travel back a few decades in time.

---

2   All translations are provided by the author, unless otherwise indicated.
3   See also (Vailly 2004).

Until the mid 1980s, CF garnered very little attention in Brittany. Where clinicians were concerned, a general feeling of powerlessness prevailed, and when paediatricians would mention the disease it was in dark and resigned terms. The discovery of the disease represented a veritable catastrophe because, more often than not, it was a death sentence for the children it affected: many of them would die from respiratory failure at a very early age. Moreover, the disease was a subject of biomedical study that held little value and promise because 'it did not enable publications' according to one paediatrician I met. Whether the lack of interest in the disease should be analyzed purely in terms of career plans, or whether these very real professional strategies should be considered in combination with a more general context that will be discussed later, the number of publications on CF in Brittany testify to its low level of interest at the time: the main bank of biomedical data (PubMed) mentions practically no publications prior to 1990. And CF did not have a higher profile among the general public. Generally, its name meant nothing to people and it was sometimes confused with other conditions, including veterinary diseases. As for the families confronted with the condition, they withdrew into their shells, often reticent to talk about it with others, or even amongst themselves, because the idea of having a hereditary 'defect' lingered. This is not that surprising, given that the term – used in a relatively commonplace fashion by doctors at least until the 1950s-1960s – was still employed by certain clinicians. One patient organization board member, shocked by both the expedient manner in which the disease was announced to him and the words used, recounts that he learned about his son's condition in a corridor: 'Your son has a defect, and the disease is the CF of the pancreas [former name of CF]'. In sum, these testimonies combine to illustrate that CF had not yet entered the public sphere.

Less than a decade later, the landscape was very different and the contrast was striking. If we take up each of the different points, first, resignation had given way to action: doctors and parents were now in the frame of mind that they had to fight for these children, who would do better with treatment. Second, the disease was now the subject of several biomedical research programmes in the area, illustrated in particular by publications. In contrast with the void described above, the same bibliographical search shows seven articles for the period 1990-1999 and 16 articles for the period 2000-2009, mostly in international and renowned journals. Moreover, a health care network specific to CF had consolidated. It allowed professionals involved in treating the condition to hold regional meetings every semester, bringing together around 30 people – mainly paediatricians, along with a few biologists. On an institutional level, from 1996 onwards, CF numbered among the priorities of several Regional Health Conferences, under the aegis of different public institutions. [4] However, we will see that this is not where

---

4   These institutions were the *Direction régionale des affaires sanitaires et sociales* (DRASS – Regional Department for Health and Social Affairs), the Ministry of Employment and Solidarity and the Préfecture of Brittany. The Regional Health Conferences were

the main initiatives and support lay. Finally, CF had become much more widely known among the population, especially towards the Western tip of Brittany. This sudden emergence was not, of course, due to a rise in the number of cases. Rather, it could be suggested that it was the result of the collective definition of a new social problem. In other words, CF went from the status of 'condition' to that of 'problem': rather than a physical state about which little could be done, it had become a problem that needed to be addressed. If the 'success' of solving a problem is measured by the amount of attention it receives, then this one seemed to be doing reasonably well, particularly in West Brittany. The approach combining realism and constructionism offers a way of considering how the 'problem' (CF) and the actors' solution (newborn screening) were able to find their place in the public sphere in Brittany. Indeed, the reality of the disease appears to have become social because of the way it was constructed by the relevant actors. This approach can also shed light upon how the issue was selected among other possibilities, in a context where this was by no means self-evident, before stabilizing over more than ten years until screening became generalized nationally. As we well know, a great many harmful or dramatic situations do not necessarily become so high profile in the public sphere and 'public attention is a scarce resource, allocated through competition in a system of public arenas' (Hilgartner and Bosk 1988: 55). Moreover, in order to result in a regional programme, this problematization of the issue alone was not enough – it also had to be placed on the agenda, not in the sense of a generalized policy in France, but on a regional level and on the institutional sidelines. So let us now turn to the role of regional actors as policy entrepreneurs and look at the first condition for screening.

Professionals as Policy Entrepreneurs

Between the years during which CF was invisible in Brittany and its rise to the forefront of health concerns, particularly in the Finistère *département*[5] (the Western part of the region), a new element intervened in the social world of genetics; an element of the kind that can contribute to forming a social problem. First, it should be noted that the disease had bit by bit become a 'craze' among biologists of different countries, making it emblematic among genetic diseases. Researchers and, to a lesser degree, health professionals and certain patient families, joined in what became a veritable hunt for the gene involved in the etiology of CF. International research on its molecular foundations succeeded in locating it in 1985, and, better still, in isolating it in 1989. This was important for biologists and had consequences reaching far beyond the social world of CF. Indeed, this was one

---

introduced as a space for debate and suggestions to contribute towards developing a regional health policy. They comprised elected officials, actors in the health systems, patient representatives and patients.

5   A *département* is an administrative division. Metropolitan France comprises 96 *départements*, with a further 5 located overseas.

of the first genes to be isolated for a genetic disease – and not just any disease, as outlined in the introduction. In theory, this was therefore likely to pave the way for other genetic approaches as the discipline reached its peak. Above all, these discoveries gave rise to a wave of hope among patients and their families who, encouraged by researchers, thought that a treatment would be available on the horizon by the year 2000. While this hope was dashed, research nonetheless had practical effects and it is no coincidence that the idea of launching NSCF formed in 1985, the very year that the gene was located.

Another decisive scientific factor, more local than global this time, also weighed in on the process. Epidemiological studies had captured the attention of the region's biomedical sphere. From as early as the 1970s, analyses had testified to the presence of CF 'hotspots' in some districts of the Finistère. International comparisons, refined over time, suggested that, alongside other regions in the world, Brittany was part of a group with the highest incidence. At the end of the 1980s, the incidence in Brittany was estimated at 1 in 1,800 compared to between 1 in 2,500 and 1 in 4,900 elsewhere in France, depending on estimations – in other words, the rate in Brittany was roughly twice that in France. It should be specified that, as absolute values, the figures remained modest as they translated into approximately 10 to 15 new cases per year in Brittany. However, these trend data constituted what political scientists call a powerful 'indicator' (Kingdon 1984) likely to fuel public action, that is to say they were part of the deciding factors in the emergence of CF as a social problem, contributing to bringing it out of the shadows. The question of frequency was indeed taken up in a presentation leaflet about the disease, designed to forge links between the instigators of the NSCF programme in the Finistère and potential partners, particularly the media. It emphasized the fact that CF was 'particularly rife in Brittany'. It is therefore easy to see how the idea that the region was 'strongly hit' by the disease was able to spread.

These various structural and situational elements remind us that NSCF would not have been possible without a frame of reference linked to knowledge: what Ian Hacking (1999), following on from Foucault, calls a 'form of knowledge'. According to this theory, the form taken by knowledge leads, at a given moment, to the emergence of a set of declarative sentences and questions considered to be thinkable or possible. Scientific questions that had no meaning in one historical period, as they were simply unthinkable, took on meaning at a given time. Furthermore, this knowledge was not confined to scholarly circles, it became disseminated throughout society, becoming a form of – albeit only partly – shared knowledge. This permeated commonplace discourse (we often hear the expression 'it's in my genes'), but also the media, where it found strong support with the yearly French Téléthon. NSCF therefore depended upon a form of knowledge that, in general, presents at least two characteristics (Hacking 1999). First, the temporal dimension is very important, as it provides a way of grasping the evolution of ideas and epistemological discontinuities throughout history. Second, knowledge is recognized as being constrained by extra-scientific factors of a social nature, rather than being autonomous. It is not simply the product of an unveiling of nature, provided by scholarly research. Taking this theory and the history of ideas one stage further, it should be noted that this idea of constraint links in with the vaster Foulcauldian notion of *episteme* according to which knowledge obeys rules of construction (Gros 1996). In short, this would mean thought is subject to arbitrary rule systems, which can appear in very varied fields, thus raising the question of scientific modes and epistemological simultaneity. To illustrate this, Michel Foucault (2001a) identifies the proximity between two seemingly distant theories, the first drawn from biology, by Darwin, and the second from physics, by Boltzmann: Darwin was the first to treat living beings at the level of population and no longer at the level of individuals, while Boltzmann began treating physical particles not as individual elements but also on the level of populations, that is to say statistically measurable possibilities. It should be noted that the statistical approach developed dramatically from the eighteenth century onwards, affecting a variety of fields, including epidemiology (Hacking 2006). The statistical studies on the incidence of CF in Brittany should be understood within the continuation of this *episteme*, of which they offer a recent illustration.

The first condition necessary for this screening policy thus emerges from this digression. In order for this policy to be carried out, it first had to be grounded upon 'the world of mind and technique in which [it was] devised' (Hacking 1999: 185), allowing certain questions to be asked: 'how many sick people are there?' but also 'what is the gene involved in CF?', 'how can patients' states be improved?', 'how can they be diagnosed at birth?', etc. This initial condition, linked to a general cognitive and technical universe (that is, genetics and statistics), was punctuated by high points (the isolation of the gene) and the appearance of indicators (incidence). However, it is also obvious that the actors involved were not simply rational individuals weighing up each decision on the basis of purely scientific arguments – they were also caught up in interactions with institutions and groups. In this vein, then, the second condition for NSCF was the way in which these actors came together – their 'configuration' in the sense of the dynamic relationships between members of a group forging both alliances and conflicts (Elias 1978).

For the purposes of clarifying this Breton history, it should be noted that Brittany is divided into four administrative *départements*. The main city in the most Western *département*, the Finistère, is Brest, while the main city in the central *département* is Rennes. In 1985, two biologists from Brest instigated the idea of newborn screening for CF in the Finistère. This was due to the presentation of new scientific data and was based upon biomedical arguments linked to the incidence of the disease, to related prenatal diagnosis and above all, to patient care. I will come back to these in greater detail in the next chapter. The first biologist, Michel Cladic, was a young pharmacist at the time, and later went on to complete medical training and a doctorate in science. Like many of the biologists and doctors encountered during this study, he was involved in a patient organization and was later a member of the Scientific Board of the *Association française de lutte contre la mucoviscidose* (AFLM – the French Association against CF) that went on to become VLM. Michel Cladic was still young and relatively inexperienced in the mid 1980s when he launched newborn screening. He had just brought together a small research team, which went on to obtain substantial recognition from scientific peers but did not enjoy any institutional affiliation or recognition at the time. In an interview Michel Cladic described his situation during this period as that of a 'maverick', which should be taken as meaning that he benefited from a certain amount of professional leeway. According to him, this opened up new possibilities that allowed him to move forward, even though this independence did entail the need to obtain funding, something to which we will return later. The second biologist was a biophysicist and pharmacist at the head of a nuclear medicine laboratory within a big hospital. He had met the main promoter of NSCF in Normandy (Brittany's neighbouring region) at a conference. The latter was a biochemist, and the former had conducted some screening trials in North Finistère. With a view to defending his laboratory's position among the other hospital laboratories (a position he perceived as peripheral), this second biologist was concerned with developing the laboratory and 'giving it a certain calibre' as he explained in an interview. Combining their scientific legitimacy with medical legitimacy, the two biologists from Brest received particularly active support from François Coat, a paediatrician working in a health care centre in Roscoff (a port in North Finistère), who was also an active member of the Board of Directors of the patient organization VLM. Shortly after his arrival in 1986, he became head doctor at the health care centre, a private non-profit establishment that had acquired a solid national reputation. The slightly higher number of affected children in their region had drawn his superiors' attention to CF. They had therefore created a specialized unit for treating the disease in the 1960s. This unit progressively became a centre of reference in the field, while remaining peripheral in institutional terms because it was not part of the hospital system. This should be linked to how François Coat describes himself in interview. Setting little store by the idea of a university career, he places the emphasis on his professional leeway – much like the molecular biologist from Brest. And it is true that when one arrives at the centre that he runs, nested between kelp and rocks, there is almost a sense of being at the 'end of the earth'. However, this geographical isolation is deceptive. The paediatrician became progressively interested in issues of health care organization that were, as we shall see, closely linked to NSCF and led him to become the main driving force behind a network of Breton paediatricians specializing in CF. Over three years, along with a few other doctors and biologists from Brest and, as we shall see, the energetic support of the president of a patient organization, the Finisterians organized information meetings about screening with many paediatricians and particularly heads of maternity units. Their efforts to publicize the idea of NSCF brought it out of the shadows and into the limelight. On the strength of this information campaign and the financial support provided by various partners – both public (hospital, etc.) and private (banks, etc.) – screening was launched in 1988 in the Finistère, to the enthusiasm of its instigators.

In order to understand this initiative from a sociological point of view, it is necessary to underline the saliency of the social position occupied by the three professionals at the origin of the screening: for different reasons, they all shared an institutionally peripheral position. One belonged to a new molecular biology team with no affiliations; another ran a nuclear medicine laboratory looking to defend its position; and the third worked in a health care centre outside the hospital system. This influenced the fact that NSCF was launched autonomously with regard to the official regional centre in Rennes, in charge of other newborn screening programmes. Indeed, one of these actors added in an interview: 'X [he cites a renowned doctor, linked with the screening centre in Rennes] had told me that it wasn't right to do that [launch NSCF] but I was free'. This position afforded them a certain leeway while also encouraging them to steadfastly develop their activities and highlight their skills. In this sense, while they were able to anticipate and decide as actors, they were also under the dual influence of their social positions and more general factors such as the cognitive world mentioned previously. Due to their relative marginality, their position regarding NSCF was similar to that of young researchers who, in general, can afford to argue in favour of a new scientific theory: on the one hand because the 'exit costs' of a recognized theory and 'entry costs' of a new theory are minimal, and, on the other, because the latter can provide them with an opportunity to carve out a professional space for themselves (Feuer 1974). Nonetheless, the stakes were not simply linked to research – far from it, they were also biomedical. These professionals' logics of action were therefore marked just as much by their scientific and medical arguments as by their social positions.

However, without the intervention of another type of professional policy entrepreneurs, this alone would not have sufficed to develop regional screening. Spurred on by the Finisterians' initiative, the directors of the regional centre for newborn screening in Rennes, under the authority of the national association in charge of newborn screening (AFDPHE), followed in their footsteps eight months later leading all of Brittany's medical actors with them. The centre in Rennes had two characteristics. First, as regional correspondent for the AFDPHE, it had been organizing newborn screening for different conditions throughout Brittany for several years. In this capacity, it held an intermediary position at the intersection between the initiatives in the Finistère and the AFDPHE's points of view and represented the most institutional element among the Breton policy entrepreneurs. Second, its history was marked by the development of public health as a discipline, to which the founding of the National School for Public Health in Rennes can testify. Current and previous directors of newborn screening across Brittany clearly laid claim to the legacy of this training, which offers insight into their professional and personal links. Moreover, this momentum in public health concerns instigated in Rennes led to regional paediatrics meetings, where all kinds of preventative approaches and screening were debated. The tradition of exchange in the field of paediatrics was therefore an established one.

When NSCF was launched in Brittany, paediatrician Christian Perret represented newborn screening in Rennes, where he was appointed director of the regional centre in 1990. He was particularly interested in the social and preventative aspects to paediatrics, as well as in the comprehensive dimension to treating children affected by CF, which involves nutrition, pneumology and gastro-enterology but also family support and public health, through screening. He was also involved in the patient organization VLM and later became vice president of its Medical Board. Furthermore, in 2002 he joined the AFDPHE's national office, thus finding himself at the intersection of the regional and national levels. In his view, Rennes' former responsibilities in the field of newborn screening gave the centre certain prerogatives for organizing the first stage of NSCF, a blood assay called the 'trypsin' test. In fact, the social and institutional positions of the main leaders of the Brest and Rennes groups led from the very start to a persistent conflict of legitimacy regarding who was to carry out the NSCF tests. In short, for each laboratory it was out of the question to let the other do this. Where the Brest group was concerned, they had three advantages: the fact that they had been the first to launch NSCF in the region; their drive and impetus (as we shall see later, they organized huge public campaigns); and the scientific legitimacy of the molecular biology laboratory, which increased progressively. On the other hand, the advantages for those in Rennes were also threefold: the legitimacy of the official AFDPHE centre; their experience in organizing newborn screening; and the practical and financial advantages of receiving the blood tests, because they were responsible for the other newborn screening tests. As with the biology laboratories, tensions also arose between the different health care providers of varying sizes regarding which centre patients should be sent to after screening. Aside from these competitive rationales, screening gave rise to a regional coordination structure, thanks to the creation of a network of paediatricians specialized in CF that met twice a year to review screening and its results, as well as to agree on health care protocol. The logics of action at work were therefore characterized, on the one hand, by tension between the two large regional groups and, on the other, by cooperation regarding health care protocols, as competition did not prevent the standardization of practice and regular reviews thus conferring greater scientific and medical value upon the initiative.

So far, we have identified a second condition for the emergence and development of this regional health policy: the configuration of professional actors with their own legitimacy, fields of competence and logics of action. The third condition did not have the same catalyzing role as the previous two, but its absence would have stopped the whole process in its tracks.

This condition was a moral one, taking morality to mean a set of values allowing actions to be evaluated on the basis of notions of good and bad. More specifically, this set of values includes, first, a prescriptive element, expressed by values, rules and codes, second, the way an individual behaves with regard to these and third, the way in which one conducts oneself (Foucault 1985). Before continuing further, I shall make a slight digression: I could also qualify this condition as being of an ethical order, given the ambiguity of the distinction between morality and ethics. As sociologist Patrick Pharo (2004) explains, it is usual to give a less prescriptive meaning to the Greek root (ethics) than to the Latin root (morality). However, he adds that there is also a deontological use of ethics, which, on the contrary, seems to refer more to strict, prescriptive rules than to the orientations of subjects considered as free in their actions. The sociologist concludes that it is necessary both to avoid tightening the semantic oppositions between these close terms and to take into account the words' usage (we talk about ethics committees and not morality committees). Moreover, the term 'ethics' is often associated today with professional practices, primarily in medicine, with bioethics, but also further afield. The two terms will therefore be used indistinctly here, bearing in mind that biomedical actors tend to speak of 'ethics'. In this part of the study, it is a question of an anthropology and sociology of morals with medical ethics as its object. It has been established that the increasing prominence of medical ethics and bioethics within biomedical concerns originates, at least in part, with the Nuremberg Trial brought against Nazi doctors at the end of the Second World War. The two main texts regulating these ethical principles are the Nuremberg Code, decreed in 1947, and the Declaration of Helsinki, adopted in 1964 and periodically revised. While they aim to embody universal values, their moral consequences and the conceptions covered by these are in the fact the result of multiple facets. An episode from the early 1990s can perhaps allow us to take the measure of these differences.

The differences between the regional and national levels appeared most clearly during a new pilot experiment launched by the Finisterians in 1992. First, it is worth recalling the distinction between the different types of screening: newborn screening (on neonates), prenatal screening (before birth, on foetuses) and heterozygote screening (on adults). The term 'heterozygote' or 'carrier' refers to people who carry one single copy of the mutated gene and who are not ill, given that CF is a recessive disease. Until the mid 1980s, prenatal diagnosis of CF depended on an enzyme assay during pregnancy, judged as being of low reliability. The real shift took place from the 1990s onwards when the gene involved – known as CFTR (Cystic fibrosis Transmembrane Conductance Regulator) – was isolated and the first mutations linked with CF were identified. Furthermore, a new method of DNA analysis called Polymerase Chain Reaction (PCR) came into play at this time, which allowed biologists to work on very small samples. The latter therefore had a quick and reliable method for prenatal diagnosis at their disposal. However, we will see that the search for mutations facilitated by PCR also contributed to NSCF's acceptability, due to the increased accuracy it afforded. In sum, NSCF and prenatal diagnosis were born from the same revolution in genetics and molecular biology.

In 1992, on the strength of these developments and in association with a small group of GPs, Michel Cladic launched a programme in North Finistère screening for adult 'heterozygotes'. The test was offered to all couples when they had their pre-marital health check. The aim was to detect those at risk of giving birth to children with CF and to offer them prenatal tests and pregnancy terminations on medical grounds where necessary. On a practical level, the pre-marital health check was considered to be an opportune moment to provide information to couples. During the check-up, this information was given by the GP, who would take a drop of blood on filter paper and send it to the laboratory in Brest. The potential parents received the results by post and were then invited to attend a genetic counselling appointment if a mutation was identified. On a financial level, this experiment was facilitated by the funds collected through a CF awareness campaign, run in collaboration with a daily newspaper and which we will return to later. All the doctors interviewed spoke of how favourably this was received by the couples concerned. The arguments in favour of this programme provided in interviews by its main promoters were threefold. First, there was the reasonably high frequency of the disease in North Finistère and the existence of CF 'hotspots' with a higher incidence of heterozygotes (around 1 in 10 rather than 1 in 35) in this part of the region. Second, there was the availability of technical tools, made easier by the relative homogeneity of mutations in the region. These two arguments overlap with those that have been and will be presented regarding NSCF and I will therefore analyze them later when discussing the latter. The third argument, more specific to heterozygote screening, emphasized the difficult living conditions linked to the disease. The explanation provided in an interview by one of the GPs involved illustrates this:

> I saw the work and the problems that CF meant for parents. ... It's a real task, you know, I don't know if you realize, it's crazy, to see a child who gets up in the morning and who coughs and coughs and coughs and coughs and who doesn't know what it's like to be healthy... It's dreadful to see a child like that. ... The kid with CF, he's sad, he's unhappy. And the boy I'm telling you about, ... sometimes, I'd have to wait 4-5 minutes until the coughing fit was over, because he was expectorating, it's awful. Awful. ... So, how could I not be, I'd say, tempted, to encourage people to do the test to eliminate this? There you go... so, it's probably because of having this real-life experience of the people I was treating, so it's, ... the real-life experience [*le vécu* in French], let's say. I think I am tempted to encourage people to do it (General Practitioner 1, 20.9.04).

This argument therefore rested upon the experience of following families' progress, sometimes bolstered by the use of examples. It was 'com-passionate' in the etymological sense of 'suffering with' and, to paraphrase Philippe Corcuff (1995), was part of a regime of ethical interpellation in the face-to-face and in bodily proximity. The system of values defended includes avoiding suffering, such as that observed by the doctor above in a face-to-face encounter that generates emotion on his part. Under these conditions, these professionals considered their action above all as 'help provided to families'. They were there to 'help them' and 'inform' them. They insisted, moreover, on the fact that the people taking the test did so voluntarily: the professionals' role was limited to offering the possibility, it was up to the parents to take the decision and it was also their responsibility to decide whether or not to continue with the pregnancy. In general, many social science studies have examined the non-directive nature of choice in genetic counselling and I will return to these in Chapters 3 and 4. Here the GPs took up this principle forged in the 1960s, which served as an ethical safeguard. As Michel Cladic stated in a press article at the time, 'we did not think it was valid to consult a bioethical body, as this would have been a waste of time. All the guarantees were present: it was a voluntary test in an at-risk region'. However, this took things too far. The initiative met with an angry response from the AFDPHE who saw something akin to eugenics at work. In 1993, it referred the case to the National Academy of Medicine, asking for a verdict on newborn and heterozygote screening.[6] Regarding the latter, the association considered that it would be inefficient if it remained individual, but that if it became collective and compulsory, it would represent a new form of eugenics that set little store by people's freedom and dignity. In the end, the promoters of this adult screening retreated in the face of these moral considerations, but also due to technical and organizational difficulties. They had underestimated changes in family structure – the increasing number of children born outside of marriage – that impeded their initiative. The project also suffered from recurrent funding problems and the fact that there were not enough geneticists to explain the results to the heterozygotes, as this notion was not that simple. After four to five years and a thousand tests, the instigators of heterozygote screening brought it to an end, even though, encouraged by the centre in Brest, certain GPs continued to occasionally offer the possibility to couples in the regions in question.

This episode takes us into the complex relationship between newborn and prenatal screening in a particularly informative manner, and this topic will be the focus of the last section of this book. For the moment, the latent accusation of eugenics should be noted and in this regard it is necessary to understand the moral grounds defended by the different parties. In West Brittany, screening of newborns and of heterozygotes for the same illness went hand-in-hand and were not antagonistic: in both cases it was a question of dealing with the suffering of the ill and their families, whether before or after birth. In 1988, a research project led by the new team from Brest directed by Michel Cladic stated: 'If the screening of heterozygotes within the population becomes feasible on a large scale, in the long term this will be the best prevention of the disease and its incidence will be greatly reduced'. This shows to what degree the aim of substantially reducing the disease's incidence in the population did not seem reprehensible in the eyes of these biologists and clinicians, and was even part of a value system centred on avoiding suffering. This value system was part of the foundations of action for which emotion could act as the catalyst. I will return to the AFDPHE's position on the national level later. I should specify from the outset that I have no intention of taking position in the never-ending debate in the social sciences about the existence of neo-eugenics, given that the term eugenics is in itself polysemic,

---

6   This request was not followed up.

taking on different meanings depending on whether it is compulsory, generalized, compassionate (etc.) or not... (Paul 1994, Koch 2004). However, the history of eugenics in France is enlightening as the originality of its foundations is twofold. It was carried forward by doctors rather than by statisticians or biologists, as was the case in other countries (Carol 1995). This explains in part why it developed so little in France. First, on a moral level, the deontology and personal convictions of the professionals were directly opposed to the strictest form of eugenics, that is the exclusion of the ill. Second, on a professional level, State eugenics went against their independent practice, endangering their freedom of action, prestige and income (Carol 1995). As for private, family eugenics, this had limited prospects. The irony is that the pre-marital health check, introduced in 1942 during the collaborative regime with Germany during the Second World War, was precisely one of the only eugenics-type measures implemented in France. In any case, the relatively weak presence of eugenics in France, historically, can afford us a partial understanding of a context in which it remains a sensitive subject capable of forging another ethos. This foray into heterozygote screening makes it clear why the whole political, but also moral, sphere in which these screening procedures took place warrants further questioning.

This 'aborted' screening programme, so to speak, implicitly sheds light on how, in order to develop, a social problem must acquire 'a necessary degree of respectability which entitles it to consideration in the recognized arenas of public discussion' (Blumer 1971: 303). The screening of heterozygotes did not achieve a sufficient degree of legitimacy to allow it to develop. As for NSCF, it fulfilled a moral condition allowing it to be, if not defended, at least tolerated, by the national bodies.

This tolerance involved the AFDPHE taking a back seat in regional matters. In 1989, the national association organized an experimental NSCF programme extended to a few regions in France (the Parisian region, the North, etc.) thus opening a 'window of opportunity', as political scientists put it (Kingdon 1984), for NSCF. However, 15 months later, they judged the experiment unconvincing and ended it. As we will see when we look the national level, this withdrawal can be explained by the fact that the AFDPHE considered the gap between the problem (CF) and the solution (newborn screening) as too great. However, encouraged by their own momentum, the Breton policy entrepreneurs forged on regardless and decided to pursue their own NSCF programme. This did not go without creating tensions. One of the Breton professionals explained explicitly in an interview: 'We were shot down in flames by the Parisians'. On a legal level, there was no particular regulation to stop them because screening tests, unlike medicines, are not subject to any codified authorization process.[7] In their view, NSCF was perfectly satisfactory and the experiment carried out in the other regions had essentially suffered from technical and organizational problems (badly prepared centres, etc.). This showed

---

7   Today still, nothing forbids regional initiatives of this type, providing they respect the law and bioethics decrees.

a refusal of what some of them perceived as Parisian centralism, and while this was certainly not what drove their action, it does contextualize it within the history of the region: in general, Brittany is marked by an age-old dispute regarding the 'Parisian' policy deciders who took so long to show any concern for the region's economic development. This is how newborn screening came to continue in both Normandy and Brittany, as well as, a little later, in other regions in central France. The regional health institutions intervened very little in NSCF during this period even if, at the end of the 1990s, they began to make their presence felt (through regional health conferences that included CF among their priorities, for example). Without leaning on State intermediaries, NSCF began from a local configuration of actors and mediums: it was therefore possible to talk about the local and then regional production of a health policy grounded in global concerns. It was as if the meso-social levels had been set aside. Finally, NSCF depended upon the constitution of coalitions of actors from a variety of horizons.

Coalitions as Resources

NSCF was easier to put in place than heterozygote screening and, above all, met with greater moral consensus, so the Breton professionals continued with this programme. And yet screening cost 2.3 Euros per child (85,000 Euros per year for the whole region) and without support from the Cnamts and the AFDPHE, they found themselves obliged to look for allies, particularly financial ones, in order to pursue and expand their action. Heterogeneous social networks had to be created that extended beyond simply the laboratory or the hospital department and this constituted an area of analysis with particular relevance for the social sciences. The fourth condition for NSCF therefore relied upon the constitution of coalitions of actors with a shared community of interests, if not shared aims.

From its inception in the 1980s, the newborn screening project was strongly supported by the Finistère delegate of the patient organization AFLM/VLM. He was a technician in an industrial company and, as well as his activities within the patient organization, had been a union activist since the 1950s and was also an administrator at the CAF (National Family Allowance Fund). He therefore had a strong activist background. He was convinced of the usefulness of prenatal diagnosis and medical abortions for parents confronted with the experience and suffering of the birth of a first sick child. Indeed, in his own personal life, following the birth of a first daughter affected with CF, he and his wife were strongly dissuaded by doctors from taking the risk of having other children: 'We were told: "You mustn't have any more children at all"' he recounts. For him, newborn screening was a necessary stage in ensuring the development of medical activity around the disease and in making prenatal diagnosis available. This is what led him to encourage the medical and scientific community to move forward with newborn screening.

As allies, the patient organizations therefore played an active role in these initiatives in West Brittany from their very inception. However, not only was

NSCF initially launched in Brittany solely by professionals (biologists and paediatricians), but also, with a few exceptions, NSCF was not at the heart of the preoccupations of patient families and organizations until the end of the 1990s. In their eyes, although newborn screening presented the apparent advantage of offering parents the possibility of prenatal diagnosis, in the end it did not really seem to make any fundamental difference to their daily lives. As a regional AFLM/VLM board member explained in interview:

> The parents, the families, have one essential, major concern, with a recurrent question, which is: 'What can you offer us to cure our children?' … Carrying out screening is good, it has to be done, but that's not the central issue. Because, anyway, screening is for those to come. But when you're the family of a sick child, [the question] is: 'What do I do to treat my child? And will they maybe be cured in the future?'… So you can understand that certain parents weren't really interested in the question (Patient organization board member 1, 17.2.03).

In this sense, without the professionals, the patient organizations would probably have adopted a different approach to the problem of CF or a different 'frame' to take up the term used by Hilgartner and Bosk (1988). Attentive to anything that could bring the disease into the limelight, the organizations accompanied the professionals in their initiative, with more or less enthusiasm depending on the *département*. They were sometimes particularly active on issues that included NSCF but also extended beyond it. In this way, a coalition of interests formed, with CF as the foundation, but with reasonable flexibility concerning the modes of intervention surrounding the illness. This aspect was reinforced by the role of another partner, from the media this time.

At the intersection between potential funders and biomedical professionals, the latter found a major ally, in the West of the region at least, in the shape of a daily newspaper – it should be noted that in the Finistère, there is a high rate of daily press readership per home (Charon 1996). In the winter of 1990-1991, the management of the regional daily, *Le Courrier du Finistère*[8] decided to launch a big fundraising campaign for the centres in Brest and Roscoff, and to take up CF as the paper's 'cause', to use the term chosen by one of its editors. Various elements contributed to this decision. First, a precedent had been set a few years prior when, following a case of cancer in his family, one of the main heads of the newspaper had become aware of the lack of appropriate equipment in Brest and launched a campaign entitled 'A Scanner for Brest'. This led to a vast mobilization to redress what was seen as a shortcoming of the State, obtaining rapid funding for the machine. This success had made an impression on the heads of the newspaper. Another reason lay with the institutional links between the Brest and Roscoff centres and, respectively, a Nobel Prize winner in medicine and an internationally renowned surgeon, who advocated helping the health care centre in Roscoff to better prepare

---

8   The name of the newspaper has been changed.

children for transplants. These two figures contributed to legitimizing the two centres, particularly as both agreed to spearhead the sponsorship committee of the funding campaign. Moreover, the question of the incidence of CF in Brittany was an important factor, exacerbated by the contradiction with the relative silence surrounding the condition at the time. More generally, health concerns – that were prevalent in society – had to be taken into account and allowed this silence to be broken. From a more strategic point of view, successful fundraising from readers was a way of increasing the daily's credibility and its 'power' in the eyes of impressed advertisers, as one of the newspaper's editors put it, in a context of rare competition between two regional dailies. The last important element to note is that the head of the *Courrier du Finistère* was friends with the director of the Roscoff centre, who was also a senator and who had made the financial needs of the centre clear to him.

Two of the driving forces behind the campaign – on the one hand, the sensitive issue of children's health and, on the other, what was seen as the particular relationship between Brittany and CF due to the 'high' incidence there – appear as the key threads running through the various articles involved in this intense campaign raising awareness – '*Opération Mucovicidose*' (Cystic Fibrosis Campaign). This translated into a page and half of articles published daily for three months. The first element, children's health, was expressed by particular turns of phrase (such as 'children's health has no price')[9] but even more by the fact that, predictably, it was at the core of the texts' subject matter. This was logical in face of the corporal reality of suffering children; it went without saying and was rooted in the historical process of sanitizing the contemporary world. The efficient foundation of the campaign (health) relates to what Didier Fassin (2009) calls 'biolegitimacy', which places health at the heart of societal concerns and determines the recognition received by many problems on the basis of health issues. The chosen cause therefore went far beyond screening itself insofar as it concerned children suffering from CF. Furthermore, and this will come as no surprise, a compassionate and affective dimension sometimes showed through ('this unjustified evil that attacks the innocent'). As underlined by the editor of the daily in an interview, the newspaper thrives in part on readers' emotions and their responsiveness in the face of these tragedies. This should be linked to the fact that more generally, according to Max Weber (1968), social activity can de determined in four ways: instrumentally rational, value-rational, traditional, and, in the case in hand, affectual (or emotional), in other words working through affects and feelings. On the other hand, there are many health problems and yet the public's attention is not infinite. In this perspective, constructionist sociologists look at how one cause can retain attention rather than another. The second element, the link between CF and Brittany, offers a way of understanding how the selection process between all possible causes worked. It was expressed by the campaign's

---

9   Unless otherwise specified, the quotations in this part of the text are taken from articles in the *Courrier du Finistère* in winter 1990-1991.

subheading ('The Breton Challenge') and expressions such as 'Cystic fibrosis strikes twice more in Brittany than elsewhere'. The higher incidence of the disease in limited geographical areas sometimes led to a shift between the figures noted in West Brittany and in the rest of the region. In certain cases, the effect of the figures was exacerbated by the ambiguity that led to a shift between the notion of being 'ill' and being a 'carrier'. The rate of healthy carriers of the mutated gene reached much higher levels, approximately 1 in 25: 'In each class, at least one child is a carrier of the gene. Yes, in Brittany CF is a disease ... that threatens us all, or at least our descendants'. The following remark from a paediatrician remembering this period is therefore unsurprising: 'When I said that CF was one or two children [born per year] in the *département* and that that was already a lot, when you saw CF everywhere, people sometimes felt there was a bit of a discrepancy' (Paediatrician 1, 9.9.02).

Thus, in a more or less diffuse and implicit fashion, the Breton regional sentiment found both an echo and a new source in a genetic disease: the scientific and medical centres concerned were in Brittany, the money collected remained in Brittany, and above all 'more' people were affected there. This feeling, sometimes bolstered by the media or patient organizations disseminating epidemiological studies showing greater frequency of the condition among populations of Celtic origin, also contributed to the mobilization. Another paediatrician explained: 'We were able to mobilize by saying "Cystic fibrosis is frequent, the gene is frequent in the Celts"' (Paediatrician 2, 27.8.02).

A partly constructed relationship was therefore established between Brittany and CF. Two remarks should be made about the 'Celts' and this 'frequency'. First, it was as if 'Celtic' Brittany (the Western part of the region) had come to know a new local variation of the stamp of genetics in the perception of origins and communities; in a way, a 'bioidentity' built upon genetics (I am adapting Paul Rabinow's (1996) famous expression of 'biosociality', a form of sociability grouping together individuals according to their biological, and notably genetic, traits). And it was as if this variant had influenced the rest of the region, which was not only historically distinct but also analyzed by epidemiologists as being genetically different (Scotet 2001), in carrying out this regional policy. Through this bioidentity and this regional policy, there was a veritable process of biopoliticization, the constitution of politics and policy on biological foundations. However, this bioidentity was much weaker than in the case of sickle-cell disease in the United States, to take another example of a genetic condition. This is unsurprising insofar as that sickle-cell disease is mainly associated with populations of African origin, whereas CF is of course far from specific to the Celts. In the United States, it has been shown that the test for sickle-cell disease largely reinforced a social and racial categorization of 'Blacks' (Fullwiley 1998). It was even considered that having the disease belied the presence of at least a 'drop' of Black blood in the genealogy of the affected subject, although the condition was obviously not absent from other populations. However, the context of racial discrimination linked with this illness and the populations it affected obviously had nothing in common with the Celtic sentiment as expressed often in West Brittany.

My second remark concerns frequency: we saw its cognitive origin earlier and now can better understand its effects. To paraphrase Ian Hacking (1999), the CF 'numbers' (that is, the statistical studies on the matter) played an important role in the construction not of CF but of the 'idea' of CF among the Bretons as well as in justifying NSCF. Let us look at the raw data. Newborn screening gave a more precise measure, showing that the incidence in Brittany was 1 in 2,900, with an increasing gradient from East to West, bearing in mind that NSCF allows us now to specify that the incidence in France as a whole is 1 in 4,400. This indicates that the ratio of difference between France and Brittany is roughly 1:1.5, which is not uncommon from an epidemiological perspective. Of course, differences in the regional incidence of genetic diseases are widespread and not specific to CF. Genetically speaking, France, like almost all countries, is a patchwork of different populations. So no matter how objective evaluating incidence can seem, there remains an element of subjectivity and construction and this contributed to how the issue was problematized.

Comparison with other health policies can shed further light. In general, there are many examples where statistical studies play a role in the recognition of a social problem. Even though it does not explain everything, Didier Fassin (1999: 8) underlines that 'putting reality into numbers is a way of constructing it and even simply of making it exist'. A good example is provided by the case of infantile lead poisoning where, thanks to epidemiological studies, the disease went from being a rare condition to ranking as an epidemic in France. Indeed, through the actions of a few health professionals, what began as a few isolated clinical cases became, over ten years, a public health problem affecting mainly immigrant families (Fassin 2004). In this regard, from a constructionist perspective it is interesting to note certain points of comparison between the two policies. First, for CF like for lead poisoning, the main people affected were children (the 'innocent', as the newspaper put it), most likely to elicit compassion. However, while in the first case, the regional policy of NSCF was constructed and took root rapidly, in the other it met with incredulity and resistance (Fassin 2004). Constructionist sociologists have tended to focus more on studying the conditions for the emergence of a problem than the speed with which this happens. Two elements at least could have contributed to this difference between CF and lead poisoning. First, in the case of CF, the figures (statistics on incidence) had largely been collected before the issue was problematized, whereas in the case of lead poisoning, the two went hand-in-hand with the numbers coming to light through epidemiological data at the same time as the issue emerged as a problem. The difference in speed was a direct and logical result of this. Second, the extension of social networks that took place in one case did not in the other. The families affected by lead poisoning were not active in the process; as immigrants, sometimes undocumented, they did not have much room for manoeuvre. Finally, in terms of social and political legitimacy, the fact that the disease affected Bretons above all was a factor in mobilizing people, which did not come into play regarding infantile lead poisoning: it was a case of 'us' (as we have seen) and 'them'. This effect of proximity increased the speed of the process and counterbalanced the limited differences between incidence in Brittany and in France.

Let us now pick up the narrative where we left it. What did this 'campaign' consist of in reality for the readers of the newspaper? There was no doubt that it was a great success in the West of the region (the campaign did not extend to the East). This success was demonstrated in financial terms, as 760,000 Euros were collected for the team of molecular biologists in Brest and the centre in Roscoff, contributing, far beyond NSCF, to acquiring equipment and paying staff. The success was also expressed by the rapid rise of real enthusiasm, widely shared by the various local actors. Several initiatives, all in aid of the campaign, can allow us to measure this. On one particular day, nearly 120 mayors put their political differences aside in order to sing in unison; another day, a meal was organized by the best chefs; yet another, a horse trek was set up. Sport was often placed at the forefront, along with the respiration that sick children so terribly lacked, and generally the events basked in an atmosphere that was genuinely cheerful and playful, but that could become tinged with gravity in the face of the suffering and difficulties of patients' families. While this recalled traditional fundraising events, these 'campaigns' were striking in their size and regional nature. The latter distinguished them from the Téléthon, while having many characteristics in common (Cardon et al. 1998). As with the Téléthon, the atmosphere was supposed to be festive. Above all, this action created the link between the participants, both individual (participants' names were mentioned in the newspaper) and collective (everyone joined in together and was fundamentally a member of a common humanity). The policy entrepreneurs, who must now include the journalists, gave moral legitimacy to their cause by foregrounding values such as solidarity. Under these conditions, many actors, and in particular local political leaders, expressed the self-evident nature of supporting the campaign. Solidarity with the fight against CF was simply unquestionable. This activism around CF affected NSCF and ensured its longevity. Far from being a flash in the pan, the strong friendships born during this period contributed to the strength of the network, and the *Courrier du Finistère*'s support for CF has not waned since. As an example, a statistical search for the term 'cystic fibrosis' in the newspaper's archives shows that in 2002 the term appeared no less than 3-4 times per day, on average. Many other events to raise awareness followed suit and the 'Cystic Fibrosis Campaign' of winter 1990-1991 acted as a catalyst giving impetus to a string of other initiatives, which slowly took root in the West of the region.

What were the limitations of these networks and this line of thinking? First, the situation was different in each of the Breton *départements*. The Finistère was in the best position because it combined expert resources, thanks to the professionals, militant resources, thanks to the patient organizations, and financial resources, thanks to media support. Elsewhere, the same notion of supporting NSCF being self-evident sometimes came to bear upon local councillors. In this way, the *Conseil général* (Departmental Council) of another *département* provided full funding for NSCF during all the years between the launch of the regional screening programme and the decision for generalized nationwide screening. And this decision was taken 'without any scruples' and 'without even thinking two hours about it', as the councillor in charge of the case put it when interviewed. This can be explained by the fact that he had encountered a few cases of CF during his previous career as a GP and that his attention had therefore been drawn to the disease. He also explained that a tenth of the elected members of the *Conseil général* were doctors who were easily sensitized to the disease and that the funding in question (around 20,000 Euros per year) remained low in comparison to the *département*'s overall budget. As for the third *département,* it contrived to find private and public funding (from donations, and the Rennes Town hall/*Conseil général*, respectively). The last *département* was the least well off, as it lacked both financial and militant resources, even though the momentum elsewhere encouraged it to follow suit. The other limitation was that, over the years, this funding became more and more problematic across the four *départements,* with local councillors in particular considering that it should be provided by the *Assurance maladie,* the state body that funds social security. In other words, the aim remained legitimate but the source of material funding was called into question. This shows to what extent this regional production of a health policy varied geographically according to *département,* but also over time as the goodwill of funders shifted. This created its uncertain nature and its main limitation.

Nonetheless, these initiatives allowed NSCF, as a response to a social problem, to survive throughout these years without withering out. This is how, 12 years after having been launched, screening had led to 118 children being identified as suffering from CF out of the 350,000 births in the region. The principles presiding over this extended action fit in with the outline drawn up by Stephen Hilgartner and Charles Bosk (1988): there was a 'dramatic' dimension (CF is a serious disease affecting children), a 'new' dimension (genetic diseases were a recent issue), 'organizational' characteristics (the two initiating centres were located in the distribution zone of the daily newspaper, and the director of the Roscoff centre was a friend of the head of the newspaper) and a recognized 'cultural' aspect (health is a major issue in our societies and the influence of genetics is extending). This satisfies the principles put forward to explain why some situations generate attention at a particular time when other, equally painful, situations do not. However, the sequential and linear view of a model of construction passing through different phases (Blumer 1971) is now outdated and should be modified. While there was, of course, a phase in which the problematization emerged and then developed, what should be retained is rather a dynamic with several dimensions and interrelated strategies and rationales at play. Moreover, this collective action was grounded on another principle linked to its dilution: the more the movement grew, the more the question of NSCF, put forward by professionals, became diluted in the wider issue of CF. Indeed, screening took on varying degrees of importance for the three groups of actors (biomedical, associative and media): it was central for the first, secondary for the second and not particularly highlighted by the third. Similarly, their logics of action were different but complementary. For biomedical actors, competition and cooperation were important; for the patient organization members it was a case of providing more or less energetic support to the professionals' initiative; and for the media actors, the issue was choosing a 'cause'. Contrary to other local health policies where the heterogeneous nature of the frameworks of action could lead to incomprehension (Hassenteufel et al. 1998), here their complementary nature was a help not a hindrance. This was probably the condition that enabled each party to support the initial project so strongly. The fact that everyone benefited from the network (the biologists and doctors from the support, the patient organizations from the enhanced visibility of the disease and the paper from reinforced credibility) contributed to its strength. There may have been conflicts, but these were between members of the same group, for instance between the biologists or between the health care providers.

Another feature of the research presented here is that the press played a major role in amplifying the issue and extending it to circles as varied as business leaders, sports personalities, political leaders and artists, etc. It is well known that the media often play a key role in selecting the problems of the public arena, to the extent that certain sociologists describe them as 'gatekeepers' (Hilgartner and Bosk 1988). More specifically, the role of the media is subject to differing points of view. Looking at a situation of 'tragic choices', Sébastien Dalgalarrondo and Philippe Urfalino (2000) studied the controversy caused by the suggestion of the National AIDS Council to draw lots to choose patients to benefit from new medication (protease inhibitors) at the end of the 1990s in France. At the end of their study, they relativized the power of the media and concluded: 'The temptation to ascribe the power to define social reality to the media soon seems unfounded when the sequential and interactive dimensions to a whole scandal or controversy are taken into account' (Dalgalarrondo and Urfalino 2000: 155). In my view, their study presents the advantage of insisting on the role of interactions between actors (clinicians or patient organization members) and the media, and advocating an analysis that is both internal (examining the content and work of the media) and external (examining the argumentative strategies and the mobilization as a whole). Nonetheless, it seems to me that overemphasizing interactions runs the risk of neglecting the specific roles of each party. In this chapter, we have seen that through its editorial choices the daily paper played an active role in constructing CF as a problem in West Brittany. I will not take this sociology of the media any further because, as we will see, the media was mainly involved at the beginning of the process. And this is logical. Often (although not always), public opinion is called upon through the media when it is not possible to appeal to institutions. Groups then manage to transform their issue into a cause of public interest, to build coalitions and in short to generate a form of 'external mobilization'. In contrast, groups with sufficient institutional links to allow them to put issues on the agenda without any media coverage constitute a form of 'internal mobilization'. In the case of the generalization of NSCF nationally, we will see that the latter prevailed.

Regarding Brittany, however, does this mean we should talk about a policy that was no longer reserved to professionals but open to the participation of the population? Regarding campaigns about the health of the 'excluded', Patrick Hassenteufel and colleagues (1998: 99) note:

> This campaign calls largely upon inhabitants' participation … . This way of working seems to constitute a break with the perception of public action in the field of health, insofar as it is no longer reserved to the medical profession but open to both new professionals and new actors, such as inhabitants.

While the inhabitants of the West of the region joined in with mobilization out of solidarity and compassion, the history retraced here shows that this health policy was above all piloted by professionals, sometimes with the support of patient organizations. The collective mobilization was organized much less in favour of screening as public action than around raising awareness about a disease. In a way, this mobilization was political, due to the favourable public opinion it generated, but in another, it was depoliticized, if we understand political to mean participation in the decision-making process. Moreover, due to its targeted nature and the fact it was relatively autonomous in institutional terms, it is necessary to question how it was made to fit in with a more general regional policy. For nearly the whole decade covered by regional screening, NSCF did not enter much in the hierarchical mechanisms of health issues. On the one hand, local actors took initiatives and invented forms of collaboration on the ground; on the other, this action took place at the margins of political arbitration. It should be noted, however, that this was partly redressed by the Regional Health Conference that placed genetic diseases among regional priorities in 1996, as we have seen, and expressed the desire to pursue initiatives surrounding CF. This went in the direction of the democratization of health, but occurred quite late in the process.

In conclusion, NSCF in Brittany has enabled us to see the necessary conditions and logics of action underpinning a regional health policy for a genetic disease, which seemed to be self-evident once its technical feasibility had been demonstrated. In contrast with the national and international debates to which NSCF gave rise, it is noteworthy that it did not lead to any fundamental opposition in the region. While the heuristic value of examining controversies has been proved on many occasions (Vinck 2010), what is striking here is the relative ease with which this health policy established itself. This was enabled by the lack of professional opposition on a regional level and the support of the general public. The conditions of possibility for this regionally consensual policy were linked to a number of elements: first, knowledge geared towards genetic diseases (originating notably in research on CF) and technical know-how; second, actors' logics of action (competition and cooperation); and third, processes of exchange with external social groups (the media, patient organizations and inhabitants). The role of the State was thus relativized and instead the emphasis was placed on local and regional levels of actors due to the specific nature of the issue (that is to say, CF in Brittany). Or rather due to its apparent specificity, given the actual and quite small difference in incidence between regions mentioned earlier. However, the effects of this policy were not simply regional because, in general, when a problem emerges it can then potentially spread into other arenas (Hilgartner and Bosk 1988) and it is common practice to attempt to influence these other arenas, although the success of such endeavours can vary.

History of a National Debate

Given the international debates fuelled by NSCF, it is not surprising that there were doubts in France about whether it was a good idea. What is more striking for the observer, however, is how a consensus was reached.

Institutional Intersections

In order to understand how solutions are chosen, it is essential to understand the groups that have the legitimacy to define the problems. The aim of this section is to retrace the formation of such a group, through the constitution of the AFDPHE. This association is not an institutional group belonging to the political and administrative apparatus, nor is it an interest group in the strictest sense of the word. Rather, from the point of view of constructionist sociology, it can be considered as the 'owner' of the field, a gatekeeper 'exert[ing] great control over the interpretation of situations and conditions deemed to fall under [its] jurisdiction' (Hilgartner and Bosk 1988: 69). From the point of view of the sociology of public action, in terms of newborn screening it could be compared, without any pejorative connotations, to a 'neo-corporatist' sub-group, not in relation to the State directly, but to the Cnamts. The label 'neo-corporatist' designates those who have the monopoly of representation in a system of sustained exchange with institutions (Chagnollaud 1999). Their main characteristics are often that they are responsible for implementing measures and establish tight contacts with institutions and the State, but have little involvement in lobbying members of parliament or political parties. And indeed, the AFDPHE had substantial responsibilities where the implementation of newborn screening was concerned and it developed institutional and personal links with Cnamts representatives, but set up few campaigns to raise awareness and influence decisions, and carried out little political lobbying. Let us look at how this group formed.

   The history of the association is based on the catalyzing role of a small group of paediatricians and geneticists working in the field of metabolic diseases. From the 1960s, they began screening babies for phenylketonuria, a rare hereditary disease (40 births per year in France) using urine and blood samples (Guthrie test).[10] Initially, it was a limited research and health care project that entailed identifying patients and offering them follow-up care, but progressively came the idea of a much wider scheme. This became all the easier to envisage given

_____

   10   At this time, the American doctor Robert Guthrie put forward a technique for collecting babies' blood on filter paper in order to carry out tests.

that other regional screening tests had been established, particularly in the North of France, where Bertrand Robin, the president of the AFDPHE at the time of my study, had also carried out tests of this type. Strongly involved in newborn screening, Bernard Robin became president of the AFDPHE in 1996 a few years before NSCF was launched in France. He initially trained as a paediatrician but he was also a geneticist with a particular interest in hereditary metabolic diseases, which were a new subject of study in paediatrics in the 1960s and 1970s, and was responsible for setting up an enzymology laboratory. He also gave consultations in genetic counselling and, for ten years, was head of a laboratory carrying out prenatal karyotype analysis, in other words the analysis of foetal chromosomes. He thus combined clinical, teaching and research activities, as well as responsibilities with the AFDPHE. He was also a member of the Medical Board for VLM. During my study, he had been 'retired' for around ten years, but his retirement had been extremely active as he was president of the national association and its regional branch in the North of France. He had a strong personality and did not mince his words, but as president of the association he also had to take into account its members' different points of view and approaches.

The hypothesis of these doctors was that phenylketonuria, which leads to severe mental handicaps, could be prevented by an appropriate diet. In 1972, they created a professional association – the AFDPHE – and structured the organization of newborn screening. The first problem, however, was funding. In 1978, they established a national convention for newborn screening with the Cnamts, which was the funding body. This brought into line various regional conventions that had been established on an ad hoc basis. The AFDPHE acquired definite legitimacy with the Cnamts and as such was not only in charge of running newborn screening but also able to suggest screening for additional diseases when deemed appropriate. It was therefore able to carry out and obtain funding for experimental programmes for new techniques or diseases, prior to any potential generalization. In return, its responsibilities entailed acting as an interface between the funding organization and the regional associations carrying out screening. Indeed, the AFDPHE constituted a federation of regional associations (the ARDPHE – *Association régionale pour le dépistage et la prévention des handicaps de l'enfant*/Regional Association for Screening for and Preventing of Handicaps in Children – of the Breton, Normandy and Centre regions...). The regions remained responsible for screening in their zone, after organizing the collection of samples in maternity units and co-opting laboratories to analyze them, and also for establishing registers of the babies tested. The national association remained responsible for drawing up accounts each trimester so that the Cnamts could reimburse the costs incurred, for establishing national statistics and for ensuring that the children identified as ill received medical treatment. AFDPHE commissions relating to technical or ethical aspects were also created. The DGS, which intervened less, was the other organization upon which the professional association depended.

This all allows us to understand the amount of energy necessary on the part of these professionals so that each of the 800,000 babies born in France every year could be screened for one, and then several, diseases in the few days following their birth. The smooth running of the association meant it had the stability to make its work long-term, until the nationwide implementation of NSCF, for the case in hand. In this way, the professional organization not only organized but also mediated newborn screening due to its strategic position, allowing it to define the principles for screening.

And what were these principles? The association's main aim was not only to identify the ill but also to direct them towards appropriate medical treatment. In other words, screening had to be not only efficient in identifying the affected subjects, it also had to be useful, with the guarantee that the ill would receive good treatment and would benefit directly from it. This was no doubt an ethos more than simply a principle; a system of values defended energetically, particularly by Hélène Ravenel, one of the key figures of the association, who contributed to its foundation. Originally a paediatrician, Hélène Ravenel soon turned to genetics and contributed to the fledgling stages of genetic counselling that she then went on to develop. Within the AFDPHE, she filled the roles of Treasurer and careful guardian of ethics. Her conception of ethics consisted in beginning with practice, as she had a certain suspicion of 'professional ethicists' disconnected from the reality of the field. She also created a national association of information about genetic diseases, aimed in particular at families affected by these illnesses, which gave her experience of parents' knowledge and concerns. This career path, along with those of the other founders of the AFDPHE, shows that paediatrics and genetics were intertwined. And although the association endeavoured to organize newborn screening, from its inception it was also concerned with prenatal diagnoses of chromosomal abnormalities and various genetic diseases. More than newborn screening alone, it was perinatal health that originally concerned these paediatricians/geneticists and I will return to this aspect later. For the case at hand here, it is becoming clear how the AFDPHE was able to contribute actively to creating an institutional trend in favour of implementing NSCF. Another association also had a role to play, albeit more marginal. We have seen how the patient organization intervened in West Brittany. On the national level, the patient organization was also present and intervened, indirectly, in the debate.

VLM (formerly the AFLM) was created in the 1960s mainly on the initiative of doctors and a few families. At the time of my study, it brought together roughly 4,500 members, a third of whom were families of patients or adult sufferers, while the remaining two thirds were sympathizers. It contributed to funding health care centres and laboratories, was involved in staff training, and offered help and advice to patient families. In terms of organization, it had a Board of Directors made up of a large majority of families, patients and sympathizers, as well as a Medical Board and a Scientific Board. As in Brittany until the end of the 1990s, generally speaking NSCF was not at the heart of the patient organization's preoccupations, even though some members and representatives were in favour of it and a few individuals here and there had made it into a cause. However, in 1999, when the AFDPHE was working on the question of whether screening was a good idea and how it could be implemented, the association came out in favour of screening as we shall see. So what happened between those two dates? At the end of 1998, the patient organization took on a new and dynamic general director, Marc Coudray, who was not the parent of sick child. After training in law and political science, he had worked for 15 years in asset analysis for a major bank. He had then worked for several years as a financial advisor to the archdiocese of Paris. His skills therefore went far beyond those expected for a patient organization. Keen to enter the associative sector, he had turned to the management of VLM where he saw his work as 'building bridges' between requirements, analyzable requests and methods to address these. Very early on, he considered that the organization was lacking a strategic base. End 1998, during a meeting of the Board of Directors, he brought up screening for CF, which he saw as a possible basis for developing the organization's activity. However, the suggestion was not really taken up at this time. It is only later that the idea grew on the basis of medical and political arguments that I will develop further when we look at those of the professionals. In any case, the link (the 'bridge') had to be created between the doctors' suggestions and the patients' problems.

The other major factor was that the organization's Medical Board came down in favour of NSCF in 1999, on the basis of arguments that will be outlined in the next section. It is important to specify that this reflection was due to the fact that several members of the AFLM/VLM's Medical Board were part of a working group instigated by the AFDPHE to look at whether NSCF was a good idea. In a more direct fashion, the patient organization acted as a pressure group working on public authorities, through various political leaders, including ministers. As for the Cnamts, it was able to see that the organization was in favour of screening and this showed that it had the backing of the main people affected – the families of patients. At first glance, then, the organization's role seems relatively complex and low-key. However, a number of questions remain unanswered, particularly concerning the power relations between professionals and non-professionals, and the circulation of information between regional and national levels. These will be taken up further on.

The first condition for the generalization of NSCF was therefore the formation of a solid group at the interface between institutions, with, on the one hand, a mediating association and, on the other, a patient organization able to provide a form of backing to NSCF. However, other conditions had to be met, particularly linked to technical and epidemiological questions. The AFDPHE was the institutional guardian of newborn screening and NSCF had to be perfected in order to be accepted by the professional association. In this sense, one of the 'streams' that fuel public policies had to be advanced (Kingdon 1984): that of solutions.

Epistemo-Political Conditions

In general, technical evolution testifies to two developments that are intertwined. The first is the conjunction, or even the co-production, of science and technology, which has led us to talk about 'technoscience' (Latour 1987). The second is the enrolment of technoscientific practices at the heart of current medicine, which had led social scientists to talk about the 'technoscientization' of medicine (Clarke et al. 2010). Medical techniques are the material form taken when science and medicine mix, but they are far from being simply pure scientific applications without any contingency or social consequences. And so what of these social factors? Wiebe Bijker (1995: 254) suggests a periodization of the different conceptions of the relationship between technology and society. The author indicates a pendulum swing between an initial period, before the 1940s, when the technical aspects of societal evolution were neglected, and a second period that went so far in the opposite direction that it considered technology as 'an autonomous factor to which society had to bow'. This was then followed by a third period, again in opposition with the previous one, in which technology appeared as nothing more than a social construct. More recently, he argues, technology has recaptured some of its intrinsic abilities, without completely losing its socially constructed nature, and within some of these new conceptions, the boundaries between social and technical factors have disappeared. In the case in hand, let us look at the interactions between socio-political factors and use of technology.

In 1979, a publication by a New Zealand biologist reported a rise in the blood levels of a protein called immuno-reactive trypsin (IRT) in young patients suffering from CF, compared to a control group. This observation offered an initial way of sorting through the population of newborns in order to identify those for whom the diagnosis of CF needed to be confirmed or contradicted by what is known as a sweat test (because it consists in testing the levels of chloride in the child's sweat). Immediately, a biochemist from Normandy with a strong interest in technical challenges and who was convinced of the benefits of NSCF for patients, decided to launch screening in part of Normandy in 1980, eight years before it was launched in the Finistère and 20 years before it was generalized in France. He was helped in this endeavour by [X], a biological and pharmaceutical products company, which provided him with the adequate reagents, pleased to have found a potential outlet for their IRT assay method, which had been little developed thus far. Screening in Normandy continued for many years, thanks to the tenacity of its promoter and consistent help from the company. It was reasonably isolated within France, however, with one exception. The Finisterians, as we have seen, launched their screening in 1988 after having established contacts with their colleague in Normandy and led their whole region to follow in their footsteps. The rest is history.

So what position did the AFDPHE officials take in 1987-1988 with regard to these regional initiatives? They accepted that the IRT marker was reliable, while expressing practical, psychological and medical reservations. First, from a practical point of view, they regretted the absence of a 'kit', that is a set of commercialized products ensuring a simple and standardized test method. This problem disappeared once [X], the company that had helped fund the Normandy screening, launched a 'kit' on the market in 1988. In turn, the firm had received help from the biochemist in Normandy, who had explained to the company's representative, now a friend, that this technical ease was a prerequisite for the generalization of screening. The biochemist had even played an active role (on a voluntary basis, he specifies), going into the company to outline the necessary specifications. The 'kit' problem was resolved, but a second, psychological, factor had a negative effect on the opinions of the AFDPHE officials, who were worried about the need to call back newborns with an initial positive result for a confirmation test. The method used was not sufficiently precise and had an estimated rate of false positives (results above a certain level in the first test that were clearly negative in the second) of between 0.5 and 1 per cent. There was a risk that this follow-up test would not always be carried out because a substantial portion of families might fall by the wayside and be impossible to contact. Moreover, it also ran the risk of worrying families unnecessarily, by alerting them to an initial positive result when the second would be completely reassuring. In the 1990s, CF was becoming relatively well known in the public space and it frightened people. It was no longer possible for parents to take the suspicion of CF in a child lightly. The third main remark made by the AFDPHE officials concerned the medical benefits of screening, considering that they needed to be better demonstrated. With a view to this, and partly under pressure from the groups in Brittany and Normandy, they promoted a pilot study that was numerically sufficient to evaluate technical feasibility and long-term efficiency in terms of health. In this spirit, in 1989, they launched the experimental NSCF programme mentioned previously that was extended to several regions, including Brittany and Normandy, and funded by the Cnamts. Fifteen months later, however, they decided to end the programme, considering that it was too difficult to evaluate the rate of 'false negatives' and that there were too many 'false positives'. These were classic problems of feasibility in screening. Above all, the national association viewed with caution the studies tending to show a medical advantage for children screened in comparison with a control group, pointing out methodological bias. The AFDPHE enjoined the biologists and doctors, particularly in Brittany, to end their programme but, as we have seen, the latter were not particularly inclined to bow down in the face of national orders, and tensions rose.

However, the question of test methods saw a sudden new development shortly after, with the perfection of genetic tests. The early 1990s corresponded to the period of excitement within the 'segment'[11] of the social world of CF that preceded and followed the isolation of the CFTR gene. In Brittany, where screening had continued against all odds, this research progressively transformed its procedures. From 1992 onwards, in cases where the IRT assay gave an initial positive result, a more precise DNA test was then carried out. It should be underlined that this was the first time the search for a mutation was included in a screening strategy on a population in France. Although the process was cumbersome, it had the advantage

---

11   The term 'segment' is borrowed from Anselm Strauss (1961), who uses it to designate the groups that emerge within a profession.

of reducing the rate of false positives. Consequently, the families' worries appeared to be limited, particularly given that the DNA test could be carried out on the same drop of blood as the first test, thus avoiding the need to take a new sample from the child. These changes undoubtedly contributed to making screening more socially acceptable in France. One of the paediatricians, who later participated in the discussions on NSCF organized by the AFDPHE, specified:

> The psychological repercussions of false positives were really too serious. ... Without MB [molecular biology], they wouldn't have followed on a national level, I don't think. ... In particular, MB allows fewer children to be called back, there are still false positives, but they are a lot fewer now (Paediatrician 2, 4.2.03).

In short, from the early 1990s onwards, genetics provided the necessary tools for constructing this health policy on a national level: alone they were not sufficient, but without them NSCF would not have been generalized. The second condition for generalization lay with the available techniques. The sum of social factors influencing the use of the IRT assay, and the search for mutations on a large scale, was such that the role played by social elements in fashioning technology leaves no room for doubt. The following elements have already been noted, among others: professional career paths (of biologists and doctors); technical challenges to be met and know-how to be acquired (by the biologists); social networks (in the West) and controversies (between the local and the national levels); instruments for national management and regulation (the national association's checks); economic interests of multinational corporations (the pharmaceutical company). Conversely, though, and in my opinion more importantly, what was the impact of the technical on the social? This question will be addressed throughout this book, focusing particularly on the political issues raised by this technology, on how these tests were able to influence the way people were categorized and on the moral objections to which they gave rise. Where this first chapter is concerned, let us note that while technical progress was necessary, it was far from being sufficient in the eyes of the AFDPHE. They wanted consistent medical arguments in favour of the benefits of NSCF for the children concerned. We must remember that this related to their very principles of action: screening for screening's sake was out of the question. From this point of view, the situation did not evolve much until the end of the 1990s, which marked an epistemic turning point in the history of NSCF.

In 1997, a new element came to bear allowing the policy entrepreneurs in Normandy and Brittany to push forward their favourite solution. Namely, the publication of the results of a vast study carried out in the United States comparing the health of sick children diagnosed after newborn screening with the health of those diagnosed using traditional methods (Farrell et al. 1997). The methodology used met with large agreement among health professionals, particularly in France. Indeed, the study fulfilled all the standards of evidence-based medicine, that is to say the medicine based on scientific criteria and statistics that developed during the twentieth century (Marks 1997). The study showed an advantage in terms of the height and weight of the children diagnosed through screening, but it did not provide any positive elements in respiratory terms despite this being the most important factor. It nonetheless contributed to the idea that NSCF could have a positive impact, perhaps low but quantifiable. A series of other articles were then published, which were less consensual in terms of methodology, suggesting that there was a clinical advantage for children diagnosed through screening. Some of these were presented at an international conference held in Normandy. The Breton paediatricians and biologists involved in NSCF were present, but also the national AFDPHE officials. Discussions regarding screening began to take a new turn, especially given the intervention of another element, which was even more important in the decision-making process behind NSCF. From the mid 1990s, international comparisons of life expectancy for CF sufferers developed. At the end of the decade, the idea became established that France was one of the countries in Europe where this was lowest. Between, on the one hand, comparative studies about the clinical state of children diagnosed through screening versus those diagnosed from symptoms, and, on the other, international comparisons of patient life expectancy, there was much food for thought. And things began to move more quickly.

Before delving any further into this history, it is necessary to question the significance of this particular moment in the history of NSCF in France. My analysis of the Breton programme placed the emphasis on its 'problematization', in other words on the construction of a public problem rallying support from part of the population. On the national level, the situation was different. While screening in Brittany had not led to any real resistance from the region's professionals, generalization was far from self-evident (the main historical architects of newborn screening were long opposed to it). There is no doubt that scientifically grounded studies provided support for the Breton professionals' initiative – genetic studies on the etiology of CF and epidemiological studies on its incidence played a crucial role. However, it is just as clear that these were considered notoriously insufficient to justify a national programme. The national and regional situations differed in particular in their relationship to knowledge: further biomedical studies were necessary in order to begin reflection about generalized NSCF. In this sense, on the national level, it was not only a question of the constitution of a public problem, as was the case in Brittany. Here, a problem was constituted but the actors had further requirements where the solutions were concerned. It was a question of 'problematization' not only in the sense of constructionist sociology, but also in Michel Foucault's sense of the word (1989: 296). He did not use the term much, but defined it as 'the set of discursive and non-discursive practices that make something enter into the play of the true and false and constitutes it as an object for thought'. And it is precisely this 'play of the true and the false', or in other words what is considered as scientifically reliable, that formed one of the differences between the regional and national situations. Grasping this nuance between the two variants of problematization is not simply an academic exercise; it also affords a more precise understanding of the third condition for the generalization of screening – the shift towards a different kind of scientific rationality.

This brings us to the final stage in the process leading to the decision to generalize NSCF in France. In spring 1999, the AFDPHE invited a working group to a meeting in order to consider whether or not NSCF was a good idea. Discussions were organized within the group, which comprised 11 professionals. With the exception of the national association's representatives, the majority were paediatric clinicians (some also held responsibilities within the AFDPHE) and there were also a few biologists and geneticists. The group included policy entrepreneurs from the Breton and Normandy screening policies, who had been pushing their solution for a long time. I will come back to the arguments in favour of screening, as well as their political stakes, later. In the meantime, I should specify that, in addition to the epistemic data presented above, the members of the group shared the idea that it should not be a question of screening alone but of combining screening with reorganized health care provision. The fourth condition for screening was therefore of an organizational nature. And this idea seemed to unite everyone's points of view, even those the most against NSCF: in November 1999, the working group sent a report to the Cnamts and the DGS, the two supervisory bodies, concluding that it henceforth recommended that systematic screening for CF be included in the French newborn screening programme (AFDPHE 1999).

In October 2000, the president of the AFDPHE presented the project before the members of the Cnamts commission in charge of newborn screening. In view of the arguments put forward, the commission agreed in principle to provide funding at an estimated cost of 1.8 million Euros per year[12] without objection, while enjoining the AFDPHE to continue reflecting upon the practical elements involved in its implementation. In December 2000, the Cnamts and the AFDPHE held a joint press conference about the decision to generalize screening in France. NSCF led to greater mobilization than other newborn screening: given how widely it was debated and even contested internationally, everyone was aware of how complex this measure was to put in place. In order to resolve the numerous practical questions raised, the AFDPHE and the working group set up different commissions. These extended to other actors, mainly biologists and paediatricians but also a representative from the Cnamts, a legal specialist, etc. After a period of substantial work, the protocols for screening, paediatric follow-up care and information were established. Moreover, the Ministry of Health did not want to be left by the wayside, considering that the question of health care went beyond the issue of screening and thus fell under its remit. In parallel to the work undertaken by the commissions, in 2001 the *Direction de l'hospitalisation et de l'organisation des soins* (DHOS – Department of Hospitalization and Health Care Organization) and the DGS, both under the authority of the Ministry, organized working meetings with various medical professionals and representatives from health care bodies, in order to prepare a Circular regarding health care centres for

---

12   This cost does not include the funds allocated (budgets and/or creation of jobs) by the Ministry of Health to the health care centres set up when screening was put in place, nor the financial support provided to the molecular biology laboratories.

CF.[13] It came out end 2001 and emphasized both multidisciplinary and specialist treatment for the disease. The organization of treatment and prevention was an opportunity to consolidate the positions of the professionals specializing in the field of CF and raise their profiles. All this work had the effect of reinforcing the position of the big health care centres and hospitals specializing in the disease. Finally, as the working commissions had given their conclusions to the Cnamts, an agreement was signed regarding the funding of NSCF. Early 2002, everything was finally ready and generalized screening was progressively set up across France.

In conclusion, this chapter has offered an initial insight into the definition of a policy in which life was the key issue and suffering served as a sign, while genes acted as the medium. The conditions of possibility for legitimate public action surrounding a genetic disease have been underlined, in a situation where the benefits were uncertain. The study of the links between the local, regional and national levels has shown that it is necessary to deconstruct the top-to-bottom view of political decisions, moving from the State to the local level. Rather, the public action here was multi-level and carried forward by local actors, who made their voices heard and negotiated regulations on a national level.

What can this history of how NSCF was set up teach us about the specificities of public action involving genetics? In order to answer this question, I will begin with a paradox. Cystic fibrosis, as we have seen, has a very particular position among so-called monogenic diseases (those affecting mainly one gene). The paradox is that it is both the most frequent genetic condition to affect European populations and yet, at the same time, it is a 'rare disease', by definition affecting less than one newborn in 2,000. And it is indeed rare, because in France it affects 180 newborns and causes 50 deaths per year. Without detracting from the often devastating effect it has upon the families concerned, in quantitative terms it cannot be considered a major health problem. As we have seen, CF was foregrounded just as much due to the endeavours of scientific, medical and other actors as because it was a self-evident priority. However, these endeavours would not have taken hold and would simply have been unimaginable had another element, reaching beyond the French context, not come into play. It is important to remember that in the twentieth century, the genetic approach became one of the leading disciplines within the sciences (Fox Keller 2000). From the point of view of sociological theory, remembering this allows us to situate local concerns within global ones, even though the latter obviously include many aspects other than knowledge (international political relations, the globalized economy, etc.). Indeed, on the one hand, actors can contribute to producing cognitive matrixes on their own level, and, on the other, these are also imposed upon them as models through which to interpret and understand the world. The more specific element that came to bear on this situation was a form of knowledge that seemed not only increasingly

---

13   The Circular in question is the DHOS-DGS n° 502 of October 22, 2001. It suggested a network of care provision, under the responsibility of the health care centres.

prevalent within scientific approaches, but also capable of spreading throughout the population. An initial specificity of this public action was therefore that while its object was a rare disease, it was grounded in genetics, a cognitive matrix that permeates many aspects of our lives.

The second point concerned the question of geographical origins. In this regard, a significant anecdote is worth mentioning. When NSCF was launched in Paris and the surrounding region, the incidence of the disease in the North of the region was ten times lower than expected by the screening promoters, whereas the rate of sickle-cell disease was much higher. After having initially thought there had been an error with the test, they realized that this was simply a reflection of the population tested, which included a much higher proportion of people of African origin than other areas. In other words, while the importance of geographical origin within the history of the Breton programme has been analyzed as a breeding ground for the sentiment of belonging to a biological community facing a common health problem, on a national level this impact was more diffuse. It did, however, remain relevant insofar as NSCF concerned a disease that is much more prevalent amongst European, or 'Caucasian', populations than African or Asian ones. The opposite situation prevailed in the case of sickle-cell disease, for which newborn screening had also been put in place, as it mainly affects populations of African origin. This screening was carried out for all newborns in the French overseas *départements* and territories, as well as those whose parents were of African origin, or from the Mediterranean basin. The biological links between genetic diseases and populations therefore had practical consequences in terms of categorizing the populations to be screened. Moreover, screening magnified the differences inherent to the biological nature of the various groups within the population ('Celts', 'Caucasians', etc.).[14] The second feature was therefore that people were categorized according to origin and this brought to the forefront the question of belonging to a population group according to origin and based on biological grounds.

The third set of features was more specifically linked to the DNA test. In the case of CF, the test increased the precision of screening and contributed to making it acceptable in the eyes of those responsible for organizing it. Genetics was therefore a bonus in terms of the public health criteria which such policies have to meet. In terms of organization, in order for the test to be carried out by the analysis laboratories, parents had to give their consent by signing the card on which the baby's blood sample was collected in the maternity unit. Since the 1994 bioethics laws in France, any DNA test requires the written consent of the person concerned, or the parents in the case of children. The ensuing practices and implications will be examined later. For the moment, it is important to underscore that, on a legislative level, one of the characteristics of these public actions was that they constituted legal subjects, in other words people who, at least theoretically, should be able to make choices within a legal framework.

———————————

14   Regarding the evolution of the link between genetics and geographical origin, see in particular the special number of the journal *Social Studies of Science* on this topic (2008).

Finally, the last feature of this public action was that it resulted from the transmission of a gene between parents and children, potentially conferring upon the latter that most precious commodity in society today – health. However, the genetic test put in place for NSCF called partly upon the same technique as screening of parent carriers and prenatal diagnoses of foetuses: the search for a possible mutation. It was no coincidence that the search for mutations was added to newborn screening in Brittany at the beginning of the 1990s, at the same time as the heterozygote screening trial was carried out in North Finistère. In both cases, this depended on the isolation of the gene responsible for CF and the characterization of the first genetic mutations. One of the features of these public actions was that they were more or less closely linked to the questions and moral protests raised about the selection of foetuses. While all public actions must respect a certain number of values in order to be adopted and to last, the particular sensitivity surrounding the issue of eugenics in France gave greater importance to this dimension here.

These different features are an integral part of the field of experience of medical genetics, as defined in the introduction, and will be analyzed along with others throughout this book. They define the framework within which genetics is likely to enter into a public policy, with its legitimacy (regarding health and knowledge), its effects (biological origin), its constraints (written parental consent) and its points of contention (the debates on eugenics). Above and beyond its sociological interest, this framework fuels the debates outlined in the introduction regarding the principles and modes of this emergence of genetics. From this point of view, we have seen that a major difference between the regional and national levels was due to the relationship to scientific knowledge. I shall now turn to this dimension and examine it in greater detail. Let us therefore enter the scientific dimension of the field of experience.

Chapter 2

On Scientific Grounds

The summary of the history of screening presented in Chapter 1 has allowed us trace its main stages and identify the conditions that made it possible. It is now necessary to analyze in more detail how the decision-making process leading to screening was underpinned by knowledge and thinking. What are the means of expertise and calculation, the knowledge and the rationalities deployed by this particular activity of government (in the sense defined in the introduction)? Although formulated differently, these questions are similar to the traditional questions of epistemology. And the question of defining truth – when does knowledge establish something to be true? – is central among these. However, while this question can fuel thinking about the place and use of truth in scientific practice, this truth should not be normative or confused with the kind that would consist in establishing whether science attains 'the' truth in its disembodied and overarching form. Rather, the truth that interests us here is defined by the set of rules and procedures that enable utterances to be produced or put into play that people then consider as true at a given moment (Foucault 2001b). More widely, these rules and procedures are part of a 'regime of truth' that covers at the same time the 'types of discourse that a society accepts and makes function as true', 'the techniques and procedures accorded value in the acquisition of truth' and 'the status of those who are charged with saying what counts as true' (Foucault, in Rabinow 1984: 73). What is of interest here is analyzing how this long-standing question was reconfigured at a given historical period, and in a given environment, because every society, but also every field of knowledge within a given society, has its own regime of truth.

At a time of recurrent controversies about the use of new technologies, one of the issues at stake is clarifying the relationships between this use and the criteria for something to be considered as scientific. An example, among many others, illustrating both the scope and topicality of the issue can be found in a field both close to and far from screening: the French debate surrounding genetically modified organisms (GMOs). This debate opposes those in favour of GMO development, those who contest the policy of the *fait accompli*, and those who believe in experiments – but which ones? – validating or invalidating the use of GMOs.

Over the past three decades, the social sciences of science have seen substantial development, both in qualitative and quantitative terms. I will not present the various key questions and numerous trends here (see in particular Vinck 1995, Hacking 1999, Bourdieu 2004), but will rather identify a few key points that can help us understand the scientific stakes of screening. Traditionally, rationalist sociologies tend to defend the idea that scientific assertions that are valid independently of social context do exist (Vinck 2010). Others, spurred on by followers of the 'Strong Programme' in the sociology of science, are more inclined towards relativism and refuse the absolute criteria of rationality. In the same vein, some reverse a commonly accepted assertion and argue that a statement becomes true because it is stabilized as a scientific fact, rather than the opposite (Latour and Woolgar 1979). This reversal is strongly contested due to its 'effect of derealization' that seems to indicate that facts are entirely fictional (Bourdieu 2004). That said, many researchers lay claim to a position that explains the stability of science by combining internal explanations (which can be attributed to nature itself) and external explanations (which depend on social and economic factors, etc.) (Hacking 1999). I shall take this position myself, as it seems to account best for what can be observed.

The question of evidence is at the heart of what is considered to be true. Indeed, according to the dictionary definition, evidence is 'Ground for belief; testimony or facts tending to prove or disprove any conclusion' (OED). However, evidence is certainly not established in the same way in physics, the natural sciences or medicine. While there are points of convergence linked to the *episteme* mentioned previously, each discipline has its own regime of truth. And each regime of truth interacts differently with regimes of power and values. We can therefore see what examining NSCF can bring to this already fruitful set of studies. The specificity of this analysis lies in the fact that it not only concerns a public action applied to a country, but is also at the interface between science and medicine. Therefore, more than other issues, it is prone to combining scientific, political and moral questions. Let us now see more specifically how evidence is constituted within medicine.

The current role of evidence in medicine has its origins at the end of the eighteenth century and during the nineteenth century among the circles of French clinicians and 'hygienists', such as Philippe Pinel, Pierre Louis, Louis Villermé, Adolphe Bertillon and Claude Bernard.[1] From the beginning of the twentieth century, as Harry Marks (1997) underlines, 'therapeutic reformers' – a set of actors ranging from doctors and statisticians to administrators and journal editors – mainly from North America sought to develop an extensive project implementing a scientifically grounded approach to medicine. After the Second World War, the orientation of practice towards epidemiology and statistics clearly expanded. In Great Britain, this movement could also be seen in the work of epidemiologists such as Bradford Hill, who established a statistical link between tobacco and lung cancer, and Archibald Cochrane, who advocated introducing greater rigour and more experimentation into medical practice. The reformers suggested an evaluation criterion intended to be reliable and universal, based on a

---

1   For more information on this subject, the reader can consult another work of mine (Vailly 2011).

type of trial named the double blind randomized controlled trial (RCT).[2] This was typically the trial advocated by the group of doctors defending what was called 'evidence-based medicine' (EBM). This group formed at the end of the 1980s around a Canadian team who published a series of articles in the *Journal of the American Medical Association*, aimed in particular at helped clinicians evaluate the reliability of studies. According to the co-authors of the founding text of this series, it was necessary to produce nothing less than a 'new paradigm for medical practice' thus relegating non-systemized clinical experience to the rank of insufficient foundation (Evidence-Based Medicine Working Group 1992). EBM generated a certain amount of enthusiasm within part of the academic elite and its precepts were disseminated in particular throughout the United States and Europe. Increasingly, not only clinical practice but also health care policy were subject to this requirement to provide evidence of efficacy. And the strictest proponents of EBM hunted down bias, and errors in methodology or reasoning.

Through the history retraced here, we can better understand the place held by evidence among the rules necessary to constitute the 'truth' in biomedicine today. However, this should not give the impression that the movement developed without resistance from the medical community. Their criticisms of EBM concerned in particular the difficulty of reconciling evidence drawn from populations with individual approaches to patients, and also the failure to take the patient's point of view into account in therapeutic decisions (Lambert 2006).

These debates and developments have given rise to a series of social science analyses focusing broadly on how evidence is produced, how it is used – or the links between production and use – and the effects of these new forms of rationality in medicine. Here, we will look above all at the studies concerned more specifically with how evidence is produced, or the links between the production and use of evidence.[3] Judith Green (2000), in particular, conducted a study on the social construction of evidence within accident alliances (organizations created for road traffic accident prevention) that bring together representatives of health authorities, police officers, firemen, etc. She showed that evidence is constructed differently according to the goals and practices of the actors involved, in correlation with their own professional identity. Very often, personal experience and common sense are considered as evidence and more so than the scientific evidence established in specialized journals. Raymond De Vries and Trudo Lemmens (2005) carried out a bibliographical study on the significant influence

---

2   The RCT consists in constituting two groups of individuals separated *at random*, one following the treatment that is the subject of evaluation, the other treated by a placebo or control molecule. Another principle is the fact that clinician and patient are not told about the nature of treatment during the trial (*double blind*).

3   Other studies concern the stances adopted towards EBM by different actors and how they appropriate its precepts in different countries in Europe or North America (see in particular Dodier and Barbot 2000, Timmermans and Angell 2001, Dobrow et al. 2006, Blume and Trump 2010, Kelly et al. 2010).

of pharmaceutical companies' commercial interests on the way clinical trials are conducted and their results reported. Furthermore, they showed the role of culture and presuppositions in the statistical battle engaged in by obstetricians in favour of, or opposed to, home birth in the Netherlands. These two studies do not delve into the depths of scientific data because they focus rather on the processes through which this data is circumvented. Tiago Moreira's study (2007) focuses more closely on scientific data because it looks at how knowledge is composed in laboratories that compile systematic reviews and meta-analyses, and how this knowledge comes to mediate the relationship between health research and health policies. In describing the daily practice of reviewers, Moreira shows how they deconstruct evidence and recalculate it using an approach that seeks to be as rigorous as possible. Some of these studies underline that the kind of objectivity characterizing biomedicine has less to do with truth as such than with the pragmatic adjustments that allow facts and evidence to be made compatible between increasingly interconnected medical institutions (Moreira 2005, Knaapen et al. 2010).[4] In this spirit, Peter Keating and Alberto Cambrosio (2009: 326) suggest that the advent of clinical trials is linked to the emergence of a new form of objectivity in biomedicine – 'regulatory objectivity' which 'produces schemes, guidelines and models of action that seek to submit the evolution of uncertainty to commonly shared rules of action'. Regulatory objectivity is not 'restricted to the use of standard measures. It incorporates the use of these measures and the entities measured as a basis for clinical judgment' (Cambrosio et al. 2006: 194). In the case of markers for leukaemia and cancer, for example, rather than the 'truth' of what these markers represent, what seems to be at stake is their compatibility between different laboratories. In short, what emerges from these studies is the contrast between the strength of evidence displayed in EBM according to the precepts of its founders and the more complex and ambiguous way in which clinical practice, measures and judgments are entangled in developing standards and forms of regulation.

I should specify that my own position regarding NSCF is closer to the epistemic stance of EBM, which values experimentation, than to the clinicians' stance, where the importance of their clinical experience predominates. EBM, for its best part, has historically consisted in demolishing notions that are taken for granted, treatments that are prescribed too lightly and pressures that are brought to bear on types of treatment by the advertising of pharmaceutical companies. I uphold this position until the critical point at which EBM neglects the patient's point of view and, of course, when it leads to trials that are dangerous for the populations being tested as occurred in Africa (Angell 1997). It seems to me that in the case of NSCF, the situation is sufficiently complex to warrant a complete study of the therapeutic effects reaching beyond the observation of a few clinicians. This is why, while I recognize the value of the studies referred to above and will use them as a basis for

---

4   I would like to thank the anonymous reviewer who pointed out this remark to me.

my own work, I would like to return to an analysis that looks more at how what is considered to be 'true' is constituted, without lapsing into rationalism.

In studying NSCF, my aim is therefore to examine a public action that mobilizes several kinds of actors around the question of evidence and its dissemination in the population. Above all, this study analyzes the moment at which their point of view can change. It is not only a question of the *epistemic frameworks of actors involved in public action*, but also of *how these frameworks are constructed and deconstructed*; in short, it is a question of *the dynamics of evidence*. In order to answer these questions, this part of the study is based on interview excerpts, but also on the material form taken by the different arguments: figures, tables and particularly texts. Indeed, EBM rests heavily on the production and circulation of such texts. My analysis will show the different conceptions held on a regional and national level regarding the nature and legitimacy of knowledge concerning screening. I will present and analyze the scientific elements that contributed to changes in points of view about NSCF. This, in turn, will enable me to show the relative place held by EBM in this process, bringing together knowledge, rumours and emotions. And all this will later allow me to better link together mobilization of knowledge and practices of power. First, I will outline the epistemic framework underpinned by the arguments of the Breton professionals, before then analyzing the scientific arguments that prevailed in order to encourage the generalization of screening. The other kinds of argument in favour of this generalization, more political than scientific in nature, will be discussed in Chapter 3.

When Conviction Prevails

At the end of the 1980s, EBM did not yet enjoy the importance it took on from the end of the 1990s. As for NSCF, the studies on its value for sick children were few and far between, lacked substantiation and gave contradictory results. When Breton screening began in 1988, a few comparative studies had been carried out in various countries between children diagnosed through screening and children diagnosed from symptoms (Gilly, Barbier and Garcia 1987). Overall, these were criticized in biomedical publications due to the small numbers of patients studied, the differences in treatment between groups, the lack of distance in terms of time, and the heterogeneity of the groups analyzed. On the basis of data linked in particular to pulmonary status, two stated they had not been able to show any clinical effect of screening or early diagnosis, while two concluded that there were beneficial tendencies. Moreover, two unpublished conference papers also came to the latter conclusion. Another study in favour of screening had been published in the prestigious journal *The Lancet,* but was strongly contested due to the methodology used, as it compared groups of children treated at different periods and was based on only a portion of the populations concerned. Above all, although its title announced a 'decrease in morbidity' in children screened at birth, it only focused on the length of hospital stays for children under the age of two.

In order to better understand the epistemic attitude of the Breton entrepreneurs, it is therefore important to know which arguments they were using and to analyze them. However, before addressing this question, it is necessary to mention that, before this stage, a certain dynamic had already been created by the tool itself.

In general, innovative technology tends to compel recognition in and of itself. In the field of neonatal resuscitation, in particular, Anne Paillet (2000) has shown that doctors consider it to be mandatory and self-evident to use all innovative means possible to resuscitate premature babies and that they introduce a moral dimension to justify this. Technology therefore seems to sometimes have a dynamic capacity in itself. Remaining within the history of Breton NSCF, it would be inappropriate to overstate its importance but naïve to ignore it. One of the paediatricians to whom NSCF was suggested spoke about it in an interview as follows: 'There is the fact that teams are interested in the technology that makes screening possible. Naturally, immediately afterwards, there's a desire to make this available' (Paediatrician 3, 28.8.02). We must remember that biologists, not clinicians, were the first to suggest screening, in Brittany and Normandy alike. They had developed a technology that they wanted to see put to use insofar as they considered that it could only be beneficial to patients.

Of course the Breton biologists and clinicians developed less technological and less immediate arguments in favour of screening. Three kinds of arguments were put forward in the interviews. They relied on, in order of increasing importance, the prenatal diagnosis that sometimes came with newborn screening, the incidence of CF in Brittany and the presumed therapeutic impact of screening.

Familial and Epidemiological Arguments

A good half of the Breton biomedical professionals spontaneously mentioned in interview an initial argument in favour of newborn screening that was based on prenatal diagnosis. Before NSCF was put in place, when two children were born close together in a family, a second sick child could be born when the first had not yet been diagnosed. Newborn screening allowed early diagnosis of the first child, and therefore made it possible to offer prenatal diagnosis for a second pregnancy, before the first child had even started having symptoms. In support of this idea, one of the paediatricians gave the example, on a compassionate register, of parents 'who are a complete wreck' finding it difficult to 'get back on their feet again' when, in the absence of NSCF, two children in a row were diagnosed with CF. Conversely, newborn screening therefore made it possible to avoid families with several children suffering from the condition. This possibility went even further because, given the familial nature of genetic diseases, prenatal diagnosis could also concern more distant members of the family with a child diagnosed through screening (uncles and aunts, etc.).

This argument testifies to a more or less complex intertwining between prenatal diagnosis and newborn screening, illustrating how difficult it can sometimes be to separate these two approaches, therapeutic on the one hand, selective on the other.

This observation brings us to a remark made by sociologists Vololona Rabeharisoa and Michel Callon (1999: 179). They suggested (but did not develop, as this was not their main focus) a separation between two kinds of gene. On the one hand, the 'domesticated, civilized gene', in other words the 'moral gene' (which would help treat the disease), and, on the other, the 'gene that is the source of discord, such as in doctrines advocating eugenics', in other words the 'immoral gene' (which would lead to prenatal diagnosis). Through this first justification for NSCF in Brittany, it becomes clear that the distinction between the two approaches is not that simple. In our case, the same technology, based on identifying mutations by examining DNA, both allowed newborn screening to be seen as more acceptable and offered the possibility of reliable prenatal diagnosis. Moreover, prenatal diagnosis itself was an argument in favour of newborn screening. This strict distinction between a gene considered to be moral and another considered to be immoral is even less tenable given the ambiguous status of CF: it is both a serious disease (it is hard for families to cope with several sick children) and one for which life expectancy is increasing (the hope of treatment remains present). This disease is therefore situated in an 'in-between' position in terms both of how serious it is and of its medical perspectives, which can simultaneously justify both approaches. Furthermore, prenatal diagnosis belongs to the regime of compassion, where the relationship with 'morality' and 'immorality' cannot be dealt with in a simple fashion. The first biomedical argument in favour of NSCF is therefore both simple in its reasoning and complex in its implications. It shifts the stakes from epistemology to morality, which will be the subject of the last part of this book.

The second argument, epidemiological this time, relied on how CF cases in Brittany were quantified, compared and interpreted. The previous chapter analyzed the studies on the incidence of the disease in the region as reflecting the weight of statistical approaches in our society. It should be underlined that they were not only a motor for the extended mobilization in Brittany, they also stoked the professionals' action, particularly in the Finistère. This question of incidence was at the heart of Michel Cladic's concerns when he began to take an interest in CF. He considered that if a genetic disease should be worked on, it was this one, because in his view it represented a public health problem in Brittany. This should be linked to the fact that regional screening was launched in the Finistère, the *département* where the incidence was the highest, relatively speaking. Moreover, these epidemiological data gave the professionals a scientifically legitimate objectivation of reality. Thus when I mentioned the particular, and partly constructed, link between Brittany and the disease, one of these professionals took care to ground this link in 'reality':

> First of all there was a reality … . It is one newborn in 2,000 in the Finistère, I mean it's not a rare genetic disease. … What we brought to people … , it's that it was really the region, in the world probably, where the incidence was highest … . We gave this information, by confirming that it was indeed a disease that was frequent in the Finistère (Biologist 1, 5.9.02).

Beyond the case of Brest, these figures were highlighted in interviews by different professionals practising in other parts of the region. When they were questioned on the reasons why regional screening was pursued when the AFDPHE had stopped its programme, the first reply was linked to incidence. This argument is based both on scientific grounds and on the fact that the epidemiological results were seen as being very particular to the local area in question. We have seen the part of reality and of construction that brought this argument into the interplay of what is true and false. As this was largely discussed in the previous chapter, I will not come back to it here. The third argument was also traditional, but presents interesting features concerning its relationship to knowledge.

Medical Arguments

The most important argument in the eyes of the Breton doctors and biologists, but also the most complex, was of a therapeutic nature. On the one hand, NSCF did not lead to a cure for the children concerned and this was at the origin of the international debate to which it gave rise. On the other hand, for the Breton professionals, NSCF was justified by the idea of the supposed therapeutic benefits for children diagnosed through screening. It is important therefore to elucidate the kinds of theories implicitly mobilized in this actual case.

Where the biologists were concerned, a technique had been developed that they wanted to see put to use given that they considered it could only be beneficial to patients. The need to offer screening was even seen as self-evident. As one of them put it: 'It seemed self-evident to all of us that early screening of this disease was one of the first things to build up' (Biologist 1, 5.9.02). The reader will recall that this same sentiment of self-evidence was seen in some of the support provided for the CF 'cause' in the *Courrier du Finistère,* and for screening itself through fund-raising. And this will come up once again when we look at the parents of newborns to whom screening is offered in maternity units. It is interesting for two reasons. First, because the nineteenth-century doctor-statisticians who were the forerunners of EBM fought precisely against this notion of the self-evident, or rather what they considered to be ideas taken for granted. According to them, it was necessary to move away from intuition and establish facts. Second, because, as Mitchell Dean (1999) reminds us, a social science analysis of government seeks to show that the elements that seem to be obvious in our ways of thinking and acting are in fact not totally self-evident or necessary. Let us now take this a little further by analyzing the mechanisms through which self-evidence functions.

First, this sentiment of self-evidence was grounded in an inductive type of reasoning. In other words, it was based on other cases or other diseases, considering that what had been true in the past would be true in the future. Pushing this reasoning to the extreme, this means that if diagnosing one disease early has allowed an improvement in health, then all diseases must be diagnosed and treated early. It is worth underlining that this inductive approach does not detract from the value of the argument. After all, most acts in life are in fact grounded in this reasoning and validated on a daily basis. Second, this self-evidence had the power of common sense behind it. By definition, this means it was based on intuitions that seemed sufficiently obvious to be shared by everyone. People all have examples around them of cancers diagnosed too late or of lesions that were allowed to become infected and that then became more difficult to treat. Henceforth, it was what Paul Atkinson (1984), following Alfred Schütz, calls a 'natural attitude' to advocate early care provision for these patients, with immediate treatment in order to prevent conditions from worsening as soon as possible. However, unlike the Schützian point of view where common sense is characteristic of the man in the street and contrasted with informed expert knowledge, the common sense in question here was also shared by expert biologists. In other words, the experts also had their 'natural' response, oriented towards newborn screening. Third, the corollary to this sentiment of self-evidence, to this shared common sense, was conviction. The Normand biologist who launched NSCF in the region in 1980, the year after the assay method was published, unsurprisingly defended the Weberian ideal-type, in other words the archetype of this position. As he explained in an interview: 'I started with the firm conviction, and for what it's worth I think it's something we deny scientists too much today, firm conviction. ... I started with the firm conviction that in principle it was useful for patients' (Biologist 2, 20.4.04). This firm conviction is similar to the more traditional firm belief of doctors. And indeed, medical conviction was also explicitly foregrounded.

As for the clinicians, they thought they would 'work better' if the disease were caught earlier. What did they mean by this assertion? First of all, screening allowed early diagnosis, a few weeks after birth rather than around the age of one or sometimes even several years later (at the end of the 1980s, roughly 60% of children suffering from CF were diagnosed before the age of one). Situations where the diagnosis was beyond the experience of one of their colleagues had made their mark on paediatricians. In interviews, they explained these late diagnoses by the unspecific nature of the symptoms, often displayed by recurrent bronchitis, a condition that is common in young children. Sometimes, they explained this delay by what, in this case, became the 'rare' nature of the disease. They underlined the fact that non-specialist paediatricians or GPs only encounter a small number of cases in their career (2 or 3 cases, more often than not). This explains the fact that they do not necessarily make the link between run-of-the-mill bronchitis and the genetic disease. Moreover, the parents confronted with 'serial misdiagnosis', in other words long periods during which no one knows the real origin of their child's problems, could lose faith in health professionals, which could later compromise the quality of treatment obtained by their child.

An initial dimension to this therapeutic argument therefore lay in the question of early diagnosis and, although this is rarely mentioned, the trust between patients and health care practitioners. However, screening would have been of little use if afterwards the child were 'let loose and disappeared' as one of the professionals put it. Another therapeutic aspect was that NSCF could give rise to immediate care provision, before complications appeared, such as irreversible pulmonary infections, and before the general worsening of the patient's state. It was a question of quickly setting up a care programme, with the idea that 'we treat all the better when we treat early', as one of the paediatricians said. Another, who played a driving role in this, explained:

> We wanted to believe, we don't have any evidence, but we wanted to believe that by catching the children early enough, by putting treatment in place from the start, we would avoid complications. ... [We had] the conviction that we would work better. And that, implicitly, the results, the quality of care and the results, would follow (Paediatrician 3, 28.8.02).

In short, the uncertainty that scientific knowledge was unable to counter at this stage did not lead in turn to uncertain attitudes. To a certain extent, this is similar to what Paul Atkinson (1984) showed in highlighting the certainty of clinicians making personal judgments on the basis of uncertain knowledge. More specifically, this sociologist defends the idea that medical students are trained for certainty, even on an uncertain breeding ground. By separating the different kinds of uncertainty in question (existential doubts, uncertain knowledge, moral and emotion uncertainty, etc.) the author counters the idea defended by Renée Fox (1957, 2000), namely that uncertainty is an all-pervasive feature of medical practice. Nonetheless, as I underline the diversity of situations encountered, I will also go on to show that other clinicians were in fact closer to this second register linked to uncertainty.

How can we explain, in these conditions, that the Breton clinicians subscribed to ideas of uncertain validity? It seems that recourse to a form of 'subjective rationality' (Boudon 1992) prevailed; indeed, it is possible to find certain reasons behind this 'belief' in the value of NSCF. Going beyond the common sense mentioned in the case of the biologists, the clinicians' conviction was rooted in the medical obsession with early diagnosis, which is ubiquitous today (Grimes and Schulz 2002) and which we will see once again with the history of screening on a national level. Above and beyond this general movement, the paediatricians sometimes also based their views on a few rare theories which they had reasons to believe in. For example, at the end of the 1970s, a scientific article had argued that the absence of pulmonary lesions when CF patients received care seemed to be a determining factor in how life-threatening the disease was. Above all, the Breton paediatricians were able to ground their views in their own clinical experience, as evidenced when they mention the problems linked to parents' loss of trust following a late diagnosis. Their clinical knowledge could, in part, compensate for the scientific arguments. There was therefore a form of rationality at work. At the same time, this rationality was subjective because it did not rely upon objective arguments regarding the value of screening for children. As one of the paediatricians put it, 'evidence' of the benefits for patients was far from established. And their position also included implicit statements, which were not necessarily problematic but could sometimes weaken their arguments. First, there was the idea that the therapeutic arguments outweighed the disadvantages, which included, in particular, serious and difficult treatment from a very young age and the impossibility of predicting the severity of the illness. Second, there was the presupposition that there was no negative correlation between care provision after screening and risks of morbidity. To my knowledge, the risks of cross infection between screened babies and older patients within the health care centres were not mentioned by the Breton professionals at this period, or very little. We will see later how this problem nonetheless became one of the crucial issues at stake in the debate. This shows how *a priori* notions can be more or less efficient depending on the situation and how the therapeutic benefits expected from NSCF were themselves not as 'self-evident' as they might seem at first glance.

To complete this section concerning the therapeutic arguments, a second kind of argument must be mentioned. While the first focused how useful NSCF was in terms of achieving the final aim, that is to say an improvement in children's prognosis, the second focused rather on how useful it was in terms of the means for providing care for screened children, even though this distinction between aims and means is partly artificial. Let me explain. Shortly after NSCF was launched in Brittany, the directors of the newborn screening centre in Rennes wanted to begin to organize their centre to provide follow-up care for children suffering from CF. With a view to this, the new director Christian Perret visited Canada, which had a good reputation in this regard. This visit contributed to forming the idea of directing patients towards specialized health care centres, taking inspiration from other countries organized around such centres. It should be noted, however, that these countries did not carry out NSCF: organization of care provision and screening were separate. In short, the prevailing idea, which appeared not immediately but over time, was to use screening to direct patients towards health care centres with greater experience of treating CF than doctors who only encountered a few cases in their careers. As this approach is similar to the one developed on a national level, I will return to it later. At this stage, let me just note that it is interesting to underline that these premises can be identified in Brittany from the early 1990s.

One last point relates to dissemination in the public space. The small group behind screening in the Finistère indicated in their information leaflet aimed at potential partners: 'Knowing from birth makes it possibly to progress fast and predicts the child's future: early diagnosis through screening allows faster care provision, which is an essential factor for a good prognosis. Knowing early changes everything...' The link between screening and an improved prognosis was expressed without reservations. Consequently, it is not surprising that the media took up this idea even though, as we have seen, the 'cause' chosen by the *Courrier du Finistère* went far beyond screening itself. However, a few articles dating from the fund-raising campaign in the winter of 1990-1991 were devoted to NSCF itself. We can read in one of these articles: 'Early care provision for children limits the consequences and the human and financial costs of the disease. The improvement in children's quality of life and chances of living to adulthood are indisputable. However, in order to achieve this aim, systematic screening must be put in place.' What began above all as a conviction became a fact. The now classic study by Bruno Latour and Steve Woolgar (1979) shows how results mixed with beliefs can slowly become established as scientific 'facts' when there is a progressive shift transforming a lively debate into a recognized, and unremarkable and uncontroversial, fact. This fact becomes a 'black box' when it is taken as read and when knowledge of the stages that led to it disappears. The research in question here presents different aspects, however: it covers more medical aspects than Latour and Woolgar's study, which is oriented towards laboratories, and reveals biomedical actors open to a wider set of varied resources, including the media.

To summarize, although the biomedical evidence in favour of NSCF was not established, the scientific arguments in its favour were essentially of three kinds: familial, establishing a link with prenatal diagnosis; epidemiological, allowing the idea of a particularly high incidence of the disease to be constructed; and medical, resting on the expected therapeutic benefits. In the end, the Breton professionals set more store by clinical experience than scientific experimentation. Furthermore, we should remember that, in general, the tenants of the strictest form of EBM differed from their opponents precisely regarding the issue of taking into account what patients had to say and their individual experience of the disease, as well as that of the clinicians. Certain criticisms formulated against EBM by its opponents are based on the fear that its advocates take a dehumanized view of medicine (Mykhalovskiy and Weir 2004). In reality, the Breton doctors distinguished themselves from both epidemiologists and medical humanists who emphasize patients' discourse to the extent that it becomes clinical evidence. Indeed, while the Breton doctors based their arguments on data from their own experience, to which they gave enough value to justify a screening policy, they never put forward the idea that this was in itself sufficient to provide evidence for the medical value of screening. The 'argument' underpinning the credibility of their position, often based on experience, was always explicitly distinguished from scientific 'evidence'. In other words, for them self-evidence was not evidence. In this way, they testify to their dual position as clinicians and researchers influenced by the standards of EBM, who not only treated patients but also read international biomedical literature, participated in conferences and published articles, etc. And they reveal an initial register of relationships between clinical and scientific practice, grounded in the pre-eminence of conviction and clinical experience over evidence, even if the latter is clearly distinguished from the former. Other professionals, on a national level, however, show a different relationship between the two.

Looking for Evidence

During all the years of regional screening, the long-standing officials of the AFDPHE were strongly opposed to NSCF. One of them had even proclaimed that screening for CF would be funded over his dead body. The controversy that existed between regional and national actors allows us to study the range of epistemic stances adopted. So what were the grounds for the reservations expressed by the professionals on a national level?

First of all, for the national AFDPHE officials, although the argument relating to prenatal diagnosis could not be completely rejected, alone it could not suffice to justify newborn screening. More specifically, their point of view was based on two aspects. First, the principle of efficiency was underlined: it had been calculated that newborn screening only avoided 18% of births of sick children. This relatively low rate can be attributed to the fact that most sick children were born into families who had never known the disease and who therefore did not use prenatal diagnosis. Then, and above all, a moral principle weighed in, as according to these officials it was not morally justifiable to use newborn screening in order to avoid further births of sick children within a family. They said: 'You don't screen a child in order to provide genetic counselling. If you want to do genetic counselling, you identify couples at risk, you don't do it through the child' (Geneticist-Paediatrician 1, 31.1.03). This argument could also be coupled with a legal principle, because the law states that a genetic test should benefit the individual being tested (in this instance, the baby). And it was above all the moral argument that prevailed. Worse, in the eyes of the AFDPHE officials, was the position consisting in using NSCF to identify heterozygote children (those carrying a mutation) with the aim of alerting the child's relatives, offering them prenatal diagnosis and, in the end, eradicating the illness. And yet this was what the Finisterian biologists were putting forward. In the same way as the generalized screening of heterozygotes in North Finistère, this question gave rise to tensions, which were more moral than scientific in nature. For the national officials, this verged on eugenics and some even used extreme terms in interviews, qualifying this approach as 'exterminating' children with CF. More generally, their position should be linked with their principles of action, which considered that newborn screening should be put in place for the benefit of the child screened. In this they took up one of the international criteria for screening, known as the Wilson and Jungner criterion. Their arguments were underpinned by a traditional conception of medicine, recalled in the Helsinki declaration adopted in 1964, which stipulates 'The health of my patient will be my first consideration'.[5] They claimed to adhere to 'ethical practices' (Dean 1999) – in other words to aims – that remained rooted in a therapeutic perspective (treating sick children). This question will come up again in the last chapter.

What was the situation more widely on the national level? Beyond what we could call the first circle of the national association, the members of the working group considering NSCF at the end of the 1990s did not, with the exception of the Breton professionals, spontaneously mention prenatal diagnosis in interviews as an argument justifying newborn screening, or very rarely. When they were

---

5 Cf. the website of the World Medical Association (http://www.wma.net/en/30publications/10policies/b3/).

asked the question directly, more than the moral principle, it was the principle of efficiency that was put forward (newborn screening only allowed 18% of births of sick children to be avoided). Occasionally, certain paediatricians did nonetheless say that they understood the argument. As in Brittany, the arguments of humanity and the clinician's experience in the face of families of sick children were called upon, in statements such as: 'Having experience as a clinician [etc.]' and 'On a human level, it's not completely without interest' (Paediatrician 4, 17.8.04). However, this type of remark was much more rare among the working group than in Brittany.

Above all, the major stumbling block for NSCF was the fact that the AFDPHE officials questioned its usefulness for the patients. During all the years of Breton screening, what prevailed for them was scepticism regarding its medical benefits for the child diagnosed through screening. In their view, there were no scientific arguments and no publications presenting unquestionable evidence that the child diagnosed through screening drew an immediate and personal benefit from it. In short, what the officials were waiting for was evidence of the efficiency of screening. And they continued to wait as time went by. During this part of my study (2002-2004), they still expressed questions or doubts on a number of occasions, whether in interviews or in informal conversations. These were sometimes explicit: '[X] has always been very dubious about the value of cystic fibrosis screening, even today. And I understand his point of view, I'm also dubious' (early 2004). The reservations that were expressed sometimes, paradoxically, even came from the main officials of the association in charge of newborn screening. It should be noted that the other members of the national working group, who were not among the founding officials of the AFDPHE, did not express these same doubts. I will return to this distinction in the following chapter. At any rate, the doubts expressed within the AFDPHE meant that at the time of this study the question of NSCF had not yet become a 'black box': it was still a 'grey box', so to speak, in other words, still at the stage where it was subject to questioning and was not yet accepted as a scientific fact. In comparison with the situation in Brittany, the relationship to the uncertainty of knowledge about the medical benefits of NSCF was very different. Even with a gap of several years during which, as we will see, several studies were published, there was an attitude of uncertainty rather than an 'attitude of certainty' (Atkinson 1984), to make an analogy with the studies about medical students and clinical practice. There was no process reducing uncertainty and this brought us back to a situation closer to that described by Renée Fox (1957, 2000). She devoted a substantial part of her work to analyzing the ubiquity of the notion of uncertainty in various biomedical contexts, considering uncertainty as characteristic of culture and medical knowledge, particularly in the case of experimental innovation. The Breton professionals and the AFDPHE officials therefore combined the two points of view. Similarly, Stefan Timmermans and Alison Angell (2001) describe two attitudes towards uncertainty and EBM among paediatrics residents: 'librarians' follow the instructions of the literature and are little affected by uncertainty, while 'researchers' take uncertainty on board and are inclined to provide their own scientific evaluation of research. Due to its socio-historical nature, the study presented here builds on this by affording an understanding of the social dynamics at play. While the AFDPHE officials were more aligned with the second group, their doubts had to be sufficiently allayed in order for the process deciding in favour of NSCF in France to play out. So at what point and under what conditions did they change their point of view? How did they reach if not a consensus at least an agreement regarding how to approach the issue of screening? The next stage of my analysis will look at the role played by methods of comparison among the arguments that eventually won out. I will not only focus on how evidence was produced (or not) but also on how it was disseminated and received, and here I will look beyond simply the circle of biomedical professionals because evidence cannot be considered as such unless it is widely accepted. The role of EBM will be revealed in the kind of studies from which information was drawn, and in the perceived credibility of this information.

The Twists and Turns of Evidence-Based Medicine

Newborn screening was no exception to the movement towards legitimizing 'evidence' that was seen in biomedicine throughout the twentieth century. And while the first newborn screening programme (phenylketonuria) was launched in the 1960s without many prior scientific studies, such an approach would no longer be possible today, particularly in France. Among the different studies arguing in favour of NSCF, the one with the most resonance in France and abroad was the vast analysis carried out by RCT between 1985 and 1994 in the State of Wisconsin in the United States. The project looked at 650,000 children, of which 120 suffered from CF (Farrell et al. 1997). It consisted in comparing the health of sick children diagnosed after newborn screening with the health of those diagnosed using traditional measures. More specifically, two groups of newborns were created at random (a screened group and a control group). Children belonging to the screened group who tested positive were taken on by a health care centre; in the case of children belonging to the control group, the positive result was kept secret and the diagnosis was established in the traditional fashion. If the patient was not diagnosed by the age of four, anonymity was lifted in order to avoid a potential lack of treatment. The initial results were published in the prestigious *New England Journal of Medicine*, thus conferring even greater legitimacy upon them due to the very strong links between the success of a 'scientific fact' and the type of publication in which it appears. This context allows us to better understand why this publication met with unanimous approval amongst the French professionals interviewed, who referred to it as 'remarkable' and 'ideal', 'with perfect methodology'.

So what were the conclusions of such an exemplary study? In 1997, it showed that the height and weight of the screened children were significantly greater than those of the children diagnosed through symptoms alone, concluding that NSCF provides the opportunity to prevent malnutrition in affected children, and it confirmed this in 2001 (Farrell et al. 1997, 2001). At this stage, the benefits for screened children seemed relatively limited, as they were restricted to nutritional criteria. However, it is probably necessary to situate the results within the context of the particular role of height and weight development in the overall evaluation of children's health; many traces of this can be found in social science studies. For David Armstrong (1995), the weight and growth charts that became part of health policy in the early decades of the twentieth century captured the nature of a certain 'surveillance medicine'. I would be inclined to say rather that they produce the 'sign' of a certain state of normal health in children, the sign being that which 'is further away, below, later. It concerns the outcome ... , not that immobile truth, that given, hidden truth that the symptoms restore to their transparency as phenomena' (Foucault 2003: 110). We can therefore understand why these parameters took on such importance in the eyes of paediatricians. However, the North American project did not bring forward any elements concerning the evolution of screened children in terms of respiratory function. Furthermore, studies on the relationship between nutritional status and pulmonary status brought contradictory results. And yet, as one of the paediatricians I encountered put it, children suffering from CF do not die from malnutrition, they die from respiratory problems. The North American project then provided new results. In 2002 and 2003, those promoting this project showed that the radiograph scores – which reflect pulmonary status – were better for the screened children in the first years of life than for the control group but that, from the age of 10-12, screened children had a lower score (West et al. 2002, Farrell and Farrell 2003). In short, from that age onwards, the lungs of children screened were on average in a *worse* state than those of children in whom the disease was identified through traditional diagnostic measures. Furthermore, they showed that this negative result was due to a higher level of infection with the terrible *pseudomonas aeruginosa* germ in screened children. This germ is known to significantly lower life expectancy at the stage of chronic infection (Farrell and Farrell 2003). More specifically, a sub-group of screened children, treated in one of the two health care centres involved in the study, had been infected by the germ much earlier than those being treated in the other centre. The problem resided in the fact that the centre was old, had a fairly small waiting room in which the young patients came into contact with older infected patients and had limited hand-washing facilities for doctors (West et al. 2002). The authors of the study concluded at the time that *pseudomonas aeruginosa* infection had a greater influence upon pulmonary status than age of diagnosis and that screening did not automatically lead to more good than harm (Farrell and Farrell 2003). However, in 2005, there was an odd turnaround in events as the researchers took up the data again, this time only taking into account the more serious forms of the illness. They suggested that infections were confounders, and that therefore it was the pre-infection period that should be considered in analysis (Farrell et al. 2005). They concluded that nutritional effects were in favour of screening, that respiratory effects were the same in both cases (until infection, interpreted as a confounding factor, in short an artefact) and that the evidence in favour of the benefits of NSCF was thus established. QED.

I have outlined this study in detail because its developments were followed closely by the clinicians and members of the AFDPHE involved in NSCF in France. Screening was decided upon in 1999-2000, so just after the first publication regarding the positive effects of screening in nutritional terms. As one of the members of the working group, who was very involved in this case on both a local and national level, recounted: 'Farrell's work disturbed everyone' (Paediatrician 2, 27.8.02). In other words, the AFDPHE officials' opposition to screening was slightly undermined by the initial positive results of the study. As for the question of germs, even before the more alarming results in 2002-2003, the French professionals were concerned about this aspect. When the working groups set up by the AFDPHE outlined recommendations and delivered them to the Cnamts in 2001, they insisted upon the rules of hygiene applicable to newborns in hospitals. However in France, as elsewhere, clinicians had not anticipated the negative effect of the infection of young patients in ill-conceived health care centres that came to light in the United States. As for the general mindset that prevailed at the time of my study (2002-2004), according to the respondents, the North American study highlighted advantages in nutritional terms but not in respiratory terms. As for the question of cross contamination, it was sometimes mentioned in interviews:

> When Farrell looked at our posters at last year's European Conference, he said: 'You've structured screening well, no problem at all, and have you thought about protecting the children from possible contamination by pseudomonas, etc.? Have you structured your care facilities well?' So he drew a lot of attention to that, and rightly so (Paediatrician 5, 9.2.04).

Certain clinicians pointed out the difficulties in avoiding the risk of cross contamination in centres. I will come back to this aspect when I outline the field study carried out in a hospital setting, as its actual impact today depends on both collective and individual practices.

This North American study, and above all how it was perceived by social actors, is interesting on a number of levels. First, on a *medical* level, it shows that screening was not inherently good (as the authors claimed) or inherently bad (as a hasty judgement could lead to suppose), but that the level of hygiene in health care centres was just as important as, if not more important than, screening itself. Second, on a *socio-historical* level, it reveals the clash between an approach based on simple long-standing foundations (avoiding cross-contamination) and another based on technoscience and modernity (screening at birth). From the eighteenth century, continuing on from the concept of salubrity that was so dear to the hygienists, particular attention was paid to the problem of the circulation of air to avoid the propagation of diseases within the hospital itself. These changes were part of a wider complete shift in perspective regarding hospital medicine: the hospital had to act as a 'healing machine' and not simply a regulatory space where one came to die (Foucault 1980: 166-182). Bryan Turner (2000) reminds us that this evolution did not occur without some resistance and disbelief on the part of doctors, particularly in late nineteenth century Austria, when it was proved that germs could be spread through contaminated surgical material. These problems were also encountered in France at the end of the 1940s when the coexistence of serious infectious illnesses and more innocuous pathologies within the same establishment led to severe hospital-acquired infections (Pinell 2004b). This shows to what extent iatrogenic diseases have been a constant problem since the inception of the hospital, even if they were not always given due consideration. Where sociologists are concerned, this problem has contributed, alongside many other aspects, to the social critique of the negative consequences of the medicalization of society (Illich 1974). For some, it even seems as if the more efficiently medicine takes responsibility for patients, the more it places the latter at risk – or rather, I would add, the more it exposes them to the perception of risks. This is what sociologist Renée Fox (2000: 416) calls the 'irony of iatrogenesis'. In the case of CF, it would be more accurate to mention that changes in health care provision have considerably improved prognoses because, under their influence, patient life expectancy has increased by 30 years in the last 40 years.

In addition to the medical and socio-historical levels, the *sociological* level must also be considered. The publications in question also offer a good example of practices in interpreting data, particularly where the issue of germs was concerned. Generally, when a new result does not fit in well with a theory, either the theory resists and the new result is ignored, or the result compels recognition and leads to the theory being modified. The North American study is a variant of the first situation in which the new result is reinterpreted as an artefact. It should be underlined that the practice consisting in selecting data from experimental results is quite common in the sciences: data is eliminated because the conditions for good observation are not considered to have been met. In any event, data are not registered passively; they call upon researchers' judgment. And EBM is not the fixed science leading to the mechanical application of principles that is sometimes described (Lambert 2006). Experimenters can also set results aside because they are not in keeping with their expectations. Could one not therefore refer to 'escaping refutation'? Classically, for epistemologist Karl Popper (1963: 37) this theoretical rescuing operation that he refers to as a 'conventionalist stratagem', partially obliterates the scientific nature of a theory, which relies, in particular, upon its refutability. To my mind, the epistemological turnaround carried out in the North American study resulted in those promoting it failing to draw the necessary conclusions from the experiment (that is to say that hygiene in centres was at least as important as screening). They should have placed more emphasis on recommendations in this area and perhaps launched another study on this subject, rather than considering it as an artefact and continuing to emphasize screening. This is why I would tend to suggest a variant on the Popperian position, with the notion of 'escaping conclusion'. More generally, this shows the need to reconsider the most demanding EBM on its own ground, that of evidence, even if I have already specified that my own position regarding NSCF is closer to EBM than clinical judgment. It remains necessary to take the experiment to its logical end and draw the right conclusions.

The issues raised by EBM are not simply scientific: when experiments are carried out on people, they also become moral. Those promoting the North American study availed themselves of a series of legal, ethical, administrative and professional guarantees in order to set up their experimental protocol. As we saw above, this protocol led them to keep screening results secret for half of those screened until anonymity was lifted. This could delay treatment and lead to the organizers being morally as well as legally responsible for a potential deterioration in the health of the children involved. This moral dimension to conducting trials should come as no surprise given the extent to which moral questions have crossed the entire history of EBM (Marks 1997). Interestingly, these questions were to be found just as much among those in favour of a clinical-based flexible approach as among their opponents in favour of a statistically grounded approach. The former defended providing treatment as soon as possible, claiming it was morally questionable to not allow patients to benefit from a new treatment. The latter defended a cautious and scientifically grounded position, arguing that it was morally reprehensible not to check for evidence of the efficiency of a molecule or treatment before providing it on a wide scale. However, it is at the end of the 1990s that an awareness of abuses seemed to really spread through the biomedical sphere, following a series of medical trials carried out in Southern countries, mainly on poor African populations. The trials for AIDS treatments in particular gave rise to heated debates in the medical community, because the clinical trials were carried out on vast African populations against a placebo rather than against another known treatment (Angell 1997). The North American study on NSCF, launched in 1985, therefore obtained authorization before this rise in awareness. Would it have been accepted in France by the ethics committees responsible for providing authorization for such practices? The biomedical actors I encountered expressed doubts not only about the legal possibility of such a trial in France, but also about the moral scruples of the clinicians. This rendered a RCT study on newborn screening impossible in France and made experimental detours essential. Other kinds of studies, less rigorous from the point of view of EBM but more ethically acceptable, were therefore carried out. Their approach was in line with that of other studies carried out elsewhere in the world and they contributed to building the scientific 'truth'.

My intention here is not to summarize all the biomedical studies carried out worldwide comparing the state of screened and unscreened children. In this section, my analysis will be limited to those quoted by the working group report submitted to the Cnamts at the end of 1999, which played a key role in the history of screening in France because it concluded in its favour. More specifically, I will give two significant examples that illustrate how elements of evidence are interwoven with the contingent details of practice. The authors of this report made a distinction between the studies that had provided 'decisive arguments in favour of the medium-term benefits provided by newborn screening' and those that had provided 'supplementary arguments' (AFDPHE 1999). Among those providing 'decisive arguments', the authors summarized, on the one hand, the North American study discussed above and, on the other, an Australian study that had just published its results. The latter compared the nutritional and respiratory status of children suffering from CF born during the three years following the implementation of screening in an Australian region with those of children suffering from the illness born in the three years prior to screening being implemented (Waters et al. 1999). It observed that the group of screened patients showed greater growth and better respiratory function than those of the non-screened patients, and that these differences were statistically significant. It all seemed extremely promising. However, closer analysis of the methodological part of the study reveals that therapeutic follow-up care was substantially altered during the two years following the implementation of screening. Thus the two groups did indeed present different states of health, but these could clearly be the result of changes in treatment rather than screening. For those advocating scientifically rigorous medicine, this was a typical case of substantial bias. The French paediatricians involved in NSCF that I encountered adopted a more nuanced position towards this study. They were able to point out its failings and yet remain convinced by its findings, as illustrated by the following interview excerpt:

> Methodologically speaking, it's very borderline because you can always discuss the fact that, during these three years, therapeutic progress was made such that the cases were no longer comparable. Nonetheless, this work also provided arguments in favour of nutritional benefits ... as well as arguments showing that respiratory function was better in screened children (Paediatrician 4, 17.8.04).

The extent of the ambiguity of the relationship towards EBM can be seen in these remarks. The bias is substantial and recognized as such, but the conclusions of the study are nonetheless considered to be established. A second example reinforces this observation and affords supplementary material for analysis. It also illustrates the value of looking at different facets of knowledge, depending on the actor concerned and above all the 'context' (Dobrow et al. 2006) in which the latter finds themselves. Among the studies that had provided 'supplementary arguments' in favour of NSCF, a study had been carried out in France, more specifically in the West of the country. It included the promoters of screening in Brittany. Once again, the study consisted in comparing the health of children screened (in Brittany) with that of children diagnosed using traditional methods (in the Loire-Atlantique region, bordering Brittany, where screening was not yet used but where health care procedures were comparable). The results seemed favourable to screening in terms of the proportion of children admitted to hospital at least once, growth (height and weight) and pulmonary status, but it had the disadvantage of only looking at a small number of patients receiving care in different regions. Moreover, it was liable to involve recruitment bias because the less serious forms of the disease could not be diagnosed in the Loire-Atlantique, unlike in Brittany where screening enabled all forms to be detected. We will see later how central the question of so-called borderline forms of CF is in screening today. The results of the Brittany study had been debated in 1999 during a meeting of a discussion group bringing together the people promoting regional screening. The minutes of this meeting, while underscoring the interest of the study, remain cautious in their conclusions:

> This study is retrospective, concerns a relatively small cohort of patients ... and runs the risk of a 'centre effect'. It therefore cannot claim to bring scientific arguments either in favour of newborn screening or against it and suggests a certain need for caution when drawing conclusions (Club Mucoviscidose régional [Regional Cystic Fibrosis Club], 25.3.99).

And yet, the same year, a project for an article signed by the main figures of the same discussion group in Brittany was submitted to the French journal *Archives de Pédiatrie* and provided the following summary: 'The homogeneous nature of the two populations [from Brittany and the Loire-Atlantique] and their health care provision allows clear benefits in screening to be highlighted ... which encourage us to recommend that it be generalized to the rest of the population' (1999). However, in the version published in 2000, the article came to a more cautious conclusion:

> Despite the retrospective nature of the study and the small numbers involved, the homogeneous nature of the two populations and their health care provision allows clear benefits in screening to be highlighted, which encourage us to recommend that it be generalized to the rest of the population, something that would need to go hand-in-hand with the follow-up care for children screened ... so as to ensure that the best benefits are drawn from this (2000).

At the end of 1999, the members of the national working group had become aware of this study (a few members had played a determining role in screening in Brittany). The report for the Cnamts mentioned that 'the short- and medium-term benefits of care provision [*prise en charge*[6] in French] in the first weeks of life have been amply demonstrated, both by the French regional study of the "Greater West" (Brittany, Normandy) and studies abroad, in particular the one carried out in Wisconsin' (AFDPHE 1999). Finally, one of the signatories of the Brittany study explained during an interview:

> We published the follow-up of patients screened in Brittany as opposed to that of those diagnosed clinically in the Loire-Atlantique region, but with a lot of bias;

---

6 The term *prise en charge* in French is ambiguous and can refer to both health care in general and treatment more specifically.

it was at the same period, but with a lot of bias, because it was two different
teams even though we had common protocols (Paediatrician 2, 27.8.02).

It should be specified that while they had all collaborated in the study, the person
who wrote the minutes of the meeting, the first author of the publication, the
person who wrote the report and the person I interviewed were four different
people. Nonetheless, these different stages allow us to retrace the chain of types
of discourse called upon according to different contexts: in an internal meeting
('cannot claim to bring ... arguments'), in a scientific article submitted for
publication ('allows clear benefits ... to be highlighted'), in the same article at
publication ('Despite ... allows clear benefits ... to be highlighted'), in a report
for the funding body ('the ... benefits ... have been amply demonstrated') and in
an interview ('with a lot of bias'). It has been established that there is a close link
between the success of a 'scientific fact' – for it to be considered established – and
the literary genre in which it is announced. Very specifically, the words chosen
correspond to types of language that can be classified according to their more
or less affirmative and assured nature (Latour and Woolgar 1979). What is the
significance of these discursive changes? In the introduction, I clearly dismissed
any idea of the actors' cynical manipulation. Moreover, it is necessary to take
into account the spaces in which these different assertions were made. Just as the
question of the beneficial effects of screening were simplified when they moved
into the public sphere at the beginning of the 1990s in Brittany, the assertions
about this study became firmer as the issue was disseminated in a wider space. It
was not only a question of being convinced, it was also a question of convincing
others. This firmness also increased over time as certain – although not all –
biomedical publications took up the results of the Australian and French studies
without mentioning their limitations, thus establishing a 'fact'. And can it not be
said that the success of a 'scientific fact' resides in how efficiently the different
stages of the author's work can be forgotten and how efficiently problematic issues
are smoothed over?[7] Furthermore, the question of convictions cannot be ignored
and we have seen the role these played in Brittany. As with any human activity,
the scientific process does not set convictions aside – in the case at hand, no longer
about the launch of screening, but about deciding between what is true and false.
The controversy between Louis Pasteur and Felix Pouchet in the nineteenth century
regarding spontaneous generation is a famous example of this (Farley and Geison
1974). It has been established that Pasteur, convinced of the impossibility of
spontaneous generation, carefully avoided publishing results that spoke in favour
of it and did not always bring new evidence in response to Pouchet's arguments.
In the end history proved him right, however, it shows the extent to which it can
be wise to take the analytical category of conviction into account when seeking

---

7   Beliefs are no longer controversial and are considered to be established in particular
'once the end product, an inscription, is available' as 'all intermediary steps which made its
production possible are forgotten' (Latour and Woolgar 1979: 63).

to understand how scientific truth is established. If the Breton doctors launched screening because they were convinced that it was beneficial, one can imagine that they were potentially influenced in their interpretation and desire to disseminate the results of their study, not out of a desire for manipulation, but due to a certain coherency in their position.

More generally, the serious consideration given to the North American study reveals a certain influence of the standards of EBM in France. However, this influence was not the religious cult that some publications denounce (Lambert 2006). And indeed, the working group set up on the national level did not, strictly speaking, include epidemiologists, who could have been particularly meticulous about the value of the results put forward. The influence of EBM was in fact substantially curbed by a flexible approach allowing unconvincing publications (the Australian study) or publications with methodological limitations (the Brittany study) to be included in the assessment of evidence. Rather than pertaining to *evidence*, these publications pertained to the *different levels of evidence,* as classified by the founders of EBM in the 1990s (Evidence-Based Medicine Working Group 1992). In this respect, it is telling that the people interviewed never mentioned a study published in 2001 under the aegis of the Cochrane Collaboration that would qualify for the highest classification according to EBM. The Cochrane Collaboration is a direct product of EBM and was founded in honour of Archibald Cochrane, an epidemiologist and clinician who published a book in the 1970s denouncing the self-satisfaction of doctors and the inefficacy of medicine (Kelly et al. 2010). The Cochrane Collaboration's mission is in particular to conduct systematic reviews of studies on a given question, selecting them on the basis of their methodological quality and examining the results of those selected. Applying these principles, in 2001, just as NSCF was launched in France, the Cochrane review considered that the elements advanced in its favour were tenuous and concluded: 'There is little evidence suggesting benefit from screening for cystic fibrosis in the neonatal period, although there is similarly little evidence of harm' (Mérelle et al. 2001a: 13).

This more flexible approach on the part of the French clinicians does not explain why France was the first country to generalize NSCF, but it does explain why it allowed it. And another factor shook this desire to find evidence for the benefits of screening insomuch as it undermined the very possibility of obtaining such evidence, at least in terms of reduced mortality for screened patients. In 1996, a paper given at a conference in the United States, and later published, concluded that in order to show a significant reduction in mortality, very large groups would have had to be constituted (3,500 people involved over several decades). These data, along with others reaching the same conclusion, were known to the professionals interested in NSCF in France. These results had the strength and legitimacy of mathematical reasoning. Originally, they looked at differences in lifespan, but often drifted onto the more general efficacy of screening. In the end, the idea was established that this evidence could not be obtained and it was necessary to either 'believe' in screening or not.

Shifting What Matters as Evidence

International comparisons in the lifespan of patients suffering from CF were also an important factor in the history of NSCF in France. These comparisons established, at least initially, that France was one of the European countries with the lowest figures. French paediatricians, and particularly those in the working group, incessantly repeated in meetings and conferences that the figures were mediocre in France and that the situation had to be redressed. So what were these alarming statistics and how did these bad results come to be established as true? My interview questions about the grounds for these assertions met with vague responses, even from clinicians who had otherwise shown that they followed biomedical publications closely. Let us return to the genesis of this scientific fact.

From 1992 onwards, at the behest of its medical advisors, the patient organization VLM set up the *Observatoire national de la mucoviscidose* (ONM – National Cystic Fibrosis Observatory) given the responsibility of providing doctors and patients with epidemiological knowledge about the disease. Between 1995 and 1997, studies established comparisons between mean or median lifespan based on data collected by different observatories in different countries. These studies mentioned negative results for France, but with the utmost caution regarding the value of comparisons drawn on the basis of heterogeneous data and the bias caused by the fact that surveys were not as exhaustive from one country to the next. In parallel to these studies, a big pharmaceutical conglomerate [X] that had included CF in its business and research strategy[8] had put in place an observatory called the European Epidemiologic Registry of Cystic Fibrosis (ERCF). It was international this time and therefore in theory built along the same model everywhere. In 1998, a French biomedical study was published, on the basis of the initial data from the ERCF, comparing a series of clinical data between European patients. This study established that the average age of death was 18.2 years in France compared with 20.6 years on average in Europe. However, due to the low coverage rate (only 1,500 French patients out of an estimated 5,000), the study mentioned reservations about its own conclusions. The following year, a 15-line summary in a conference report published by the ERCF explained: 'Evaluation of results was hampered by a gradual reduction in follow-up which, if not randomly distributed, could cause bias and misinterpretation … [S]urvival differed substantially between countries even when large countries were compared'.

The only studies published by the European registry were some very preliminary results and a conference report. However, this did not prevent analytical precaution from becoming more and more discrete, before disappearing altogether. Thus, in France, it became established and taken up in biomedical articles that 'the average age of death is around 20 in France and Great Britain, 23 in Germany and 31 in Denmark' (in 2000) and 'the average age of death is

---

8   This strategy took the shape of the commercial development of medicines, a research policy including the illness, financial support provided to biomedical journals on CF, etc.

lower in France than in other European countries' (in 2001). Again, the types of utterance changed semiotic categories and became more and more affirmative. However, the scientific and social conditions according to which the facts were true, notably the low coverage rate in France, disappeared to a greater degree than with the Brittany study. By setting aside all the modes of production of knowledge and by providing a conference summary as a reference in texts that would then go on to become references in the matter, the concrete stages through which this knowledge was produced became obliterated. This is precisely how scientific facts or beliefs are established. Moreover, the success of a fact is not only dependent upon the disappearance of the stages through which it was constructed, but also its dissemination, as was the case here. Henceforth, it even took on the shape of a rumour.

And this rumour spread due to several factors. First, the role of the pharmaceutical conglomerate [X] can be noted as the body funding the ERCF study. Second, the legitimacy of these uncertain results was enhanced by the fact that one of the instigators of the ERCF comparative study was a nationally renowned paediatrician: the strength of an idea is definitely linked to the credibility of the people carrying it forward (Wood, Ferlie and Fitzgerald 1998). However, it was not just a scientific fact, it was also a medical fact. In other words, these data caused quite a commotion and were probably taken up so widely and yet unthinkingly precisely because they gave a more dramatic turn to the disease. Although on a medical level the different parameters were of course linked, it was no longer a case of comparing radiograph scores and rates of infection, but rather of comparing years of life and premature deaths. This dramatic dimension must no doubt be taken into consideration in order to understand the drive of health care providers, the relevant authorities and the board members of the patient organization. It had a substantial impact, because these studies came out just before NSCF was launched in France and contributed to this decision. As one of the paediatricians from the national working group put it: 'The fact that the French figures weren't good disconcerted the national officials, including at ministerial level' (Paediatrician 2, 27.08.02).

The Cnamts, which was responsible for deciding whether to fund NSCF, was also kept informed of these results via the AFDPHE. Moreover, this worrying information was also in circulation within the patient organization VLM, causing a great deal of emotion, as can be imagined. We should remember that the majority of the most famous CF clinicians were members of the patient organization where some even played an active role as medical advisors. One of the instigators of the ERCF comparative study was both president of the Medical Board of the patient organization and a member of the national working group on NSCF. In 2000, he presented his results during a general assembly of the patient organization, shortly after the organization took a stance in favour of screening. He showed curves for life expectancy and a table mentioning average ages of death that were 10 years lower in France than in Sweden. It is noteworthy that the words 'death' or 'dying' appeared no less than five times in this table. One of the organization board members recalls the shock caused within the families:

> In terms of median lifespan ... there's a ten year gap, it's substantial. France is not bottom of the class in Europe, but it's not far off ... that was communicated to the families in general assemblies ... [he pretends to swallow] they were difficult for the families to swallow, you know ... Some Scandinavians had come and compared their score with ours, and it was... Wow... (Patient organization board member 2, 5.9.02).

And thus a scientific rumour was born. However, the fragile nature of rumours leaves them open to being eventually refuted. Shortly after, new elements came along and altered this vision of the premature death of young CF sufferers in France. In 1998, the organization AFLM/VLM had launched a call for tender to take charge of following up on the National Cystic Fibrosis Observatory and had given the job to the Ined (*Institut national d'études démographiques* – National Institute for Demographic Research). The demographers who took over the case file did not see the data on European comparisons in the same light. One of them explained in an interview how important it is to use homogeneous methods and to aim to include all the patient population when comparing life expectancy. He called into question the 'hastily drawn conclusions' about the so-called bad results in France. Through his wording, this demographer took a statement considered as true and demoted it to the rank of a dubious opinion ('to compare data ... correctly', 'to have a critical view of sources', 'to invalidate certain hastily drawn conclusions'). This new light shed on the matter shattered the idea that patients in France did not live as long as those in most other European countries. The very paediatricians involved in NSCF who had previously shown alarm retracted what they had written. One of them underlined in an interview 'the considerable uncertainty of interpretations' due to the fact that a substantial proportion of the patient population was not surveyed. Finally, as the French Observatory increased its coverage rate of patients and included data on patients less known to hospitals and health care centres and often less seriously affected, these figures rose quickly. Between the periods 1997-1999 and 1999-2001, the life expectancy of patients in France went from 33.3 years to 38.8 years and the mean age of death went from 21.1 years to 23.8 years (ONM 2001, 2004). A progression of five and a half years in life expectancy in two years could not be explained by a spectacular improvement in treatment efficacy but rather by a more complete survey of patients, some of whom were only mildly affected. The alarmist results for France had no solid foundation. And it thus transpired that France was in fact classed within the European average, while Denmark and Sweden remained the most successful countries. And yet neither of these two countries used NSCF. Henceforth, evidence shifted to a different subject.

The ERCF study did not only affect estimated life expectancies. By establishing a link between life expectancy and the size of centres in which patients were treated, it suggested that patients' respiratory function declined more rapidly when they were treated in small centres (under 50 patients) than when they were treated in larger ones (over 100 patients). In short, the results were 'bad' in France – which in fact they were not – because the organization of centres was ill conceived. For the health professionals involved in NSCF on a national level, these results were established. Or at least, the clinicians putting forward these data had to be taken at their word because the results were never published either. Each time an article referred to them, it was either via the brief conference summary mentioned previously or via an English study that did focus on centres but not on their size (Mahadeva et al. 1998). More specifically, this English study showed, on the one hand, better growth and a better respiratory status in patients treated in specialized centres, but, on the other, a higher rate of infection with the terrible pseudomonas germ. As one paediatrician summarized, these results could be understood differently depending on what you wanted to see. Here, the evidence was therefore ambivalent and could support opposing arguments. It should be noted, however, that a Dutch study also indicated a benefit linked to specialized centres, even though possible areas of bias were mentioned by the authors (Mérelle et al. 2001b, Mérelle, Meerman and Dankert-Roelse 1999). Moreover, the life expectancy of patients in Canada, a country that also centralized CF health care, seemed to be good, although the comparative elements were indirect. To summarize, what seemed relatively clear was that in the three countries where patients appeared to live the longest – Sweden, Denmark and Canada – patients were often treated in specialized centres with large numbers of patients. But this was far removed from the initial standards of EBM and RCTs. The ERCF study, which was perhaps the most significant in terms of constituting evidence at this time, was the least well documented (one brief conference summary). And yet it undoubtedly had a decisive impact on the decision regarding NSCF. The importance of providing follow-up care in large centres treating more than 100 patients was also fore-grounded as a major scientific argument in favour of NSCF in the report of the national working group delivered to the Cnamts in 1999. These results did not give rise to debate or controversy, because this time the evidence seemed more solid in the eyes of the AFDPHE. We should not forget that these results were intertwined with those that seemed to show a low life expectancy for patients in France. They were consolidated by what was considered to be established truth, which had taken a dramatic turn. Incidentally, it should also be noted that evidence had shifted from one subject to another. Insofar as that none of the three model countries used NSCF, it was no longer a question of evidence for the efficacy of screening, but rather of evidence for the efficacy of health care centres.

This train of ideas leads us, finally, to the media. It would be too lengthy to outline in detail here, but let me simply mention the fact that when the AFDPHE and the Cnamts held a press conference at the end of 2000 to announce that screening was being launched, the information was widely taken up. Although this chapter as a whole has shown the complexity of the data involved, the salient feature here was the link established in the media between screening and the expected increase in life expectancy. However, this link was expressed in two different fashions: the first was cautious (in some national dailies or during interviews with paediatricians involved in national screening), while the other was more direct (through journalists or in widely read mainstream publications). In the latter cases, no doubts were expressed and views were not at all tempered.

By way of an epilogue, we can note that after NSCF was launched in France, several other studies were published to evaluate its efficacy, but they continued to compare different periods or regions. Amid this proliferation of data, the Center for Disease Control and Prevention (CDC) in the United States, a point of reference in terms of public health, established a grid of reliability of results in order to evaluate the main studies on this subject. In 2004, it stated that the benefits of NSCF were sufficient to consider including NSCF in newborn screening in conjunction with systems ensuring access to high quality treatment. More specifically, it concluded: 'On the basis of evidence of moderate benefits and low risk of harm, CDC believes that newborn screening for CF is justified' (MMWR Recommendations and Reports 2004: 1). In 2009, the *Haute Autorité de Santé* in France, a public authority responsible for evaluating medical acts and services, produced a report indicating an improvement in growth and nutritional status thanks to NSCF, but an absence of conclusions regarding respiratory function. It stated: 'The implementation [of screening] is more the result of scientific beliefs and a societal choice than a choice based exclusively on evidence' (HAS 2009: 64).

In conclusion to this chapter, the scientific foundations underpinning the field of experience of NSCF in Brittany and in France can be said to belong schematically to two registers: on the one hand, the pre-eminence of convictions regarding evidence, involving a degree of clinical experience; on the other, the pre-eminence of scientifically established evidence in the decision-making process, also involving a degree of clinical experience. This second side can itself be divided into two variants, the first embodied by the AFDPHE officials who expressed their doubts during my study, even once the decision had been made, and the second, embodied by the members of the working group (aside from those from Normandy and Brittany) who participated in the decision-making process and did not share these doubts. Overall, the opposition between the proponents of both positions is the sign of the 'epistemic tension' described elsewhere in the case of AIDS drugs trials (Dodier and Barbot 2000). In the case of AIDS, different ways of considering the link between scientific and clinical judgments depending on the doctor are reported, with some pleading in favour of the principle of randomized controlled trials and others campaigning for protocols to be relaxed. In comparison with this article, the study of NSCF presents one difference: it was not trial philosophy that was in question here as, strictly speaking, in the first position there was no 'trial'; rather it was more profoundly the question of the relationship between knowledge and action that was at stake. Overall, the results presented here show a large range of positions and go to show how variable scientific ways of thinking through responses to a given question can be.

A second important aspect to the question concerns the processes through which the 'truth' is constituted as well as the dynamics of changing points of view. Questioning these dynamics enables analysis to go beyond the somewhat fixed approaches that tend to present medical knowledge as grounded in certainty or, on the contrary, uncertainty. The scientific elements that contributed to changing the points of view of the AFDPHE officials include the following: the initial results of a North American study complying with the most traditional standards of EBM, but which I attempted to demonstrate went on later to 'escape conclusion'; different studies situated on a whole scale of 'levels of evidence' related to more flexible forms of EBM; the idea that evidence was impossible to obtain; alarming unpublished results on patient life expectancy in France that resembled a rumour; and a shift in the subject of evidence, which linked these results with the existence or absence of health care centres treating more than 50 or 100 patients. This somewhat heterogeneous list shows that the decision was not made because of a particular event, but rather through a process involving different elements related to knowledge. In comparison with other studies (particularly Cambrosio et al. 2006), regulation relied here not on meta-analyses or the mobilization of thousands of researchers and clinicians in clinical trials, but on a range of indications and of levels of evidence from various parts of the world, that seemed to act collectively. However, as in other studies (cf. the introduction to this chapter), the role of clinical judgment and professional experience in ways of considering and fashioning evidence is also shown here: evidence not only shapes practice, it is also shaped by practice. The French doctors were under a certain amount of influence from the standards of the strictest form of EBM (that emphasizes RCTs) but in a slightly more flexible version that allowed them to make decisions about screening based on results that did not follow these standards. More generally, this kind of study leads us to question the role of experts in public policy and the criteria for what is scientific, at a time when science plays an important role within policy. Expressed learnedly, there is matter for a critique of scientific reason; expressed simply, science brings legitimacy, but not always on the grounds that we imagine. The list summarized above also shows that, whatever its ambiguous relationship to EBM, biomedicine remains invested with emotions (Mykhalovskiy and Weir 2004). The role played by statistics presented in terms of years of life lost can testify to this; the scale of measurement suddenly had very concrete resonance in terms of life or death. Finally, my analysis shows that, as underlined by other authors (particularly Dobrow et al. 2006), evidence is strongly rooted in contingency and local contexts, particularly the evaluation of life expectancies, carried out at a given moment and linked to both a given country and the organization of care provision. Indeed, sociologists underline the need to take better account of how treatment is organized in different health care systems when studying EBM (Mykhalovskiy and Weir 2004). However, this aspect relates just as much to the public health dimension – in its various clinical, but also sociological, political, etc. forms (Kelly et al. 2010) – as it does to the scientific dimension. This last point suggests a dimension that is just as political as it is scientific. And this link between how knowledge is mobilized and how power is practised remains to be explored.

Chapter 3

Governing

Forming the 'truth' about what people are, in their capacity as living beings (ill or not; 'at risk' or not; lacking treatment or not) and about what improvements could be made depending on this state (mode of therapeutic care; risk evaluation; decision about whether to know these risks or not) can lead to a series of actions. These depend on the aim at stake (treating the ill; identifying and monitoring all individuals at risk, even slightly; eradicating the illness, etc.). In other words, the constitution of knowledge considered as true can be linked to conduct and ways of acting. The people concerned by this knowledge can appear as *subjects* with hopes and needs while, at the same time, being the *objects* of decisions and techniques that escape them. This shift between subject and object therefore raises the following questions: Who is a 'subject' in a position to act, assert themselves and make choices? Who is an 'object' of public action and policies? One of the theoretical benefits of the Foucauldian conception here, in contrast to the Cartesian or Sartrean traditions, is that subjects do not result from something intrinsic to, and constitutive of, people but rather are formed through processes (Foucault 2001b). Therefore, depending on their experiences, these subjects change, take on different forms or see their powers as subjects eroded.

The 'voluntary consent of the human subject', underlined by the Nuremberg Code in the wake of the Second War World, is now one of the cornerstones of good biomedical practice in terms of research and treatment. This political/moral framework must be understood in light of the crimes committed by Nazi doctors, without forgetting the controversies generated in the 1960s by clinical trials that showed little respect for human subjects (Beecher 1966). Moreover, the question of the subject is particularly relevant in the field of genetics insofar as the weight of eugenics has made the question of patients' autonomy a sensitive issue.

Whether they express it in this way or not, many social science publications have focused on the place of the subject in genetics, either showing its limits or, on the contrary, underlining its scope. In the 1990s, certain researchers emphasized the deterministic effect of 'geneticization', seen as an approach to medical or societal questions that is excessively influenced by genetics (Lippman 1992). This deterministic vision has been increasingly called into question by other social science researchers (Kerr 2005, Rose 2007). However, they neglect to remind us that the changes in genetic knowledge – where the gene no longer holds the same central position as in the 1980s or 1990s – have probably altered patients' and doctors' conceptions of diseases, as well as the leeway available for those affected by them. The geneticization and determinism that were feared at a certain period are less relevant today, although this does not mean that their detractors should be forever relegated to that position. We now know that genetic tests do not always bring certainty, but rather an evaluation of risk, and we will see examples of this. And even in cases where things are almost certain, theoretically several options remain open (knowing or not, receiving care or not, continuing with a pregnancy or not, etc.). If we consider that types of knowledge can be linked to different types of power, a plausible hypothesis would be that the greater the diagnostic and prognostic uncertainty, the more it is possible to call upon subjects' autonomy and responsibility. For Thomas Lemke (2004), it is precisely the notion of genetic 'risk' and the uncertainty it brings that confronts people with choices and calls upon their autonomy and responsibility. Certain studies, while refuting any clear-cut distinction between what is imposed and what is accepted, argue that subjects are produced through notions of patients' responsibilities, choices and wishes in terms of genetic tests (Novas and Rose 2000, Rose 2007). This point of view has the advantage of analyzing fundamental evolutions in a reasoned manner. Since the 1950s, a non-directive approach to patients has been the norm in genetic counselling sessions, often taken up in professional discourse. However, if this rationale is analyzed more closely, this new subjectivation is far more reminiscent of the idea of full, active citizenship than of people being alternately subjects and objects. Sometimes it tends towards flattening out the disparities between social groups (who has access to information and who is a subject?), towards considering practice and rhetoric on the same level (what 'choice' is offered and under what conditions can people take it up?) and towards neglecting both structural constraints (what role do family, social, cultural and economic contexts play in these choices?) and the effects of its changes (what is the effect of giving individuals responsibility as opposed to social and political responsibility?). And yet these questions seem essential in order to deal with subjectivation and politics more widely.

Among the body of social science studies showing the practical and conceptual limitations of the principle of self-determination in biomedicine (Boulton and Parker 2007, Corrigan 2003, Dixon-Woods et al. 2007, Ducourneau 2007, Jacob 2007, Hedgecoe 2005), several studies put this notion of choice to the test where genetics is concerned. The questions of how consent is obtained for research in genetics and of the relationship between professionals and patients in situations of genetic counselling have given rise to numerous publications. Some of these highlight the dilemmas facing professionals due to their avowed neutral position or facing patients who must make a decision regarding prenatal diagnosis (Conrad and Gabe 1999). Other studies show how cultural and social constraints can weigh upon parents' decisions – such constraints include the imperatives of good health in our societies, the influence of professionals on parents who follow their advice and the lack of available social benefits for the handicapped (Kerr and Cunningham-Burley 2000). Lene Koch and Mette Nordahl Svendon (2005), in particular, analyze the case of people undergoing genetic counselling for hereditary forms of cancer in Denmark. The genetic risk of disease leads the patients to take 'responsibility', which means that they have no other choice than to opt 'freely' for prophylactic measures. This shows that it is not appropriate to make a clear-cut separation between what is chosen and what is imposed. In reality, although we cannot simply talk about things being imposed, within bioethical discourse there seem to be values and imperatives that rely on patients' 'free choice' as well as variably complex conditions for how effective choice can be, depending on the situation. Moreover, and without even mentioning the use of genetics for reasons other than the strictly medical (police, family, etc.), the viewpoint considering that people are confronted with choices in genetic counselling neglects the fact that we seem to have already entered mass genetics, and are not simply targeting people said to be at risk.

The situation of interest here, in the context of NSCF, differs from genetic counselling: individual consent for genetic testing is necessary in order to carry out screening on entire populations but without individual consultations. In the 1960s and 1970s, when the bioethical principle of autonomy was developing, screening for genetic diseases on populations of neonates appeared using blood samples. A tension arose between two principles: on the one hand, protecting children's health by carrying out screening on the widest possible scale; on the other, safeguarding parental autonomy and consent. Due to their medical benefits, many newborn screening programmes were in fact made mandatory. Today, the question of subjects within genetics is once again topical due to a rapid increase in the quantity of newborn screening tests, changes in the aims in question (some conditions are screened for without leading to any treatment) and the evolution of techniques employed (DNA tests can now be used). In short, we can see here the changes and limitations facing the individual 'genetic subject'. Let us now turn to the situation where collective subjects are concerned.

Studies on patient organizations in the context of genetic diseases can shed interesting light on subjectivation. In the United States, certain organizations developed alliances with political leaders and biomedical researchers, expressing citizens' claims in the name of sick children (Health, Rapp and Taussig 2004). More widely, the members of the different organizations for genetic diseases brought about a 'genetic citizenship' that not only made financial claims, but also demanded that their experience be respected and recognized, and that their wishes in terms of research and health policies be taken into account. In France, Vololona Rabeharisoa and Michel Callon (1999) explored the case of the French Association against Muscular Dystrophy (the AFM), which is emblematic of the 'power of the patients' over research. Indeed, this association is in a position to carry out substantial fundraising (roughly 100 million Euros per year), thanks to the Téléthon, and to weigh in directly on how research programmes are oriented, conducted and evaluated. Above all, it does this through the voices of the patients' families rather than those of its medical and scientific advisors. Should we, then, extrapolate from this and extend this particular relationship to research to other organizations? As the authors themselves admit:

similar organizations in France (like the AFLM) or in the USA ... do not seem to have developed forms of action, and in particularly of mobilization of research and the medical field, comparable to those imagined by the AFM. ... The patients progressively gave way to doctors and researchers [within the association], losing control of the definition of their research policy (Rabeharisoa and Callon 1999: 176).

A study carried out at the end of the 1990s shows that the AFLM/VLM, which is our focus here, seems to have had the ability to attract CF researchers but also difficulty in adopting a strong research policy with regard to researchers and doctors (Larédo and Kahane 1998). A key idea in this study is that the organization's therapeutic aim was strongly influenced by the hopes of gene therapy. As this could only be part of innovative science, it was therefore considered that research policy had to be decided by scientists above all. These examples of organizations can allow us to begin to draw a clearer picture of the configurations. Patient organizations, even simply within the field of genetics, could not be any more diverse in terms of scope, aim and capacity for action. The problem of political representation and equity therefore arises: certain patients manage to mobilize resources and attention that others simply cannot obtain (Bonnet et al. 1998). This also leads to the question of the political meaning that we ascribe to these groups, which hover between active citizenship and interest groups. Although in France it is considered to be against the general interest for interest groups to participate in decision-making, unlike in other countries like the United States where this is clearly integrated, in reality this participation often occurs. The use of 'influence activities', which used to be the preserve of economic interest groups, is now becoming generalized across a number of fields; for Emiliano Grossman and Sabine Saurugger (2006) this justifies the term 'society of interest groups'.

On the strength of these analyses, in this chapter I will examine the political side to the field of experience and *what governing means for a genetic disease*, understood as outlined in the introduction. More specifically, it will be a question of using the history of NSCF in France to examine *the role of genetics in how subjects conduct themselves*. This will entail looking at how different actors are constituted as governing or governable individuals (or groups), at how the entity to be governed is viewed and at the means and instruments through which this government is exercised. An initial section will focus on the subtle power relations between professionals and non-professionals in the history of this screening in France, with the notable influence of the former and a generally fragmented conception of practices. A second section will then reveal and analyze one of the major arguments in favour of NSCF in France, showing how it was partly seen as a tool through which to govern the sick in both space and time. Finally, the last section will consider government at its extremities, where it comes to resemble capillaries, that is to say with the mothers of children screened in maternity units.

Power Relations

The AFDPHE and its Institutional Partners

Max Weber (1968) underlines that action or domination are all the easier to establish when they are considered legitimate by those subjected to them. This first section will look at how the AFDPHE became a legitimate professional association in the eyes of State institutions, affording an understanding of one of the ways subjects are forged. The study of the foundations of this legitimacy will show that they consist in four elements: principles of efficiency (saving children and ensuring adequate care for those diagnosed), of economy of means (calculating expense as minimally as possible), of rigour (monitoring the work of the regional associations) and of reflexivity (knowing when to end a programme). Let us look at these in detail.

In 1999, when the AFDPHE presented the case to the Cnamts for NSCF to be added to the other screening procedures on the basis of the conclusions of the working group, the Cnamts readily agreed to provide funding. Although the relationship between the professional association and the funding body 'had not always been idyllic', as one respondent put it, the AFDPHE benefited from its legitimacy in the eyes of the Cnamts. This is evidenced by a letter from the national director of the funding body addressed to the president of the AFDPHE, proudly displayed in the AFDPHE building at the time of this study. It mentioned newborn screening as 'one of the greatest achievements of the French health care system', of which the AFDPHE officials, with their 'commitment and extraordinary personalities', could be proud. Of course, at this stage such a letter is simply a flattering indication of legitimacy at a particular moment in the association's history. If we go back in time, we can see that the first screening programme launched by the association, which concerned phenylketonuria, played a particular role in this legitimizing process. Although it was launched in the absence of 'evidence' of its efficiency, it proved emblematic of successful screening. Thanks to this, the AFDPHE could pride itself on having avoided serious mental deficiencies in hundreds, later thousands, of children. Its representative made sure to remind the Cnamts of this when submitting the funding request for NSCF. This initial success of phenylketonuria screening paved the way for other forms of newborn screening: hypothyroidism (1978), sickle-cell disease (1989 in the overseas *départements* and territories and 1995 in Metropolitan France) and adrenal hyperplasia (1995). Beyond the medical success of the initiative, from a more organizational point of view structures and practices were put in place that facilitated the launch of NSCF: there was no difficulty in adding a test concerning CF using the same blood sample. This advantage was also apparent in the coverage rate of newborns approaching 100 %: given that almost all births took place in maternity units, the population was pretty much captive. This contrasted with other screening policies and made a favourable impression on the Cnamts officials. Another significant positive element in the eyes of the funding body was that the professional association had the advantage of reducing costs. Its officials tried to calculate them as minimally as possible and worked on a voluntary basis. Moreover, the association was considered to be capable of ensuring the rigorous implementation of screening, providing national reports and monitoring regional laboratories. This allowed the association to evaluate and, if necessary, change or even stop screening programmes. This links in to the last aspect of the legitimization process. For the Cnamts officials, the fact that the association had proved itself capable of stopping programmes when it judged them unconvincing was undeniably an argument in its favour. The decision to end the experimental NSCF programme set up in 1989-1990 is a good illustration of this principle. And in fact, during the present study, the national AFDPHE officials occasionally threatened to cease NSCF if the rules established with the doctors did not lead to results and particularly if these doctors did not provide the accounts expected by the national association.

This all shows how the professional association became a legitimate institutional partner of the Cnamts, who considered that it provided efficient help in preventing rare but incapacitating diseases. Beyond the association and on a more general level, phenylketonuria also played an important role. It was – and still is – one of the rare genetic diseases for which curative treatment could – and can – be provided. It therefore contributes to validating the genetic approach in general, which, as we have seen, has been slow to show its therapeutic benefits. In other countries, such as the United States, screening for phenylketonuria was largely foregrounded by professionals to demonstrate the medical and social benefits of screening for genetic diseases (Lindee 2005). Lene Kock and Dirk Stemerding (1994) studied how a screening programme for CF carriers was set up in Denmark in the 1990s and suggested the term 'regime' to designate the technological, organizational and societal practices resulting from previous processes of 'attunement' between technological options, professional demands and social acceptability. Likewise, in France the 'regime' of newborn screening already established for phenylketonuria, and then hypothyroidism, facilitated the emergence and acceptability of other screening procedures based on the same kind of technical organization and social interaction grounded in legitimacy.

This legitimacy explains in part why the institutional partners took a backseat with regard to the professional association where newborn screening was concerned. So far, I have analyzed the AFDPHE's relationship with the Cnamts more than the relationship with the DGS, the other supervisory body. While, statutorily, the DGS was part of the board of the professional association, the attendance and involvement of its representatives on the board varied in regularity. In reality, the Ministry of Health played an accompanying role with regard to the movement more than it managed or instigated it. In an interview, one of the AFDPHE officials expressed regret about the Ministry's lack of recognition for the association's work: 'The Ministry watches…, it's a supervising body that doesn't know anything about us'. Furthermore, there were sometimes power struggles between the two supervising bodies, the Cnamts and the DGS. When

NSCF was decided upon, the Cnamts organized a press conference to announce it before the DGS had even given its approval on the matter. According to one of the institutional officials, this shows how, when the Cnamts decides to free up money and the French association organizes screening on the ground, 'it happens, with or without the DGS'. The Cnamts 'forced the DGS's hand' regarding the screening decision, she adds. However, as we have mentioned, the Ministry of Health did not want to be left by the wayside where the organization of health care was concerned and, in 2001, organized three meetings on this subject, through the DHOS. At a time (2000-2001) when providing equal treatment for patients across the country was a stated government priority, the Ministry of Health wanted to take control again. It went much further than the AFDPHE officials had anticipated, disseminating a Circular advocating that *Centres de ressource et de compétence de la mucoviscidose* (CRCM – Centres of Resources and Competence in Cystic Fibrosis) be set up; they are multidisciplinary centres, which meet a set of specific requirements.

So what can this foray into the past tell us about how roles and power were divided between professionals and institutions in this health policy? The case of the AFDPHE is significant regarding the field of health care, where the history of practice shows how multiple means – often separate from the State, ranging from charitable organizations to learned societies – come together to tackle medical problems. Generally, when it comes to contributing to the 'government of bodies' (Fassin and Memmi 2004), the French State intervenes in an accompanying role more than it gives orders. The specificity of the AFDPHE resided in the fact that it had the monopoly over policies in this domain and this therefore corresponded to a delegation of power. Although the AFDPHE's board was open to the supervisory bodies, the professionals were the real driving forces behind it. The association's role went beyond that of simply providing an assessment informing and providing an opinion for the decider before political arbitration (Lascoumes 2005), it also filled the role allotted to those who govern.

Spending time on the AFDPHE premises affords an understanding, at least in part, of what it means on a practical level to be a government association (as defined in the introduction). Depending on the day, between one and four people worked there: Hélène Ravenel, who was a more than active retired person of a respectable age; a second, younger individual, who was an epidemiologist by training; a paediatrician (one day per week); and a secretary. It is by spending time with these people that I was able to begin to understand what was later described to me as the 'screening mindset'. One of them explained to me that in a given hospital, there was too much of a 'doctors' mindset'. This meant that interest was mainly shown in the ill and in publishing about their cases, rather than focusing on organizing screening and also showing interest in those who were 'normal', that is to say the healthy children screened. A letter had even been prepared to reassure the parents of 'normal' children, but apparently 'they' were not particularly interested in that. Visibly, even if the majority of the actors in question were doctors, two approaches could be defined with, on the one side, the clinicians in charge of treating the children diagnosed through screening and, on the other, those responsible for organizing screening, the ex-founders of the national association (who have now handed over the reins to other national officials). This subtle distinction will be examined a little later on; first, it is necessary to look to the patient organization in order to complete this study of the power relations at work.

The Patient Organization

For the AFDPHE officials, screening decisions fell to the professionals, who were in the best position to evaluate how appropriate they were. According to them, these decisions were complex and parents of patients or their sympathizers did not have enough knowledge to allow them to participate in the debate; for this reason they did not wish to involve the patient organization in the working group on NSCF. This was not a position taken on principle, but the conclusion of several, more or less difficult, years of prior collaboration within the Scientific Board of the AFLM/ VLM association. This is why the latter was not involved as such in the working group set up by the AFDPHE, despite making a certain number of public statements in favour of NSCF in 2000-2001 thus ensuring a certain strategic visibility. As the director of the AFLM/VLM association recognized, the responsibility for screening had to fall to the AFDPHE: 'It's [Y, president of the AFDPHE] who deserves the credit for newborn cystic fibrosis screening … If [Y] hadn't grabbed the issue by the horns, I'd still be at it' (Patient organization board member 3, 5.12.02). However, the patient families enjoyed sufficient public and institutional legitimacy for the Cnamts to ask for their opinion on screening. For were they not the people concerned first and foremost? They had the legitimacy of real experience. For this reason, it was important to the Cnamts to meet with the patient organizations (AFLM/VLM and SOS Cystic Fibrosis), and check that they were in favour of NSCF. The working group put in place by the AFDPHE were well aware of this and made sure they mentioned 'the parents' justified request' for NSCF in their recommendations to the Cnamts. In the same spirit, but with more ambiguity, during a conference on genetic tests aimed at doctors and researchers in 2001, one AFDPHE official put forward the argument: 'The Association against cystic fibrosis is calling for this screening' (Observation 26.1.01). I only understood much later the full ambiguity of the term 'the Association against cystic fibrosis' in this kind of sentence. Who, precisely, within the patient organization was calling for screening? Parents? Adult sufferers? Doctors? Researchers? How did they influence the decision? In short, who were the active subjects where screening was concerned?

The patient organization was the locus for a subtle game of internal power relations between professionals and non-professionals. It should be remembered that, like many patient organizations, this one was created at the instigation of doctors. And yet the statutes of the AFLM/VLM association required that its Board of Directors be composed in great majority by patient families and sympathizers. This board made it a point of honour to take position in favour of NSCF before its Medical Board did. In order to underscore the prerogatives of the directors, in 1999 the president of the AFLM 'informed' the Medical Board of the 'Board of Directors' decision to launch serious reflection about newborn screening for cystic fibrosis', with the Medical Board adopting a favourable opinion shortly after. However, this anecdote is deceptive, because the professionals had a major influence, at least in terms of newborn screening. The reasons for this were twofold and linked to the weight of erudition and the relationships between actors. First, until the end of the 1990s, the Board of Directors and patient families followed the generally negative opinions of their Medical Board regarding screening, considering that it was most competent to judge this. More generally, while the members of the Board of Directors could take decisions that differed from the point of view of their 'experts', for them NSCF was not a sufficient priority to justify such action. As one of the organization board members said in an interview: 'First we listened to the specialists... they had the voice of erudition' (Patient organization board member 4, 17.2.03). The arrival of spirited new director Marc Coudray in 1998 was not unrelated to the Board of Directors' stronger positions vis-à-vis their experts. And shortly after his arrival, Marc Coudray forged links with François Coat, the director of the health care centre in Roscoff, one of the rare doctors to be a member of the Board of Directors. They worked very closely together during this period, as the new director 'had a policy', while the parents showed difficulty in freeing themselves from expert advice. Above and beyond this interplay between actors, the Board of Directors took position in favour of NSCF, when it knew that discussion was already well under way on this same topic within the Medical Board.

On a less anecdotal level, it is important to remember that several members of the Medical Board of the patient organization, including Breton actors, were part of the working group organized by the AFDPHE. The president of the Medical Board was even the head of one of the commissions set up by the AFDPHE. Moreover, in 1999 he was replaced at the head of the Medical Board by another member of the working group, who was none other than the general secretary of the AFDPHE. Under such conditions, it was unsurprising to see the viewpoints of the Medical Board and the working group converge. In this sense, one can suppose that the patient organization's medical advisors placed a certain amount of pressure on the long-standing officials of the AFDPHE, who, as we have seen, were opposed to NSCF and this did not go without creating tensions. As one of the people I interviewed put it: 'There was a lot of pressure from the AFLM/VLM on the AFDPHE, some people were in both' (13.8.02). I later understood that when people, particularly doctors, spoke of 'VLM' or 'AFLM', they were often not referring to the patient families and their representatives, as one might legitimately assume, but actually the Medical Board (or doctors) of the organization. And yet we have seen that members of this Medical Board, with the considerable support of the director of the Roscoff centre aided by the new director of the organization, did in effect weigh in on the decisions made by the AFDPHE who then negotiated with the Cnamts. The term 'patient organization' therefore emerged as ambiguous and only a detailed study could identify who were actually the active subjects in terms of newborn screening: doctors and/or families?

The patient organization not only contributed to the decision about screening, through its doctors, it was also involved after the event: first, in terms of the organization of care and, second, as a pressure group. Certain doctors from the patient organization played an active role in the professionals' reflections concerning the reorganization of health care centres. These were notably materialized in a working document written in 1997 by François Coat, the director of the Roscoff health care centre, after discussion with Christian Perret, the director of the screening and health care centre in Rennes, about setting up a care network for CF in Brittany. They were also reflected by the paediatric recommendations made in particular by a group also coordinated by François Coat and members of the Medical Board, including Christian Perret. These recommendations were published in a special number of the journal *Archives de Pédiatrie*. They stemmed from European Registry results in terms of differences in life expectancy and suggested the 'determining role of health care organization' in addressing this. In short, they justified the creation of health care centres for CF and defined what criteria should be met to qualify and how they should function. These recommendations were broadly taken up by one of the national commissions formed under the aegis of the AFDPHE following the Cnamts's agreement. They were also given to the group formed in parallel by the DHOS. The Circular distributed by the DHOS-DGS concerning the health care centres showed similar viewpoints. In sum, this circulation of ideas shows how the doctors of the AFLM/VLM association, first in Brittany then relayed on a national level, weighed in indirectly on the national reorganization of care.

More directly, the patient organization acted upon public authorities through various national political leaders, playing the role of pressure group. For although, overall, the Ministry of Health had little influence on the screening decision, we have seen how it took back control when it came to reorganizing health care. In order to make it easier to open doors, the patient organization even called upon a lobbying company to act as a mediator. As one of the board members of the organization explained, such a company is an advisory firm including former members of ministerial offices who, in exchange for payment, use their contacts to facilitate meetings with political representatives. In short, the patient organization had the social and financial resources to enable them to act and give them a certain power. Other representatives from the organization interceded directly with the Ministry of Health to alert public authorities to the difference in life expectancy between CF sufferers in France compared with neighbouring European countries. According to them, raising awareness in this way was fruitful:

> It was one of the elements that meant that [X, State Secretary for Health] …
> said that it was indeed scandalous and that, given these conditions, we had to
> move towards… And that's how the CRCM were born… We went down there

[to the Ministry], we showed the documents that had been analyzed. It was a factor in getting recognition that there was an anomaly. ... And I think this had quite a big effect. I spoke about it directly with [X, State Secretary for Health] (Paediatrician 6, 30.6.04).

In what is said here, it is possible to discern two types of action that are typical of pressure groups (Grossman and Saureregger 2006): recourse to science (producing an expertise that is considered to be objective, through measures of life expectancy) and recourse to morality (establishing data liable to scandalize or run counter to ethics, through the differences in life expectancy between countries).

A strategic dimension could also be seen in this action. The differences in patient life expectancy between the Northern countries and France was the 'most fascinating' element in the eyes of the members of the Board of Directors of the patient organization, as Marc Coudray, the director at the time, explained in an interview. According to him, this fact had even contributed strongly to shifting the Board of Directors' opinion in favour of NSCF: 'In France, someone who is born in 2002 has an average life expectancy of around 32 years, in Sweden, it's 48 years. Then, the Board of Directors voted unanimously for setting up newborn screening, I can tell you' (Patient organization board member 3, 5.12.02). From then on, the idea that began to form bit by bit was to help achieve better treatment for patients through newborn screening. This idea will be developed further later on, as it is very similar to the professionals' position. And indeed, several people more or less claimed to be at the origin of this idea, which initially circulated within a relatively small circle. More specifically, for Marc Coudray there was a dual strategic dimension to this position. While the first dimension concerned the patients, the second concerned the patient organization itself, because he saw in screening the opportunity to channel the energies within the organization. Another Medical Board member of the patient organization underlined this argument in an interview: 'It allowed the patient organization to coalesce around a key theme, which was screening and then the organization of care ... It was an opportunity for a tenable political theme' (Patient organization board member 5, 26.3.04).

Finally, the strategy defended by the general director of the AFLM/VLM association involved raising CF awareness within the whole population. This included the shift between being ill and being a 'carrier' (of a mutation, not a disease) that we also noted in Brittany and that took the number of people affected nationally from 6,000 to almost 2 million. Marc Coudray explains how he defended this idea in front of the members of the Board of Directors: the organization had to have a foundation stone and this could only be France, as otherwise the organization would represent nothing more than a corporatist interest. It was necessary to emphasize that there were almost 2 million carriers of the gene in the country. He told them, 'If we manage to demonstrate to France that this is a public health problem, then we can put your illness centre stage' (Patient organization board member 3, 5.12.02). Along the same lines, the following sentence can be found on the organization's website: 'The ['Communication'] department [within the organization] has the considerable but very gratifying task of organizing ... the recognition of cystic fibrosis as a public health issue'. It was a question of getting away from being seen as an interest or pressure group, as outlined above, because the latter do not have good press in France.

In order to find a medium for this strategic element, the patient organization published publicity inserts raising awareness for CF in mainstream newspapers. The presentation of the insert was relatively striking. It showed a foetus wearing a mask identical to those worn by CF sufferers to help them breathe, underneath the following text:

ARE YOU AMONG THE 2 MILLION FRENCH PEOPLE WITH A GENE THAT CAN PASS ON CYSTIC FIBROSIS?

... Without knowing it, you could be carrying the defective gene for cystic fibrosis. Just like 5,000 children and adults, Anne [the foetus in the photo] will suffer from serious respiratory and digestive problems that will prevent her from living like everyone else. Cystic fibrosis is the most common genetic disease affecting children in France (2001).

This condensed two social factors likely to encourage mobilization: the serious nature of the illness and its frequency, which gave the disease the particular and ambiguous status of being the most frequent rare genetic disease among European populations. The important message lies in its insidious nature, its invisibility; anyone can carry the mutation without knowing it. While the figure of the person who is ill without knowing it is a classic in medicine, the fact of using the picture of a foetus emphasized the fact that the defect could be passed down. In doing this, the organization established a link between the ill, their families and the general population, with the gene acting as the vehicle for this link. This strategy allowed everyone to be made aware of the risk of passing on the disease, while avoiding mentioning that everybody carries several silent mutations, more often than not without any effects. Specifying this would have trivialized genetic abnormality and clouded the warning message. Moreover, and this was by no means the least important of its aims, newborn screening reinforced this mode of raising awareness, because it affected all parents in maternity units.

To summarize, the role played by the AFLM/VLM association had been low-key and this undermined my hypothesis regarding its central role in the decision to generalize NSCF. Its members may have acted as subjects at certain times – they had 'acted on the actions of others' (the political leaders) – but as subjects often under medical influence. The decision-makers were therefore the professionals. While generalizations should not be made about all the organization's practices simply on the basis of the issue of screening, it would be difficult to claim that the patient families were autonomous with regard to their medical advisors. Assuming that the examples of other diseases, such as muscular dystrophies (Rabeharisoa and Callon 1999, Rabeharisoa 2003), can be extended to CF would mean overestimating the autonomy and role of 'patient' organizations. Nevertheless, the organization contrived to raise the interest of the political leaders involved in the reorganization of health care provision after screening was decided and, in this sense, managed to make itself heard. As mentioned in the introduction, this influence, albeit relative, calls into question the meaning of the political within our societies, between active citizenship and pressure groups. Indeed, this effect of lobbying testifies to the shift in the public authorities' centre of interest towards individuals or groups of individuals (an organization) as opposed to towards the population as a whole. This tendency produces a fragmentation effect that is in part reminiscent of the one that resulted from the debate about NSCF between experts, which will be examined in the next part.

Governing in Time and Space

The members of the working group set up by the AFDPHE, some of whom were members of the patient organization's Medical Board, played a leading role in the decision regarding NSCF. It is necessary, though, to understand the political grounds on which they based NSCF; in other words towards whom it was geared and to what end. Nikolas Rose (2001) underlines that the striking role of professional associations and ethics committees in how biomedical practices are carried out regarding prenatal diagnosis is linked to a particular form of 'pastoral power', which is not oriented towards the population in general but rather targets individuals 'at risk'. The metaphor of pastoral power is borrowed here from Michel Foucault (2001b), who uses it to designate a kind of power that is oriented both towards the whole flock of which the shepherd takes care and each individual sheep composing it. According to Nikolas Rose (2007), the fact that prenatal diagnoses target at risk individuals rather than entire populations largely dismisses accusations of eugenics and the somewhat exaggerated way in which some analysts insist on seeing the past in the present. Given that NSCF takes place after birth, any possible accusation of eugenics was removed, so upon what form of power was this type of intervention grounded? Upon what link between power centred on the individual and a policy aimed at the whole population did this rest? In short, what conception did its promoters have of screening as a mode of government?

The interviews carried out with members of the AFDPHE working group testify to the fact that actors differed depending on their practices (those who treated the ill/those who did not) and on how they evaluated newborn screening (in terms of purely medical benefits/broad consideration of the problems).

The words of the following paediatrician attest to the first position: 'When I talked to [X, who took the second position] about it, I'd say: "You don't know what it is to have people come in with kids age 4, 5 [that are not being monitored], it shouldn't be like that...". You start off with a statistics thing but very soon you're dealing with a family' (Paediatrician 5, 9.2.04). This respondent underlined his own clinical experience compared to those of others and highlighted the individual or the family within a population. In the same vein, those holding the second position were sometimes characterized by their abilities in terms of screening but not their clinical approach: 'Mr. [X, holder of the second position] is not really a clinician, he's above all an organizer, someone who's a real expert in terms of newborn screening' (Paediatrician 4, 17.8.04). It should be underlined that these were the same clinicians who, on a national level, did not express the doubts of the long-standing AFDPHE officials regarding screening. To come back to the question of epistemic frameworks, these clinicians were therefore both concerned with having scientific evidence of the benefits of screening and keen to ground their position in their clinical abilities. In this regard, to take up the terminology used by Stefan Timmermans and Alison Angell (2001), they were followers of 'evidence-based clinical judgments'. Nonetheless, it is important to underscore that these different conceptions were not only geared towards evidence or not. As we will see now, they determined the scope of population towards which the action was oriented. In this respect, they were just as political as they were scientific.

The second position is expressed here by one of these 'screeners', who was in fact also a paediatrician:

> The problem is that people only talk about medical evaluation, they forget all the rest. Evaluating is not just saying that the patient is doing fine or not doing fine or doing a bit better; it also means looking at the problems you might have created, the costs, everything there is around that action, informing parents, etc. … in the given population (Paediatrician-Geneticist 1, 5.2.04).

The same concern with taking into account the different aspects to screening was highlighted when, in 1991, the AFDPHE officials brought their experimental screening programme to an end. At the time, they underlined in a biomedical article that it was important not to 'ignore the serious drawbacks and the cost of useless examination of the false positives, nor the psychological and social risks, and even the consequences of treatment received too early such as repeated hospitalization … respiratory colonization by resistant germs, the toxic effects of antibiotics'. This understanding of the issue took into account not only the medical effects on the sick children, but also the other possible effects linked to children who were not ill. This is how we should understand the remark heard at the AFDPHE headquarters about the 'doctors' mindset' of those who 'were not really concerned with those who were normal' as opposed to the 'screening mindset' which led to insisting on the importance of sending letters to the parents of normal children.

While some professionals were on the brink of both positions (clinical and screening organization), for some, the kind of medicine defended relied on following patient 'cases' and, for others, on a policy technology centred on the population. Knowledge grounded in clinical experience produced power oriented towards patients, even if screening was carried out on the whole population. Knowledge based on screening produced power geared towards the population.

Overall, there were more partisans of the first approach who were clearly more in favour of screening than those of the second. In short, screening was decided upon by the paediatricians who specialized in CF, rather than by those of the AFDPHE. The former illustrate how a preventive policy applied to a population can sometimes, in reality, be based largely on a case oriented approach. This orientation should be linked to the history of medicine in France, more affected by power centred on individuals than by policy techniques exercised over populations, unlike English medicine for example. This way of viewing practice produced an effect of fragmentation, which was not specific to France or even to medicine. The working group was crossed by debates that were similar to those identified in the case of mammography in the United States, where the orientation of epidemiologists concerned with various problems (women's anxiety, cost, etc.) were in conflict with a clinical approach concerned with not letting any cases go undetected (Kaufert 2000). More generally, the 'screeners' defended a conception that appeared internationally in the 1990s, when post-war enthusiasm regarding screening gave way to a more general consideration of the problems to which screening can lead, particularly in psychological terms or regarding over-diagnosis (Armstrong 2012). So far, the main governors, their power relations and their ways of considering screening have been identified here. The techniques of government deployed now remain to be examined.

Screening as a Technique of Government

Beyond the scientific and medical debate, two decisive arguments seem to have contributed to a consensus emerging in France, whether it be among the group of professionals put together by the AFDPHE, the supervisory bodies (Cnamts, Ministry) or the associative board members.

First, as with the Breton programme, a strong concern with the moment of diagnosis was expressed on the national level. It was considered that CF was diagnosed too late in France, bearing in mind that before screening was set up, two thirds of children were diagnosed before the age of one. The professionals explained that patients diagnosed at the age of six or seven could have greatly deteriorated health, due to a lack of knowledge of the illness among unspecialized paediatricians and lack of adequate care provision. How should this argument be understood? First, one of the characteristics of the health policies that emerged in Western countries from the eighteenth century onwards was that they aimed to not only cure illness but also prevent it (Foucault, 2001b). One of the consequences of these changes was that the timeframe of disease altered: it was no longer a question of treating people after symptoms appeared but rather of anticipating disease; instead of waiting for the future, 'attempting to transform [it] by changing the health attitudes and health behaviours of the present' (Armstrong 1995: 402). However, it is probably necessary to take this even further and observe that it was a question not only of anticipating, but also of catching things as early as possible. It was as if a race against time began at birth regarding illness. This calls for two remarks. First, given the professionals' dominant role in the decision-making process and the fact that this temporal argument was theirs, the 'time' in question here was definitely that of the doctors. The patient families' 'time' and how they experienced it is another question that will be addressed later. Second, this new timeframe of contemporary medicine, which brought the future into the present by diagnosing illness from birth, enrols screening in a 'social' time. Defending this notion, Norbert Elias (1992: 8) advocates the idea that the measure of time is a practical concept and its evolution is linked to that of human societies: 'What the concept of time refers to is neither a conceptual "copy" of a flow existing objectively, nor a category of experience common to all people and existing in advance of all experience'. Today, even if other notions (certainty/risk, benefits/ disadvantages, etc.) come into play, speed and immediacy, or even anticipation, are the order of the day in medicine as elsewhere.

Where the second argument in favour of consensus is concerned, questions of space also appear in a striking manner. In general, since the emergence of hospital medicine, a new spatial organization of disease has been in place; it is no longer simply expressed by external symptoms but located in the depths of organs and tissue (Foucault 2003). And what NSCF brought about was precisely another redistribution of space, no longer concerning illness but patients themselves. Indeed, an idea emerged in relation to the data revealed previously about the differences in life expectancy between countries in Europe and the positive effect of the centralization of health care. This idea consisted in linking screening with follow-up care provided to patients by specialized centres following standardized protocols, rather than by doctors who only encounter a few cases of CF in their career or apply heterogeneous follow-up procedures. For half the people interviewed, a necessary condition for screening was that treatment then be provided by health care centres working with enough patients to be experts in this rare disease; without any guarantee that this would also happen, NSCF lost its interest. As one of the paediatricians who was part of the AFDPHE working group explained:

> We were agreed. If there was no obligation to set up a specialized centre to manage it – though at the beginning this wasn't as clear-cut as it became later – it [NSCF] wasn't worth doing. Because [otherwise] everyone would provide treatment on their own in their own way and there had to be some coherency (Paediatrician 5, 9.2.04).

Likewise, the Cnamts did not want to set up systematic screening if there was no guarantee that the children would receive good health care afterwards. The other half of people involved, a majority of the members of the AFDPHE working group, went even further in this direction, and even reversed the rationales. For them, screening was a *way* to achieve better health care: the heterogeneous nature of practices and the dispersion of facilities had to be addressed, and NSCF was a stage in the process of improving care provision. As we saw previously, this position was also defended in Brittany from the end of the 1990s onwards by the main paediatricians responsible for newborn screening. One paediatrician from the working group explained:

> I defended [this] screening by saying that a way to achieve better care for cystic fibrosis was to go through newborn screening ... . It will be very difficult to make it obligatory for health care to be provided by specialized centres and it seems to me that one of the ways to achieve this is through newborn screening (Paediatrician 2, 27.8.02).

One of the AFDPHE officials specified the importance of this argument: 'If we hadn't had that [this argument], I think we wouldn't have done it [screening] ... We took the opposite argument by saying: "We're badly organized, so we're screening to get better organized"' (5.2.04). As another member of the working group summarized, in the end screening was a powerful way of directing patients towards centres. In this sense, NSCF was just as much a tool to orient patients towards reorganized health care provision as it was an aim in itself (Vailly 2006, 2007).

More specifically, this tool had two sides; the first aimed at the patients, as we have seen, and the second at the doctors. This second side consisted in encouraging paediatricians to follow standardized treatment protocols, in other words to be 'disciplined'. However, this order sometimes met with resistance. One of the AFDPHE officials described the situation as follows in an interview:

> There was a certain discipline that we were able to impose, I apologize for the term, impose with consent, upon our colleagues regarding these questions of phenylketonuria diets. Whereas the people involved in cystic fibrosis ... , you could say that every time we signed a protocol, the ink wasn't even dry yet and they were already doing the exact opposite (Paediatrician-Geneticist 2, 22.2.05).

More than discipline, it was therefore a question of a mode of government, which was applied with the consent of the person involved and left room for resistance. This resistance to following protocol was sometimes explained by clinicians in interviews. One of them considered the health care protocol to be too rigid. He foregrounded his 'age' and 'experience, which mean that [he] no longer needed that', as well as 'the freedom' that he demanded for each patient, requiring an individualized treatment plan. Moreover, the specificity of French medical practice was often brought up to explain this resistance. One of the doctors claimed that many of his colleagues 'think that the patients belong to them, that having to fill out forms to send off to a central body is a slightly Soviet way of working and that it is necessary to respect everyone's freedom' (Paediatrician 4, 17.8.04). According to the respondents, this meant that it was not possible to organize health care in France as if they were in Scandinavian countries or in Canada, where the patients were directed in a very pro-active fashion towards a few large specialist centres (four health care centres in total throughout Sweden, two or three in Denmark, etc.). The professionals put three kinds of reasons forward, linked to the real or supposed behaviour of patients and/or doctors as well as the organization of health care in France. These reasons could be cultural (we live in a 'Latin' country not a 'disciplined Anglo-Saxon' one), psycho-social (patients are 'scared of centres and are in denial about the illness') and political/medical (there is no 'public health' momentum). Some of these arguments were taken up by officials at the Cnamts and the DGS. The only solution to direct patients towards specialized health care centres in France therefore seemed to be to set up screening. This offered a way of bypassing the paradox according to which countries where this kind of organization of health care prevailed did not actually screen. And yet there are diseases in France, like haemophilia or cancer, that are treated in centres without being subject to any generalized screening. A more trivial, but no less convincing, explanation for the fact that health care organization happened via newborn screening was more situation-based and is based on the idea that it was the AFDPHE and associated clinicians who promoted it.

In this way, the history of NSCF allows us to retrace the birth of a technique of government applied to the conduct of both 'self' (the medical ensemble enjoined to follow protocol) and above all 'others' (the patient families brought to send their children to the CRCM specialized centres). Compared to the traditional understanding of government (governing oneself and governing others), it should be noted that the first facet, government applied to oneself, relates here to a collective 'self'. Rather than calling into question individual behaviour, it was the medical ensemble to which the individual belonged that was targeted, hence the resistance that could arise. This resistance echoes research describing a tension between approaches that are grounded in scientifically based guidelines and approaches that emphasize the autonomy of clinicians on an individual and collective level (Timmermans and Angell 2001, Armstrong 2002). For David Armstrong (2002), this tension hides another one, between clinicians' autonomy as individuals and as a collective. According to him, scientifically based practice guarantees collective autonomy and the power of practitioners (as they are best placed to win over patients, institutions, etc.) and at the same time hampers the individual autonomy of the clinicians who find themselves having to follow protocols. As for the second facet of governing, applied to the conduct of others, screening for a genetic disease made the population more captive because it had the advantage of being applied to all newborns. Moreover, the fact that NSCF was in part a tool used to direct patients 'spatially' should not be surprising if we remember that historically medicine was the art of spatial distribution, through questions of hospital locations, the displacement of cemeteries, the separation of patients likely to contaminate each other, etc. But as Michel Foucault (1980: 69) underlines: 'Once knowledge can be analysed in terms of region, domain, implantation, displacement, transposition, one is able to capture the process by which knowledge functions as a form of power and disseminates the effects of power'. And this spatial reorganization of course had effects in terms of power.

Sociology and anthropology are aware that while it would be inaccurate to explain all behaviour by interests, in this case professional, much behaviour is equally impossible to explain without taking them into account. Moreover, the smaller scale of the regional context means that it is sometimes easier to understand the concrete power issues at stake at that level than in broader contexts. Let us therefore return to Brittany. Above and beyond the different actors' scientific and medical arguments, in the first chapter we saw how the non-institutional positions of the screening promoters contributed to its launch. Professional reasons and interests were both involved here. One of the Breton biologists who engaged actively in screening explained these in an interview. They were more complex than simply power issues because his explanation combined different dimensions to the desire to launch NSCF: professional ambition, with 'the concern that the laboratory should continue to work, take on a certain calibre' and have a 'serious reputation'; responsibility, with the professional's role being to 'make things work' because 'there are jobs being offered'; professional concern, with 'a certain anxiety about a decrease in work' and 'becoming a rump laboratory'; and finally, the marginalization of their work, because the laboratory did not have 'a very official position', was not invited to meetings alongside the other laboratories, etc. More generally, the biologists did not want to give up any of their field of work and the reader will remember that the directors of the screening centre in Rennes protested vigorously against what they saw as screening being monopolized. The director took the view that while the molecular biology tests could be handed over to the Brest laboratory, which enjoyed national and international recognition, it was simply out of the question to let screening for a disease as important as CF be carried out solely in Brest. It was a question of prerogatives. A number of arguments were called upon: institutional legitimacy, because the official screening laboratory was in Rennes; financial reasoning, with the streamlining of budgets and the fact of avoiding multiple laboratories; and sometimes, the employment of personnel. No agreement was reached and so for many years screening for CF in Brittany took place in two different places instead of one, unlike all other newborn screening.

These effects of power not only concerned the laboratories but also the health care centres. It is important to remember that the position of the health care centre in Roscoff, in particular, was fragile due to its geographical isolation and institutional situation. As its director explained: 'We're in an isolated place. If we don't think about what we're going to do in the coming years, we're dead. The CHU [large teaching hospitals] have a captive market, we don't...'. It was a question of developing projects so that the establishment would evolve, as it was only by evolving that it would survive. From the very beginning of Breton screening, children were directed to the main centres, and the centralizing effect of treatment and care soon made itself felt. This led to friction between the clinicians of the centres. A Breton paediatrician explained in an interview:

[X] said to me 'But why is this patient with you? Why isn't he with me?'. ... My consultant, at that time, had banged her fist on the table a bit saying ... 'If you want us to do screening, the children are going to have to come to [Y], otherwise we won't do it' (2002).

Likewise, during a meeting between Breton paediatricians, one of them, addressing his colleagues, indicated that 'all the screened children had got away from them' and that the centre [X] 'sucked up patients'. In an interview, another paediatrician was even more terse: 'Screening was a way of taking all the winnings. And taking all the winnings meant taking patients' (2002). That said, another dimension must be taken into consideration and it is important not to forget what a substantial task it was to treat patients suffering from CF, demanding considerable effort from medical professionals – it was therefore hard for them to simply turn the page just like that. One remark made by a paediatrician shows this commitment to the disease as he said in an aside to his neighbour during a meeting of Breton paediatricians: 'It's true that we put our heart and soul into it [the care of patients suffering from cystic fibrosis]' (Paediatrician 7, Observation 6.2.03). The findings of my field study presented at the end of this book are in line with this.

Certain regional directors of patient organizations judged these power games and competitions severely. One of them implored the doctors 'instead of looking out for their own interests' to 'look out for those of the patients', the only ones that mattered, 'by trusting doctors with more expertise or who are given more means'. He took a stand 'against the petty school wars, at the patients' detriment'. His words were harsh and testified to the resentment of someone who had seen too many patients suffering in conditions that, in his view, could be improved. With hindsight, a public health doctor who rubbed shoulders with paediatricians in the region during these years, analyzed the professional 'niche' that CF began to represent in the academic sphere and the conflicts that this newly formed niche could create in the context of the development of paediatrics. According to this doctor, each paediatrician 'was looked for a niche in which to practise, in which to obtain recognition in the field of paediatrics, on both a local and national level'. These paediatricians were looking for a space in which they could achieve this recognition, either from their peers or more generally in the social space.

Similar stakes could also arise on a national level. A paediatrician remembering a national meeting in which he presented the screening strategy coupled with the reorganization of treatment to his colleagues from small and large health care centres, spoke in interview, albeit elliptically, about the worried reactions of certain colleagues: 'With the criticisms that you can imagine: "The small centres, there you go, the big centres, this policy, bla bla bla, the big ones are going to eat the small ones"' (Paediatrician 6, 30.6.04). Likewise, during a meeting in one of the various services in which I carried out my study, I heard a paediatrician protesting to a colleague about the fact that a patient was receiving follow-up care in another service, concluding: 'We all need patients'. By this, we should understand that a hospital service must be fuelled with patients in order to meet the requirements of 'clinical knowledge', and even more so where low incidence diseases are concerned, hence certain power stakes at work.

However, power is not only manifest in its stakes, it is also revealed through its effects. The DHOS Circular mentioned previously stipulated that in the five years following the implementation of screening, the centres treating less than 50 children suffering from CF could no longer be considered as CRCM. At the end of the selection process for health care centres' applications, a decree was published in 2002 creating 47 CRCM around which treatment networks were to be structured. In Brittany, the Rennes and Roscoff centres were notably designated as CRCM. And on a national scale, the Ministry supported the creation of these 47 CRCM by allocating two budgets, of 4.6 million Euros each, and by ensuring the creation of permanent posts (nurse coordinators, physiotherapists, etc.). This shows to what extent CF enjoyed substantial attention and funding from the public authorities, which contrasted with the relatively restricted population affected. As a paediatrician involved in NSCF summarized with lucidity in an interview: 'Here is a disease that has enjoyed 90 millions francs for 200 cases per year'. Above and beyond these contingent explanations and the interplay between actors, this paradox can only be understood if it is put back into the context developed in the first chapter and general introduction. The form of genetic knowledge spreading in society and the scientific research that it called upon generated great media interest and was also foregrounded by the patient organizations, thus giving a real 'boost' to genetic diseases. And these elements also encouraged the selection of one of these diseases among all the possible public health causes, and we have seen how this happened. According to certain paediatricians, this gave ideas to others: 'Cystic fibrosis was given as an example: "You see what they've managed to obtain, we have to get the same for others"' (30.6.04) remarked one of them. Moreover, from 2002 onwards, the CRCM officials organized themselves into a 'Federation of CRCM' and then into the French Cystic Fibrosis Society, as an administrative structure and learned society, guaranteeing a certain scientific and medical legitimacy. As one of its officials wrote in a paediatrics journal: 'The federation ... is also a learned society ... which reinforces its legitimacy in its administrative and political vocation.'

This range of results shows that screening meant working towards the health and well-being of patients through the use of a biomedical technique, with a number of resulting consequences: care provision was structured and treatment centralized, but also means were provided and legitimacy ensured. It would be caricatural to reduce this health policy to power *strategies* on the part of professionals and this is not my intention here. There was no deliberate and preconceived strategy as such, but rather a technique for managing professionals and for directing patients that developed during the process itself. While it may have played a role, a purely utilitarian theory based solely on interests could lead us to neglect the other dimensions mentioned previously. However, this policy did have power *stakes* and *effects* namely in the rise in the cohort of patients treated in the centres, ensuring the durability and credibility of the latter, in the means provided to them and in the general visibility of the disease. An analysis of the repercussions remains to be carried out, to examine the extent to which CF served as an example, particularly within the National plan for rare diseases, adopted in 2004 in France.[1] From the point of view of the sociology of professions, the following hypothesis has been expressed (Frattini and Naiditch 2004: 69): 'Implementing screening led to national decisions ... that reinforce cystic fibrosis as a sub-specialization, understood as the institutional recognition of health services that are identified, structured and funded in a specific manner'. More generally, this is part of the substantial trend of changes in biomedicine grounded in the centralization of care (Clarke et al. 2010). Studying local policies combating AIDS, Olivier Borraz and Patricia Loncle-Moriceau (2000) notably developed the idea that rather than constituting a public health approach in the traditional sense (approaching health issues collectively and taking into account questions of prevention), these policies led to the health care model being rebuilt in a way that consolidated hierarchical structures. For both the policies fighting against AIDS and those related to NSCF, hospital facilities emerged strengthened from the process. The results presented here show that above and beyond the professional rationales at work, there was an art of leading professionals' and patients' conduct. At the same time, as we shall see, this art entailed the assent of all those involved, including the parents in maternity units.

Consenting Subjects

French bioethics laws were an integral part of a movement transferring legitimacy so that each individual could take charge of their own health and feel 'responsible' for it. And as we have seen, these laws made provision for the strict regulation of DNA tests, which required written consent from the individual being tested or, in the case of children, from their parents.[2] This precaution not only allowed all individuals to play a supposedly active role in their own health but also aimed to prevent potential abuses linked to the excessive and badly controlled use of genetics. It should be noted that this was not applicable to the study of all genetic diseases, particularly not to those that just entailed protein analysis, but only to those that involved direct DNA analysis. This detail should be linked to the representations surrounding DNA, often seen as holding all power, all danger and all virtue. It should be specified that, in reality, NSCF takes place in two stages

---

1   Rare diseases were retained as one of the five priorities of the August 9, 2004 law relative to public health policy. This plan made provision for Centres of reference given a seal of approval and bringing together a set of multidisciplinary hospital expertise organized around highly specialized teams.

2   Law n°94-654 of 29.7.94, decree n°2000-570 of 23.6.00 and law n°2004-800 of 6.8.04.

and the DNA test is not carried out on all newborns, but only those with an initial positive IRT assay. However, the screening organizers chose to collect the consent of all parents and we shall see why later. When their written consent is requested, the parents are constituted as legal subjects with a certain amount of leeway at their disposal. Within such a delicate combination between individualizing procedures (the consent of each individual) and globalizing techniques (the screening of populations), what exactly happens at this point of intersection? How do the legal subjects created in this way find their place within a procedure that is inherently objectivizing, given the size of the populations involved? What local procedures are used to pass down this government to the maternity units?

In June 2000, a decree framing tests of genetic characteristics for medical purposes stipulated: 'The [written] consent ... of the person who is prescribed a test ... must be free and informed by prior information including, in particular, indications about the range of the test'.[3] Following the publication of this decree, the AFDPHE ethics committee organized reflection about its consequences in the case of CF. The committee first asked whether the consent of all parents in maternity units should be collected, or only those whose children were concerned by the genetic test. The difference in scale was substantial, going from 800,000 consents per year in the first case to 4,000 in the second. The committee came down in favour of the first option because it avoided calling back parents in the case of an initial suspicious assay and thereby generating lots of often unwarranted anxiety (of the 4,000 tests, only 180 confirm CF). And as we have seen, the AFDPHE's action was directed towards taking into account a variety of aspects, including families' concerns. Another argument was based on the idea that collecting written consent from all parents could lead to them being provided with better quality information. The commission set up by the AFDPHE in charge of informing parents and professionals began reflection on this subject, which led to a set of recommendations being produced about this information. This commission was coordinated by the Cnamts official who was following the question of newborn screening and who was a member of the AFDPHE bureau. The reasons that had led her to become involved with this issue were linked to the fact that she regretted the lack of information given to her about screening when she gave birth to her children, aside from the fact that the test was not painful and was generally negative. This sensitivity to the information provided was heightened by the use of genetic technology. In an interview, this official implicitly expressed certain reservations about the excessive use of genetic tests on the basis of the dynamics created by the existence of the tool, or even a potentially fantasized view of the tests ('it is not because we know a new screening technique and we want to use it', 'you don't put the child through the mill'). In this spirit, the Cnamts gave its financial support to the creation and dissemination of information leaflets aimed at professionals in maternity units, on the one hand, and parents, on the other. However, the way the

---

3 Decree n°2000-570 of 23.6.00.

information was presented was not neutral, as it determined in part whether consent was given or refused. So how was this information provided in maternity units?

In order to answer this question, we studied[4] the information provided to parents of newborns as well as the way in which written consent was collected in two hospital maternity units in the Parisian region (Vailly and Ensellem 2010). These units looked after 1,800 (Maternity 1) and 2,400 (Maternity 2) births per year. They therefore had a high average, given that in France these figures can range from a few hundred to more than 4,000 births per year. The first unit had a neonatal service and the second had both a neonatal service and a neonatal intensive care unit. As the results of this study differed very little between the two maternity units, they will be presented together here, unless otherwise specified.

An information leaflet published by the AFDPHE and entitled '3 days: the age for screening' was given to parents the day after birth – the day called 'D1' by the health professionals – while written consent was collected and the baby's blood sample taken on 'D3' (or 'D4'). When parents left on D2, they were asked to return for the test and telephoned, and called back if necessary, if they did not come. The two-day interval between D1 and D3 was intended to fulfil the technical conditions for the assay (taking the blood three days after birth) and to give the mothers or parents the time to read the leaflet. For the rest, distinctions should be made between the two units. In Maternity 1, a paediatric nurse simply gave the leaflet saying something like 'Here is the leaflet for the Guthrie test, which we do at 3 days. Right, so you can read that'. Sometimes, if the mother did not understand, she would add: 'It's screening for certain diseases'. In Maternity 2, the leaflet was given out by a paediatrician, who mentioned legislative constraints, using words such as:

> Here's a little leaflet about screening for all the diseases you see on here, it's compulsory. But since last year, we've also had screening for cystic fibrosis. In the unfortunate event we find something, we do a genetic test and in France we can't carry out a genetic test on a person without their consent. So here's a card to fill in for that, for you to sign (Paediatrician 8, Observation 16.5.06).

Half of the time, he added a comment about the importance of screening and/or the serious nature of the diseases: 'It's important, it's to avoid diseases' or 'These are very rare, but very serious diseases'. The card, which would collect the blood sample and the mother or parents signature, was given on D1 with the leaflet, whereas in Maternity 1 it was given on D3 when the blood sample was taken. It should be noted that the recommendations given to professionals in maternity units, specified in a brochure for their attention, were to 'give the parents clear, accurate, precise and above all comprehensible information. Do not alarm them without cause (the diseases we are screening for are rare)' (AFPDHE 2001a: 6). In the same vein, the head of the service in Maternity 1, where the verbal

---

4   This part of the study was carried out in collaboration with Cécile Ensellem.

information was more succinct, explained in an interview that the parents are 'less anxious' when the information provided is minimal and the test less medicalized. We can therefore appreciate the difficulty of the exercise: there is a fine line between delivering relatively complex information for consent that is supposed to be 'informed' and the risk of worrying, or even terrifying, parents unnecessarily, given how rare the illness is. When people are 'at risk', it makes more sense to give them the different sides to a problem than when the risk of disease is low (here 1 in 4,400).

For Thomas Lemke (2004), as we have seen, it is the notion of genetic 'risk' and the uncertainty that it carries with it that leads people to be confronted with choices and calls upon their autonomy and responsibility. Here we need to go further, by underlining that the low risk just mentioned contributes to the succinct nature of the information provided and therefore to the limitations of the process of subjectivation. More generally, in the case of other practices, such as prenatal screening (before birth) in Great Britain, this tension between delivering information and avoiding the generation of anxiety may be the source of moral dilemmas for health professionals (Williams et al. 2005). Difficulties thus arise in adapting the procedures for obtaining consent to entire populations, leading to a sort of injunction that is contradictory within consent procedures (informing without worrying). Moreover, a further element reinforces this effect. Nancy Press and Carole Browner (1997) show how blood tests to detect developmental problems during pregnancy have become routinely accepted in the United States among other health care practices. Likewise, the newborn screening in question here is part of an economy of health care, and in a way that heightens this routine acceptance because there is no individual consultation, unlike for the prenatal test. A complex equation is formed between issues of consent, psychological well-being of parents, routinization of processes and lack of individual consultations.

The other aspect of this information concerns the material medium through which consent is given. For Marie-Andrée Jacob (2007), following Donald Brenneis (2006), the documents given to people often remain 'analytically invisible' in studies on consent, despite being just as informative as the ideas or representations that these people carry. The brief nature of the paediatric nurse and paediatricians' words shows that the essential points were in the leaflet distributed, which should encourage us to take this question all the more seriously. With its glossy paper, colour printing, photos of babies and typography, the leaflet first and foremost meets aesthetic criteria. Moreover, it is easy to read thanks to its presentation in the form of questions and answers, its typographical variations and its relatively simple style. As for the substance of the text, it gives a brief history of the different screening programmes mentioning their very positive impact. This is followed by information about the benefits of screening and practical aspects about how the tests are carried out and how the results are given. Then information is provided about the diseases being screened for. Regarding CF, this information specifies: 'With early and rigorous care, the frequency of clinical manifestations can be substantially reduced. This enables the patient to have a better quality of life, even though there is no specific treatment which can cure the disease' (AFDPHE 2001b). As for the card collecting the signatures, seemingly commonplace, it is situated more on a legal and technical plane than on an aesthetic one. It includes the following sentence: 'Having received the information, we the undersigned (surnames, forenames) …., mother, father of the child …. born on …. authorize ☐ do not authorize ☐ the physicians responsible for newborn screening to conduct, if necessary, a genetic test to screen for cystic fibrosis. Date …. Signatures ….'. This authorization is therefore limited to CF and allows protection from any unethical and unregulated use of other potential genetic tests.

Overall, the written information can be described as clear, well-presented and persuasive: who would not want their child to receive the best possible care if, unfortunately, they turned out to be ill? Through its aesthetics and its readable nature, the leaflet conforms to the common practice of 'ethical bureaucracy', which shows a concern with the form taken by consent documents (Jacob and Riles, 2007). This is how the leaflet achieves not only its respectability as the medium for moral values but also its efficacy. More specifically, this efficacy meets the aim of informing parents about the different newborn screening in question and obtaining the maximum number of signatures, more than it provides a genuine medium for 'informed consent' about NSCF. Regarding the characteristics of screening, while the possibility of a further test is mentioned, no figures or graphs are presented to show or represent the rate of people called back or of people diagnosed as ill/ not ill in a general population. Regarding its effects, the notions of benefits and risks, which remain complex, are not mentioned, despite having been at the heart of the national and international debates about whether NSCF was a good idea or not (Wilfond et al. 2005). In relation to this aspect, Angela Raffle (2001) makes a distinction between the differences in the aim of information provided for medical consent – either obtaining maximum levels of consent or ensuring informed choices by mentioning the limitations of screening – and between the drawbacks of each option. In particular, the second option can lead to screening, and in some cases access to health care, being set aside. This shows how complex it is to present medical uncertainty in an understandable manner, particularly when it has to be presented to everyone. The most balanced solution would probably consist in explaining the advantages of screening, without confining the explanation to that and without avoiding any mention of its limitations.

After the information stage, let us now consider how consent is obtained. In Maternity 1, the blood sample was taken by a paediatric nurse in a small office from a vein in the newborn's hand using a small syringe linked to a tube (rarely by pricking the baby's heel). In Maternity 2, the samples were taken by a nurse in a room only used for treatment. As the card was given on the first day (D1), it was often already signed when blood was taken.

There is not enough space here to present examples of observations but, to summarize, the exchanges were very laconic and in the vast majority of cases the signature was obtained without any difficulty or discussion. The information in the leaflet no doubt explains this in part, just as it contributes to the record level of consent for NSCF obtained nationally, which reaches no less than 99.7% (AFDPHE 2004). Of course, everything is set up to obtain as many signatures as possible. What also appears here is the vast consent of mothers who sometimes even expressed disbelief or irritation regarding those who refuse consent. In addition to this, it should be specified that in interviews or during informal conversations certain paediatricians highlighted the difficulties posed by the language barrier with foreign mothers. During our observations, this situation concerned three cases (7% of all the mothers), in which the mothers did not speak French. In two cases, the forms were signed by the mothers, who did not understand them, and in one case, they were signed by the partner, who understood that it was a question of screening for diseases. These mothers or parents are borderline cases and it is well known in the social sciences that such cases can often prove of heuristic value. On the one hand, these parents cannot be left out of a routine procedure applied to a whole population; on the other, their signature is clearly purely a formality and while they are constituted as legal subjects, this notion is void of meaning in this situation. It should also be noted that in Maternity 1, the father was usually not present the morning of D3 and only the mother signed. It was therefore the mother who played the role of legal subject, more than 'the parents' or 'the family' usually mentioned in legal texts or information leaflets. However, in Maternity 2, the card was given on the first day when the father was present and often the cards were signed by both parents. We can therefore see that subjectivation is constituted just as much through apparently trivial details as through general principles. Finally, the verbal information provided about the results insinuates that if the parents are contacted after the test, it means the baby has 'something'. Unlike the leaflet, this information does not specify that, at the screening stage, checks can be necessary or tests redone without the diagnosis being confirmed afterwards. Where the parents called back are concerned, at least, this can actually generate the anxiety that it seeks to minimize. Overall, with its both formal and trivial nature, the consent process is a formality in both senses of the word: on the one hand, a process prescribed by law and, on the other, an unimportant act that must be accomplished. It can even be said to be part of a well-oiled mechanical routine that is more self-evident than anything, a fact to which the high rates of consent can testify. But on what grounds is it felt to be self-evident? Let us now examine the rationales at work.

The interviews conducted with the mothers of newborn babies afford a more precise understanding of the conditions and reasons for their consent. These interviews focused first on the information that they retained about screening, second on the reasons why, in their opinion, they were asked for their signature and, finally, on their motives for consenting. We should remember that in 7% of cases this interview was not possible because the mothers, of African origin, did not speak French. These situations aside, 60% of the mothers interviewed said that they had read the leaflet or 'read [it] quickly' (53% of all the mothers, if we subtract those who could not read it). Forty per cent of the mothers interviewed therefore said they had not read the leaflet (47% of all the mothers). Half explained this by the fact they were tired or weak, sometimes following caesarean sections or complications during birth, while others replied that they had not had time to read it. Nonetheless, in reality we cannot discount the hypothesis that some may have had difficulty reading it or were not used to reading. Others said that they knew about screening because they had other children (often without knowing that NSCF had been set up since) and, finally, a few explained they had not received the leaflet.

Regarding the reasons behind the request for consent, two thirds of the mothers thought that the request concerned all the diseases being screened for or, conversely, that CF was the only disease being screened for (incorrect answers) while one third had understood that the request applied to CF, among other diseases being screened for (correct answer). Moreover, although the consent form did stipulate this, as we have seen, only half the mothers had understood that they had signed permission for a potential genetic test, while the other half were not aware of this. The following interview excerpt illustrates the latter situation, observed in the same way in both maternity units:

> *Did you read the information card, or did you just sign? (Interviewer).*
> I read that I was giving permission for them to take a blood sample from my child. ... (Mother 1).
> *So was the signature for any kind of blood test? (Interviewer).*
> For those diseases (Mother 1).
> *Does the term 'genetic test' mean anything to you? (Interviewer).*
> Is it for Down's Syndrome? (Mother 1).
> *No (Interviewer).*
> I don't know then (Mother 1, Operations manager, 29.6.05).

It should be specified that, conversely, some mothers had taken in all the information, although this was more rare. Regarding the conditions for accepting, written consent can involve a variety of situations, which include the possibility that the request has not been read or has been badly understood, and this concerned a substantial portion of people here (at least half). It is true that the particular moment at which consent was collected, just after birth, was not necessarily the most beneficial for the most tired mothers. Neglecting this situational dimension, like with people involved in clinical trials who have just been affected by a heart problem (Corrigan 2003), runs the risk of restricting the subjects' ability to constitute themselves as such. However, the problem raised is more general. Several studies show that a relatively substantial proportion of people concerned do not read consent forms, in situations as varied as gynaecological surgery in the UK, epidemiological genetic research in France or organ donation in the United States and in Israel (Akkad et al. 2004, Ducourneau 2007, Jacob 2007). In the case that interests us here, the reasons for consent can allow us to grasp at least in part the rationales underpinning this fact. These reasons seem to be the same for all mothers. They rely upon the idea that it is better to diagnose as early as possible to be able to receive care for a possible disease: unanimously, it is considered better to 'know' and be able to start treatment as early as possible, if necessary. For example, these mothers said in interviews:

> It's reassuring for parents to know their child probably doesn't have this disease. And that if there is something, ... it will be caught as soon as possible (Mother 2).
> *Why is early screening good? (Interviewer).*
> Maybe to get treatment more quickly. It's a disease that can't be cured, but to get it treated as quickly as possible. To have a better quality of life afterwards (Mother 2, Radiology technician, 2.6.05).

The reasons behind this consent confirm a general assent regarding screening, based on two elements. On the one hand, it relies on a transfer of information from the leaflet, where a certain implicit trust in national screening policies is expressed, as this interview illustrates, taking up some of its ideas and expressions ('it can't be treated', 'a better quality of life after'). On the other, it is based on values and presuppositions. As Mary Dixon-Woods and colleagues (2007) explain, people who give their consent do not just passively receive the information they are provided with, which they are capable of understanding or not; rather, they also come armed with their own experiences, values and presuppositions. In our case, the number who did not read the leaflet or receive verbal information and yet still gave consent allows us to measure how important these elements are, some of which coincide with the rationales or discourse of biomedical actors. First, from a structural point of view, as this screening is caught up in a rationale of care provision, it should be situated within the context described in the introduction of the increasing sensitivity to health issues in Western countries. Second, screening is based on the idea of acting early, with the temporal inversion between diagnosis and appearance of symptoms that this implies. This idea is grounded in the medical obsession with early diagnosis. Going beyond medical reasoning, it has the weight of common sense behind it, as described regarding Breton screening (early diagnosis to avoid the situation worsening). Third, this theory of common sense also includes implicit statements, grounded in the idea that there are no disadvantages to screening. However, although the North American consensus conference in 2004 did end up recommending NSCF, we have seen the risks of cross infection between babies screened and older patients in *certain* health care centres in the United States, sometimes with higher infection rates in children diagnosed through screening than in those diagnosed on symptoms. We can therefore see how the notion of informed consent raises other issues than simply a rational choice made by subjects, where values and presuppositions interweave.

Moreover, the value of this generalized assent is tempered by the conditions of the information provided and the inherent limitations of the situation (tired, busy mothers, etc.). Even though the particular care taken regarding the written information should be underlined, here we nonetheless see individualizing procedures come up against the practical difficulties raised by globalizing policies.

Legislators enthusiastically institutionalize good practice, but without considering the problematic issue of mass screening. They establish what Marie-Andrée Jacob and Annelise Riles (2007) call a 'bureaucracy of virtue'. Thus, the effects of the injunction to ensure subjectivation, expressed by the legislator to the organizers of screening, are adapted to concrete practices. However, in order to be complete, this study would need to be extended to examine how screening organizers and health professionals, particularly in maternity units, explain and justify these (fear of generating anxiety and complexity of the equation to be balanced, as we have seen, but also organizational constraints, lack of time, large amount of other information to give, etc.). In any event, it does not seem very reasonable, if only in terms of cost, to mobilize a whole medical arsenal to obtain consent for a test that, given the incidence of the disease, identifies 180 cases per year. In conclusion, the mothers in maternity units constitute subjects who may be convinced but remain limited, acting under the influence of an idea seen as self-evident, in marked contrast with the debates that have taken place, and continue to do so, within the international biomedical arena. It is as if the more screening becomes part of a health care routine at the level of a population, the less women's subjectivity is called upon.

Questioning what Ian Hacking (2005) calls a philosophical 'knot' (here the imposition of constraint versus freedom of action), this political configuration adapted to a population presents several characteristics. From a theoretical point of view, within a newborn screening policy that seems, at first glance, to meet with much consensus – it relates, after all, to taking care of sick children – it is important to be clear about how conceptions of the individual and the collective, of power relations, of types of domination and of spaces of freedom can be interrelated (Vailly 2006). The history of how screening was set up shows that patient families or their representatives, doctors from the patient organization and doctors from the professional association established reciprocal relationships of influence. These influences were reinforced by the effect of dual professional affiliations, which created a relatively limited network of experts. However, these influences and this network should not lead to the image of an a-hierarchical social micro-world where everyone was placed at the same level (patient families and professionals). This would run the risk of flattening out the depth of power relations as part of an analytics of government that is only looking for relationships between free subjects. And it should be underlined that while the originality of this framework is to go beyond the opposition between domination and freedom, it does not deny either. Moreover, on the one hand, screening revealed itself to be largely a means through which to direct patients towards health care centres, as we have seen, and on the other, the maximum percentage of consent obtained and the real assent observed in interviews is part of a form of power that runs through the social body on a productive mode. The test is not imposed as such; rather, it is a question of a productive network of power, in the Foucauldian sense, based on the approval of those that it concerns on a local level. In this sense, the process is one of acting upon others who act themselves, in a more or less active or detached fashion. And their positive response is based on an accepted norm according to which it can only be beneficial to receive the earliest possible diagnosis and care, and there are no disadvantages to this.

On a more concrete level, this analytics allows us to examine how different types of subjects are formed within this hierarchical depth. Overall, this history of NSCF shows the decisive role played by professionals, constituting them as deciding and acting subjects in their own right, whereas the patient organization was involved in a more peripheral and non-deciding manner, albeit a real one given its action as a pressure group. Here, though, it is necessary to be precise about what is meant by 'patient organization'. The detailed study of the people actually involved showed that the organization's medical advisors played a role that was at least as important as that of the non-professionals when it came to deciding about screening. Moreover, the mothers in maternity units in general are given a specific form of power: providing their signature or not. In terms of newborn screening, therefore, the professional association to which power was delegated, the pressure group and the mothers in the maternity units all had a certain specific form of more or less extensive power. They come together to form 'full subjects' (the professionals of the professional association and the Medical Board), 'subjects under influence' (the patient organization in itself) and 'limited subjects' (the mothers in maternity units). In the present case, the real subjects are the professionals. The analytics of government also allows the distinctions between those who govern and those who are governed to be put back within their own dynamics. Certain groups may have the upper hand at certain times, and lose it later on, such as the professional association, which did not play a decisive role in terms of the centralization and organization of care provision as this was neither its vocation nor its mission.

Table 3.1   Typology of the doctors and biologists involved in governing NSCF in France

	'Mavericks'	'Clinicians'	'Screeners'
Scientific stakes	Conviction	Evidence (levels of)	Evidence (levels of)
Moral stakes (relationship between prenatal and neonatal)	Linked	Separated due to principle of efficiency	Separated due to ethical principle
Political stakes	Individual, illness	Individual, illness	Population, different problems
Stance regarding NSCF	Enthusiastic	Favourable	Sceptical

Finally, as we come to the end of these first three chapters, it is possible to draw up a typology of the doctors and biologists involved in governing NSCF in France. Three profiles come to light (the 'mavericks', the 'clinicians' and the 'screeners') adopting three stances regarding screening on the basis of scientific, political and moral stakes (cf. Table 3.1).

In Brittany, the *mavericks* were enthusiastic. They were carried forward by their conviction regarding the benefits of screening and centred their contribution on the sick individual; for them, newborn screening and prenatal testing combined without any problem. On a national level, the *clinicians* came down in favour of screening at the very end of the 1990s, on the basis of different levels of proof of efficiency; they distinguished newborn screening from prenatal testing according to a principle of efficiency; and they also centred their contribution around the sick individual, whereas the *screeners* took into account the general population and different problems. The latter were the most sceptical; they also based their reasoning on different levels of evidence, but distinguished between newborn screening and prenatal testing according to a moral principle. And moral questions arise in the interstitial spaces created between the truth about what we – or others – are and the way in which we – or others – 'are responsible' and conduct ourselves – or themselves.

Chapter 4
Extending Abnormality

Various studies in the social sciences have shown an expansion of abnormality, or rather of the commonly held idea of medical abnormality in wealthy countries. Examples illustrating this abound: the definition of autism has widened leading to a rise in actual and related cases, 'normal' cholesterol levels are increasingly exacting, and childhood lead poisoning has gone from being rare to having the status of an epidemic in France, due to a decrease in the level of lead considered acceptable in the blood stream (Vailly 2008). Without seeking to provide an exhaustive account, it is possible to identify several of the *modi operandi* through which this expansion occurs. One of these is population screening, which now includes more people presenting a wider range of physical characteristics to the medical gaze (Armstrong 1995). Another is the evolution of the mental health field: Robert Castel (1991) has shown the expansion of medical practices in this area, from psychiatry to psychology, including psychoanalysis and behavioural therapies. The increasing precision of biomedical techniques constitutes yet another mechanism through which this trend operates. Among many other examples, pregnancy ultrasounds can be cited, where the detection of small anatomical abnormalities associated with an increased risk of chromosomal anomaly can lead to dilemmas for both parents and professionals regarding how to proceed, as well as to the loss of foetuses due to further, more intrusive, tests (Getz and Kirkengen 2003). Economic pressures can also play an important role when abnormality becomes a source of profit for pharmaceutical companies or a criterion for exclusion from various forms of social protection. In Belgium, in particular, Ine Van Hoyeghen and colleagues (2006) have shown how in the case of bank insurance, normality is not defined by the absence of illness but by the absence of risk, and a substantial number of people do not fall within the category of normality due to financial and banking reasons. It should, however, be noted that this expansion is partly countered by profound social and economic inequalities which can, on the contrary, lead to the people in question having a restricted conception of medical abnormality. This is the case, for example, concerning the absence of early detection of tumours in immigrant women in Australia (Markovic, Manderson and Quinn 2004). Because these women normalize abnormal signs or because their experience of bodily abnormality is not in line with medical explanations, diagnosis of gynaecological cancers is delayed or impaired for them. Furthermore, the study of social inequalities in access to Down's syndrome screening in France has revealed that there is a higher level of prenatal diagnosis in women of higher socio-economic status, which means that foetuses considered to be abnormal by these woman could be considered normal for women more distanced from the medical field (Khoshnood et al. 2006). Despite these important qualifications, generally speaking Western biomedicine appears to have more and more means at its disposal to produce medical abnormality. In this context, one of the issues at stake for the social sciences is to try to understand how this expansion is linked to societal values. In this respect, bringing down levels of detection and tolerance for illnesses is part of a larger movement rejecting bodily impairment, which is increasingly considered to be intolerable (Fassin and Bourdelais 2005). The example of newborn screening can afford us an understanding of one of the ways in which this takes place.

Let us first look at the relationship between abnormality and the norm in medicine. The notion of normality in medicine, as commonly understood, goes back to the 1820s when physiologist François Broussais put forward a new organic theory of disease according to which the latter was due to an increase or a decrease in physiological levels (Canguilhem 1978). This idea met with huge success, particularly under the influence of Auguste Comte, who went so far as to shape it into a vast political design. In Comte's view, a state of normality throughout all society was evidence of progress and should be everyone's goal. Clearly, from a very early stage, normal and abnormal phenomena suggested not only purely factual circumstances but also an attachment to a value (harmony, in Comte's case). Generally speaking, this attachment occurs through a shift from what is normal to what is the norm. In the same vein, Ian Hacking (2005: 3) recalls that the idea of normality creates a bridge between description and evaluation: 'It is an idea we ostensibly use for objective descriptions, based on facts ... It is also an idea that we use when making value judgments, instituting rules or establishing principles'. The distinction between normal and abnormal is therefore not neutral, for not only is it part of a social and moral space, it also informs us about this space. Also within the medical field, anthropologist Margaret Lock (2000) shows that far from being merely a product of biology, normality and abnormality are culturally constructed and associated with a social, political and moral order. In the case of ways of giving birth, for example, when Inuit women are enjoined to give birth according to the customs of Western medicine, the bodies of women from the United States and Europe notably are being taken as the standard for normality, which is definitely linked to political and social presuppositions. Beyond medicine, although the question is too vast to be dealt with here, sociologists and anthropologists are led to study how norms are interiorized, in relation to an obligation that sometimes takes on a moral nature. Traditionally, it is a question of thinking about the link between normality and deviance (Becker 1966, Goffman 1963). Moreover, looking simply at abnormality in the field of genetics, certain features are worth underscoring.

In the 1960s, in step with the changes in medicine, Georges Canguilhem added to his thesis by beginning to take into account what was, at the time, the very recent study of genetic mutations and relating this to the concept of error. He summed this up as follows: 'To be sick is to have been made false ... in the sense of a "false fold" [i.e. a wrinkle: *faux pli*] or a false rhyme' (Canguilhem

1978: 172). For Marc Chopplet (2001), this association with error is linked to the discovery of an increase in the rate of mutations induced by radiation: mutation became synonymous with disruption and corruption. And yet it is not a purely negative notion because it is at the root of the evolution of species: mutation allows species to adapt to changes in the environment and thus allows life to continue. It is therefore the sign of abnormality at the level of a population (when it is at the origin of a disease) but this abnormality is also in the order of things, where the temporality of species is concerned (when it drives evolution). This is part of what Giorgio Agamben (1998: 18) calls the exception: 'The exception does not subtract itself from the rule; rather, the rule, suspending itself, gives rise to the exception and, maintaining itself in relation to the exception, first constitutes itself as a rule'. This is why, at the level of the species, mutation could be said to be the exception that confirms the rule. Furthermore, there is often a second ambiguous aspect to mutations. It has now been established that they can contribute to reaching a diagnosis, by identifying the biological origin of symptoms or by revealing a major molecular anomaly. And yet as they are often unable to predict how severe the disease will be or when it might arise, they can also leave open the question of the boundary between the normal and the pathological, and similarly the resulting prognosis. They produce results in terms of tendencies (this mutation is more often linked with that effect) and therefore do not always offer the irremediable and clear picture they initially seemed to provide. In addition to their possible intrinsic ambiguity, genetic diagnostic criteria are sometimes at odds with physiological and biological criteria (Miller et al. 2005). Although uncertainty may be age-old in medicine and even inherent to clinical practice, this shows that it nonetheless takes on new shapes and finds new sources in scientific and technological changes. More specifically, the result is greater certainty about the origin of the disease, but with lots of uncertainty about the prognosis. In this context, the question arises of how clinicians actually approach this complex situation. From this point of view, CF offers an interesting perspective, because its history is characterized by the issue of its limitations. It has undergone a process of nosological expansion, with further disorders being added, such as pancreatitis and types of male infertility (called Congenital Absence of the Vas Deferens or CAVD), which are defined as mild forms of CF (Hedgecoe 2003, Kerr 2000, 2005). Indeed, in biomedical discourse, CF is often represented as a continuum ranging from forms of infertility to severe forms, with intermediate forms between the two. The disease therefore offers the possibility for a detailed study of the question of the boundaries between normality, abnormality and pathology.

Here, I shall revisit these questions anew and analyze the biomedical definition of the normal and the abnormal at work in borderline forms of genetic disease, more precisely within the context of NSCF. I shall look in particular at some of the 'consequences' of this definition, in the sense of its social and moral implications (Bowker and Star 2000). The example of newborn screening will be used to understand how biomedicine regulates its relationship to the norm. More specifically, the aim of this chapter is to answer three questions: how does NSCF *reshape the expansion of the idea of abnormality*, and how far does this abnormality extend? How, in turn, are *professional practices* altered? And does the *biomedical norm* therefore also change, and if so, in what way? A certain number of studies on classifications in biomedicine have focused on the nosological dimensions and/ or on professional practices. They rely on an analysis of the biomedical literature (Hedgecoe 2003, Kerr 2000) and on interviews (Keating and Cambrosio 2000, Kerr 2005, Miller et al. 2005) or, less frequently, on observations (Featherstone et al. 2005). The analysis presented in this chapter differs from these in that it calls upon the observation of professional practices, while also analyzing their consequences upon the norm (and the interface between the neonatal and the prenatal). However, it does not address the consequences of NSCF from the point of view of either the child categorized as ill after birth or the child's family.[1] The first part of this chapter looks at the technical limitations of NSCF that lead to a substantial rate of so-called borderline forms being identified and thus extend *biological* abnormality. The second part deals with professional approaches and attitudes, ranging from individual to standardized treatment, as well as the practices associated with paediatric follow-up care, at the root of an extension of *clinical* abnormality. Finally, the last section uses a local field study to analyze the consequences of these practices at the intersection of newborn screening and prenatal diagnosis, showing how the norm is altered, but this time in respect of the foetus.

Techniques and Biological Abnormality

The Art and Uncertainties of Screening

Broaching an anthropological or sociological question in biomedicine often entails looking at techniques. As social science researchers have long shown, these are far from being a pure application of science, independent of any social contingency. The NSCF procedure in France relies on three techniques. First, it is based on a blood assay of a protein called immuno-reactive trypsin (IRT), carried out on all newborns. If this first test is positive, a commercially available 'kit' is then used to test for the 30 most frequent mutations of the CFTR gene involved in the etiology of the disease. If one or two mutations are found or the trypsin level is above a certain level, the families are called to the CRCM so that a sweat chloride test (sweat test) can be performed on the child. This all reflects the relatively complex nature of the screening flow chart, which also includes certain checks. This complexity would remain limited if each of the techniques used gave results with no overlap between normal and pathological – generally speaking, though, this is rare in biology (Grimes and Schulz 2002) – and if they provided coherent classification systems, which is not always the case. As we shall see, each of the

---

1   For a study on this subject, see (Grob 2011).

three techniques relates to a different form of knowledge that produces its own definition of normality.

The IRT assay derives from statistical knowledge, based on the increase in IRT levels seen in young patients suffering from CF, in comparison with a control group. This knowledge is not explanatory – it does not help find the origin of the disease – because the clinical and biological significance of IRT levels has not been established. Despite its shortcomings, this assay affords the practical advantage of allowing so-called 'suspect' children to be distinguished from normal children within the overall population of neonates. At this stage, it does not yet distinguish between those who are ill and those who are normal.

The category of the suspect child testifies to a linguistic shortcut that has a peculiar ring for those unaccustomed to it. This relates to a habit among clinicians consisting in reducing a person to their state of health or their medical results (they will say 'So and so is improving' rather than 'So and so's condition is improving'). It should be noted that the term 'suspect' in question here obviously does not imply any suspicion of guilt or moral failing on the part of the individual being referred to, as in the case of a 'suspect individual'. Rather it is a question of a morally neutral medical suspicion, often even compassionate, that affects the very picture of innocence – the newborn child.

The intervention threshold, which defines the dividing line between normal and suspect, is quantitative. In general, the whole art of screening consists in reaching a compromise between sensitivity, which tends to lower the threshold and identify more suspects, and specificity, which tends to raise it and identify less. In 2003, those organizing screening raised the cut-off point of the IRT assay, considering that the number of children requiring a genetic exam was too high (roughly 6,000 per year) and represented a substantial financial cost, without identifying more sufferers. The threshold went from 60 to 65µg/ml, which may seem like a minimal difference but had considerable effects on the number of children categorized as suspect and requiring a DNA test: this number decreased from 6,000 to 4,000 per year. Nonetheless, given the number of children ultimately classified as being affected (180), the definition of abnormality for this initial test remains relatively broad. And when the result of this first test is abnormal, the DNA test comes into play.

This second stage is set in a form of knowledge – genetics – that identifies the primary cause of the disease. In scientific terms, this cause resides in a change in the sequences of nucleic acids in the gene that codes for a chloride channel of the epithelial membranes. Looking first at how this genetic test was included in the screening procedure, it is necessary to recall that it increases specificity: thanks to this test, 6,000 (and then 4,000) 'suspect' children were whittled down to 550. For this reason, as we have seen, it contributed to making NSCF socially acceptable, insofar as it contributed to lifting the AFDPHE's reservations. Nonetheless, the organizers encountered a difficulty in the fact that a large number of different mutations of the CFTR genes have been identified worldwide (more than 1,500 to date!). And it was technically impossible to test for all of these on thousands of children. So which should be chosen over others, aside from the most frequent (the famous 'ΔF508', also called 'F508del')? With the help of molecular biology laboratories, the most common mutations in the different regions of France were mapped. Once again, the 'Celtic' Breton population was set apart as more genetically homogeneous than other regions. More generally, the situation was described as follows in scientific publications: 'The Northern part [of France] appears as subdivided into at least three zones, from West to East: Brittany, comprises a Celtic population (G551D), the Nord-Pas-de-Calais is peopled with Scandinavians (394delTT) and in the North East, there is a Germanic region (R553X)' (Claustres et al. 2000). In this excerpt, each region is associated with a people and a more specific mutation. Based on these studies, and after trials with different commercially available 'kits', the commission in charge of DNA tests retained 30 mutations, including a so-called 'African' mutation detected above all in populations of African origin. The representation of the illness was therefore not limited to the so-called 'Caucasian' forms affecting mainly European populations, where the disease is clearly more frequent. These details reveal the importance of geographical origin in strategies for finding mutations. Letters and numbers are assigned to given world populations testifying to their genetic identity and mixture.

Turning now to the questions raised by this genetic test in terms of normality and abnormality, the following categories are created: normal (no mutation and an IRT below a given threshold), suspect or heterozygote (one mutation) and affected or likely to be affected (two mutations). However, it should be noted that roughly 500 heterozygote newborns are identified every year, which represents a few per cent of the total population of heterozygote newborns. This can be explained by the fact that most have an IRT level below the cut-off value and are therefore immediately categorized as normal. In cases where one or two mutations are detected, the situation becomes more complex for two reasons. First, there is the problem of transposing techniques, similar to the drawbacks identified in the case of screening for breast cancer (Kaufert 2000), which arises because the tools used were originally designed for diagnostic and not screening purposes. In the case of NSCF, the 'kit' used includes so-called severe mutations, which usually lead to serious forms of CF, and a few so-called mild mutations, which can make certain characteristics visible that are difficult to interpret on newborns in the general population. Moreover, biologists and paediatricians explain that the same mutation can lead to very different clinical signs in brothers and sisters from the same family. These limitations left the paediatricians I encountered somewhat disillusioned, judging molecular biology to be somewhat disappointing in this regard.

For instance, the mutation called 'R117H', which is the second most frequent mutation in France, can lead indiscriminately to classic forms of CF, attenuated forms, simple forms of male infertility or even, in some cases, no symptoms at all. More specifically – and the significance will become apparent later – R117H leads preferentially to CF when associated with another genetic marker called 5T, and preferentially to infertility when associated with the 7T marker. However, cases of respiratory symptoms in patients with the 7T marker have been reported in the world. Eight and a half per cent of screened patients carry this mutation, compared with only 0.3% of patients on record in health care centres before NSCF was set up (ONM 2001). Promoters of screening were surprised by this substantial increase, but it can probably be explained by the fact that most of the children in question were considered normal before screening was implemented and abnormal afterwards. The fact that this mutation is still included in the screening 'kit' remains subject to debate today in France and abroad (Thauvin-Robinet et al. 2009). A further problem in addition to transposing techniques appeared in the shape of a diversification effect. This is linked to the fact that elaborate genetic testing is carried out on the CFTR gene in cases of uncertainty, thus identifying one of the many, and often little-known, mutations that have been identified in the world. In sum, as a paediatrician explained in a meeting: 'With the kit and the technical advances [of genetics], the laboratory detects mutations more frequently and the percentage of mild forms has increased' (Paediatrician 2, Observation 1.6.05). In other words, with newborn screening the proportion of children affected with borderline forms increases in the patient population. In short, with the molecular test, the definition of abnormality may become narrower in comparison with the IRT assay but it is broader as compared with the symptom-based criteria used before newborn screening.

Another question facing the screening organizers concerned the rare children whose parents had not given consent for a DNA test and who were deemed 'suspect' by the initial IRT test. Above all, the same problem arose for the far more numerous children with no detected mutation but high levels of IRT. How should two apparently contradictory systems of classification be used? Probabilities and statistics established on the basis of regional data initially concluded that if the first assay was above a certain level (30µg/ml), families should be asked for another blood sample to carry out a second IRT assay. The child would be three weeks old at this point, so the new IRT test was called 'D21'. The parents therefore received a letter from the Screening Federation asking for a new blood sample to be taken by the GP or maternity unit. Care was taken in formulating the letter to avoid the word 'cystic fibrosis' so as not to alarm parents about quite a well-known and generally serious disease. However, despite the fact that in the overwhelming majority of cases (998/1,000) this test resulted in the child being classified as normal, being called back like this often caused parents extreme anxiety. As explained previously, this procedure was mentioned verbally to parents in maternity units just after birth, without any preparation for this routine further test ('We will contact you if there is something', etc.). The director of a centre for newborn screening in the Ile-de-France region surrounding Paris explained in an interview that she received calls on an almost daily basis from worried or even panicked parents:

> There are parents who are extremely anxious. When that's the case, it's generally crazy, there's the father, the mother, the grandfather, the grandmother, everyone calling each other. ... Sometimes I have mothers in tears on the telephone. There's really a lot of stress, because for them, it means there's something, the

kids are necessarily ill. So it's extremely hard to deal with (Screening centre director 1, 19.10.04).

She also explained how she insists that the health professionals, who emphasize 'the right to know' the reason why the child has been called back, do not worry parents by mentioning the name of the disease when the new sample is taken. She gave the example of a mother who had been told about 'cystic fibrosis screening' and who had telephoned her in tears. In short, the 'right to know' comes up against the right not to be worried, without, or almost without, reason. Then parents wait for the results or to be called back for a final test (the sweat test). Just as different rights come into conflict, so do the timeframes, from the short-term of screening to the long-term of waiting. This gives us an idea of what the timeframe of screening means for some parents, when the time saved in terms of diagnosis is also a time during which 'suspect' cases are confirmed or invalidated. Professionals can also perceive this timeframe differently. One AFDPHE official explained that, for her, informing parents of D21 test was an urgent matter, so as to be able to reassure them, whereas for the CRCM clinicians this was not urgent insofar as that group of children represented a small number of patients to monitor. According to her, the clinicians are in a hurry to screen – we have already seen the importance of timeframe as an argument justifying NSCF – but not always in a hurry to reassure. This brings us back to the eternal concern with the patients rather than with all the parents. Other more practical reasons behind this waiting period, given by the regional director of the screening centre, are grounded in the fact that the laboratories processing sweat tests are overloaded or that the babies do not yet weigh enough to collect sufficient sweat for the last test. Nonetheless, we can see here how what could be called *social hypochondria* can be created. This recalls historian Roy Porter's words when he says: 'These are strange times when we are healthier than ever but more anxious about our health' (Fox 2000: 419). This paradox only becomes apparent if we reposition it within the context of the value of health in our societies, as outlined in the introduction: treatment and anxiety work along the same logic. Between 2002 to end 2004, the D21 test concerned several thousand babies per year, representing 90% of the 'suspect' cases after the IRT and DNA tests, whereas in reality it only identified eight patients per year in France. Moreover, the procedure was extremely time-consuming for the regional screening centres. Given these results, it was decided that the procedure should be altered.

Generally speaking, it was clear – thankfully – that the flowchart and protocols should be changed given the initial results recorded, which had allowed the AFDPHE to establish statistics. The professional association applied this flexible and reflexive approach by modifying the procedure for D21 call-back at the end of 2004, during my field study. The children were now only called back when the initial IRT level at D3 was above a certain threshold (100μg/ml). This change can be estimated to have reduced the rate of call-backs tenfold; in the Ile-de-France region, for instance, this went from 100 call-backs per month to around 10. Social hypochondria was therefore reduced thanks to the professional association's adaptability. More widely, the question of cut-off values is crucial in this regard and denotes which philosophy is underpinning screening: looking to achieve maximum benefits for patients by identifying as many as possible or looking to create as few negative effects on the population as possible by generating anxiety in as few as possible.

Diagnosis and its Timeframes

The way in which categories of normal, suspect and ill change at the time of diagnosis remains to be analyzed. Historians take the history of CF back to the medieval period when the salty kisses given to children were the sign of imminent death or satanic possession. Much later, in the 1950s, a heat wave in the United States led to heat prostration in children with CF at Columbia hospital. Di Sant'Agnese, a doctor at the hospital, is said to have looked for the reason behind the salt depletion that had occurred alongside this strange exhaustion. It was several years before this physiological cause for the disease was recognized by his peers, but this paved the way for the sweat test (ST) as a diagnostic measure for CF. This test is therefore based on knowledge that is both clinical, tracing back to the physiological causes of the disease, and statistical, revealing elevated chloride levels in affected patients. It leaves the realm of screening to enter that of diagnosis, and is performed during paediatric consultations. It can rely on three distinct methods and is expressed numerically. The associated categories are normal, CF-affected, and, as we will see, a potential intermediary category, the very existence and definition of which are a major issue within NSCF. Here, normal and abnormal are differentiated on the basis of data that create not a dividing line but rather an indeterminate area delimited by two cut-off values. While this is a well-known difficulty, the situation is aggravated in the case of NSCF for two reasons. On the one hand, the value of the lower value gave rise to debate in France. At the time of my field study, there was discussion about bringing it down from 40 to 30mEq/L, so as not to let cases go undetected – a change that went on to be implemented, in keeping with certain international recommendations. On the other, this value can give slightly different results depending on the ST method used: 'My 30 may be different from yours' (Observation 2.6.05) said one paediatrician during a professional meeting. In other words, the classification is partly built on the local context of the method used and the place it is carried out (Roth 2005). Finally, a borderline result (between 30/40 and 60) should be placed not only in a local but also in a temporal context. In a presentation given before his peers, one paediatrician in charge of a CRCM explained that intermediate ST values could increase over time and the children then fall into the diseased category. For this third test, the idea of abnormality was therefore extended by lowering the cut-off value (from 40 to 30) and by projecting into the baby's future.

These difficulties should not give the impression of generalized confusion, however, as this was not what I observed. According to AFDPHE national statistics, it is estimated that 14% of affected neonates fall into the borderline category. This is therefore a high proportion and at the same time the number of children concerned is low (Munck, Houssin and Roussey 2008). Overall, the techniques implemented for NSCF lead to more children being classified as having abnormal results due to two effects. The first is a cumulative effect. In theory, the sweat test remains the test of reference but it is sometimes called into question by the genetic test. In combination, rather than cancelling each other out, the uncertainty that comes with each test tends in fact to be incremental. The second effect is linked to the fact that this approach is characterized, implicitly, by the decline of the clinic. We are far from the clinic originally defined as the activity carried out at the patient's bedside (*kline* in Greek is the bed) when called for by the patient or their loved ones. As one of the screening organizers said regretfully to the CRCM doctors: 'It has been described as a clinical disease. You erase all the symptoms … . You erase all the clinical semiotics. It's no longer the same disease' (Paediatrician-Geneticist 1, Observation 24.6.03). Conversely, other professionals sometimes defended a more biological conception of the disease. During a national meeting of the Federation of CRCM, one of them exclaimed: 'You can't start with MB [molecular biology] and then decide on a clinical basis. There are two mutations, genetically speaking there is therefore cystic fibrosis and it's your discourse that's going to modulate it. You chose for this screening to be genetic' (Observation 9.12.04). Consequently, this raises the question of the aim of screening: is it to identify a disease or a biological anomaly? Is the intention to detect affected individuals or to detect all genetic anomalies? This question was sometimes asked by paediatricians in professional meetings.

As early as 1961, sociologist Anselm Strauss spoke of the refrain of clinicians who disapproved of too great a reliance on laboratory techniques (Strauss 1961). Byron Good (1994) underlines the fact that approaching diseases more and more often in molecular terms, which involves redefining their categories, could mean a change in the medical landscape that is almost as radical as the change analyzed by Michel Foucault in French medicine between the eighteenth and nineteenth centuries. After *The Birth of the Clinic* (Foucault 2003), are we now seeing its death? Probably not, as will become clear during the field study of paediatric consultations. However, newborns with borderline forms show few if any symptoms, and this can only undermine the clinical approach. As a result, the relative weight of the 'clinic' compared to biology and genetics declines during the screening period and during the first years of the child's life. Finally, it should be noted that this decline in clinical considerations goes beyond the tension described by other authors between clinical aspects and genetic reclassification for professionals dealing with CF (Miller et al. 2005, Hedgecoe 2003). In the cases they describe, the process begins for a family when a patient shows signs of more or less serious symptoms that need to be diagnosed and treated. The situation is different when the 'patient' – but can we talk about illness at this stage? – is still very young and/or their parents have not yet actively turned to a clinician. The conception, or even the definition, of disease thus changes, or rather continues to change. It is temporally remodelled because the whole period prior to symptoms arising, when people would previously have been considered healthy (which can be 5, 10 or even 40 years for a borderline form) is now one during which they are considered to be outside of normality. The conception is also spatially remodelled by the sphere in which it circulates: more often than not, the family has never seen a case of CF or the associated symptoms, and has no experience of the disease. Moreover, while it is not rare for conceptions of diseases to change quickly over time, the fact that this is a genetic disease means that the effects of such changes extend to the whole biological family, both current and future as we shall see.

Managing Uncertainty

Clinical Abnormality

Early care provision for sick children was an argument in favour of introducing NSCF in France. However, it contributes to paediatricians' doubts in cases of babies with no symptoms, who would nonetheless enter into a demanding care programme at a very early age. However, health professionals have to respond very quickly to these ambiguous situations. What logics of action do they call upon and with what consequences? How are children with uncertain diagnoses categorized and monitored?

At the time of my field study, there was some confusion in paediatricians' discourse regarding the so-called borderline forms and particularly when it came to what to say to the parents. A few examples, taken from local and national meetings, can illustrate this: 'We are in an awkward position when we find an "unfamiliar" mutation … We lack the tools for what we're going to say' (Paediatrician 8, Observation 3.12.04); 'We don't really know what to say [to the parents]' (Biochemist 1, Observation 23.11.04). One of the paediatricians also expressed his questions in an interview:

> You have children that would have been diagnosed at age 20 … . Should we bring children who haven't asked for any of this into such a substantial and rigid care programme? … . Is it really worth bothering them at the age of one, when they won't have any symptoms until they are 40? … . What do we do with them? We don't know (Paediatrician 10, 8.2.05).

These words touch the very heart of a diagnostic dilemma. One thing biomedical innovations have in common is that they often cause dilemmas for professionals, for instance in the field of neonatal resuscitation (Paillet 2000) or in foetal medicine (Williams 2006). What practices result from this? The first choice to be made by paediatricians relates to the wording that they use.

The historical and central role played by language in clinical thinking is well known, where 'descriptive rigour will be the result of precision in the statement and of regularity in the designation' (Foucault 2003: 139). Descriptions and clinical pictures, but also classifications, are drawn up through language. And these classifications interact with the people they describe, thus contributing to 'making up people' (Hacking 2005). The stakes are considerable for those concerned because this leads to labels that have a huge social and individual impact in terms of self-perception, how others perceive them, health cost coverage, employment prospects, etc. (Bowker and Star 2000). Where the 'borderline' forms in question here are concerned the terms 'pre-cystic fibrosis' or 'CFTRopathy' were sometimes mentioned during my observations. While there might seem to be no doubt about the weight carried by the term pre-cystic fibrosis, due to the threat it conceals, the degree of importance attached to this issue differed between respondents. The following exchange between professionals, recorded during a national meeting that brought together the leading CRCM paediatricians, illustrates this:

> Should we talk about cystic fibrosis? Sometimes the term cystic fibrosis is more of a burden than the disease itself (Paediatrician X).
>
> [I would say] 'CFTRopathies'. Cystic fibrosis is maybe a bit strong (Paediatrician Y).
>
> Why use a different term [than cystic fibrosis], as long as you qualify the information? Talking about an 'anomaly of the CFTR gene' bothers me, how are the parents going to explain that to the rest of the family? (Paediatrician 4).
>
> With underprivileged people, sooner or later you have to go all in [either say cystic fibrosis or not] (Paediatrician Z).
>
> I take the entirely opposite view. It's all very well to say mild CF but ... [with another term] for the family, the child wouldn't be in the cystic fibrosis category... (Paediatrician 5).
>
> Given that it has been established that there is no phenotype-genotype [severity of the disease-genetic pattern] correlation, I don't see why we would tell them it is not a serious disease... . It's not just medical hypocrisy to say that things are unclear (Paediatrician 4).
>
> Yes, there are multiple cystic fibrosES [with emphasis], but it's a different matter if you label it as cystic fibrosis when you have good reason to believe that the only problem will be infertility (Paediatrician 5).
>
> If you label it cystic fibrosis, they'll carry that throughout their life (Paediatrician-Geneticist 1).
>
> Isn't it worse to tell them that it's cystic fibrosis later on? (Paediatrician 4).
>
> How can you know that? (Paediatrician X, Observation 24.6.03).

These exchanges highlight two things. First, they indicate that health professionals express concern about how to qualify the information they give to parents and the worry this can cause. And they hold different positions on the matter; at the time of the survey, no stable national consensus had been achieved and this remains the case.[2] Second, they show how children with an uncertain diagnosis will sometimes be classified in the generic CF category on the basis of arguments relating to language ('as long as you qualify the information', 'how are the parents going to explain that'), social presuppositions ('with underprivileged people') and biomedical knowledge ('Given that there is no phenotype-genotype correlation'). In 2004, an AFDPHE study showed that a CF diagnosis had been established for 18 children carrying a R117H mutation (two identical or different mutations) while presenting a normal sweat test. These children are now no longer just carriers of a biological anomaly; they have an illness that is generally serious, irrespective of their own particular status. Of course, professionals anticipate the worry that they cause and 'qualify' the information provided to the parents. However, as with all conditions, the truth of the disease is expressed through words and the term 'cystic fibrosis' is part of this. Yet unlike other conditions, the link between symptoms and words is broken, and once the term has been uttered, it can take on an even more brutal resonance.

On a deeper level, health professionals are in two minds about whether to adopt a standardized or individually based approach. On the one hand, a preliminary assessment based on the Breton screening programme, therefore enjoying greater hindsight, was presented at a conference. This concerned approximately 30 children with so-called mild mutations who received regular medical follow-up care (at least three consultations per year and, for more than half of them, two physiotherapy appointments per week) and had good respiratory status, with the exception of one child. In establishing these initial assessments, paediatricians assembled their own local resources that could serve as a guide for classifying patients. Certain AFDPHE officials mentioned the need to gather national epidemiological data, which could bring up the level of generality. Specifically, the 'sciences that classify people' have to meet numerical imperatives: they have to 'count' and provide the quantitative data that is most suited to effective classification (Hacking 2005). However, as we have seen, genetic mutations do not lend themselves well to this exercise. They are qualitative by nature and their diversity makes it a difficult task to establish cohorts that are sufficiently large to be significant, especially when dealing with a disease that remains rare. On the other hand, professionals confronted with situations of uncertainty speak repeatedly of taking a case-by-case approach to patients, saying, for example, in a meeting: 'We had a case of mild mutation where the child died' (Pulmonologist 1, Observation 28.5.05) or 'As a rule, these patients have longer life expectancies, but if they die at the age of 12 or 20 then...' (Paediatrician 2, Observation 9.12.04). The doctors are impatient to see what they can learn in terms of expertise as these children get older, in order to orient future practice accordingly. Some discuss among themselves whether it would

2   In 2009, 8 out of a total of 50 CRCM declared that they did not retain a CF diagnosis in one of the situations leading to a borderline form (HAS 2009: 119).

not be possible, as a precaution, to wait 5 or 10 years rather than reassuring parents erroneously. Even though they are all aware that a dramatic outcome is not inevitable, they tend to underscore these adverse instances, which leave a more lasting impression than favourable outcomes. The practical consequences are that they are unwilling to run the risk of failing to detect situations where a child's condition might suddenly deteriorate and they therefore act cautiously. The study showed that these precautions led a majority of the professionals to monitor children with borderline forms, including under a more flexible regimen, rather than considering them to be healthy. On the national level, a preliminary study conducted by the clinicians themselves in 2005 showed that when a child had two mutations, one of which was mild, they were monitored every month or every three months. When a child had two classical mutations and an intermediate ST, they were monitored every month. When a child had one mutation, or none, and an intermediate ST, one third of health professionals reassured parents, while two thirds asked families to come back and did not reach a firm conclusion at that stage. A paediatrician summarized this situation in an interview as follows:

> There are definitely undetected cases of cystic fibrosis among us. But we uncover them by newborn screening. So we create stress for parents and then we'll see 10, 15 years later, that these patients are completely asymptomatic. And will maybe have bronchitis a little more often when they reach 60. ... This is one of the issues of screening, I mean we underscore a biological anomaly, that we then transpose across to a potential evolution. Whereas among those cases, it's not black, it's not white, ... there are patients who have so-called mild mutations that will be very severe ... . And the problem is that we monitor forms that would not have been diagnosed before (Paediatrician 11, 10.12.04).

The tension between assessing populations and focusing on the emergence of individual cases seems to be moving in favour of the latter. This observation should be linked with the study of the history and political stakes of the implementation of NSCF in France. This emphasized the pre-eminence of power centred on patient 'cases', in other words on the individual, rather than geared towards policy techniques exercised over populations. On a smaller scale, we can see here a more individual form of 'pastoral power', more geared towards the individual sheep than the flock, something that should be linked to the history of French medicine. Despite the fact that the French hygienists sought to establish medical statistics, medicine remained more oriented towards the relationship between the clinician and the patient than towards populations, in contrast to English medicine. More specifically, the approach towards monitoring children both derives and deviates from two medical traditions (Desrosières 1998). On the one hand, it is no longer confined to the traditional 'one-to-one consultation' (the *colloque singulier*) between doctor and patient, which leads to care provision directly linked to the individual nature of the case. On the other hand, it is not content with statistical reasoning based on averages that miss the specificity of situations. Closer to Claude Bernard's experimental medicine, the preference is for medicine that claims to be both scientific and distrustful of probabilities. Indeed, for Claude Bernard, scientific medicine should use the experimental method to find and analyze the sequence of cause and effect, but it should not treat patients 'on average' because reality is individual (Desrosières 1998). It is as if statistics were case-driven or as if a whole group with an uncertain future were influenced by what is actually happening to the individual patient. Although medical care provision is less demanding for borderline forms of CF than for classic forms – in the latter case, the average time spent on care daily is no less than two hours – abnormality has extended its influence to clinical practice where consultations and physiotherapy are concerned.

Finally, another element should be mentioned that can sometimes contribute to these care practices. The exodus of patients towards CRCM often brings them into the teaching hospital context. And some of these centres are at the intersection between clinical practice and research, especially those aiming to remain at the cutting edge. This does not mean that patients all become research objects, but this biomedical context should not be forgotten. One paediatrician, for instance, spoke up in a meeting to suggest enrolling patients with borderline forms in research programmes: 'Opinions diverge on these patients, who may or may not be ill. We're in the realm of clinical research. We need a protocol [to know] if they agree to clinical research' (Paediatrician 12, Observation 24.06.03). The research approach is contested by the AFDPHE organizers because it does not meet screening principles, that is to say screening in the interest of the newborn child. In their view, by mixing clinical practice and research clinicians run the risk of not addressing patients in the same way as when the two approaches are dissociated: 'They mix their practice and their research. ... You don't say the same thing [to patients] as [what] you would say if you didn't have a research project'.

Furthermore, as we shall see, the idea of abnormality does not just affect the screened child, it reaches beyond birth to affect the children to come. The purpose of my local study was to better grasp the stakes of this link between defining what is normal and establishing a medical norm.

From the Normal to the Norm

Situation 1: Catherine and Patrick are the parents of little Lea who was born a month and a half ago. The future seems rosy until Professor Berteau, Head of the Paediatrics Service in the hospital where I conducted my study, phones them about doing 'a trypsin level test' on the baby, and arranges for an urgent appointment the next day. The professor then explains in the consultation that Lea 'has two positive indications – a very high trypsin level and the presence of one mutation – but [that] there would have to be three [for her to be considered affected by the condition]'. The father is pale and very anxious. I go along with the parents and baby to have the sweat test. During the hour and a half that this lasts, the parents' anxiety is apparent and the atmosphere is heavy. The biochemist carries out a sweat assay. A number appears. The father asks: 'So?'. The biochemist replies: 'The first one [assay] is reassuring, but I'd rather have the other one. But I'd rather let Mr. Berteau tell you, with the clinical symptoms'. Then the biochemist explains that she does not have enough sweat to carry out the second test. When we return to his office, the professor indicates that the test is negative because it is at 25 'with the norm being 60'. He adds, saying each word quite distinctly: 'You can definitely assume that your child DOES NOT have cystic fibrosis'. The parents give a sigh of relief and everything seems to go back to normal. The professor writes on the baby's chart, reading aloud as he does so: 'Conclusion: Cystic fibrosis: No. Follow-up care: No.' and adds: 'I've finished my screening'. Then he suggests that the parents return two months later to check the trypsin level, which is decidedly very high (1,200 compared to a cut-off value of 65). He also encourages them to carry out another sweat test, as only one of the two usual methods was interpreted that day, and it was the least accepted of the two. In addition, he urges them to arrange for genetic counselling, to identify which parent is carrying the genetic mutation so as to alert their brothers and sisters. Two months later, the parents tell the geneticist in their appointment that Lea is healthy, that her weight gain curve is normal and that her final sweat test was 30 but her trypsin level remains high. The geneticist suggests performing a test to identify which of the two parents is carrier of the identified mutation and conduct a thorough exploration of the gene involved so as to detect a possible second, rarer, mutation in the child. He adds: 'Assuming that she has some form of cystic fibrosis, it would be a very mild one. ... The sweat test is normal, so in principle there is a low risk of cystic fibrosis as such; there could possibly be other genetic anomalies, although I think that is very unlikely, which could lead to pancreatitis'. Six months later, genetic investigation continues, there have been multiple consultations and tests, and the conclusion remains uncertain. In an interview, Catherine expressed her worry and bitterness:

> It's been nine months now that we've been living in a state of worry, you can't imagine. And we've been through a huge number of appointments ... . It's really destabilizing because still today we don't have a clear and precise answer ... . As soon as she would lose a gram, as soon as she was ill, it was the end of the world (Catherine, 21.9.05).

She went on to speak of what seemed to her like undeclared research. She said that she would be willing to participate in research, but considered that it should be clearly indicated as such. She added that it was inhumane to keep parents and children in such a state of anxiety. Her situation is typical of the 'patients-in-waiting' living between illness and health after screening (Timmermans and Buchbinder 2010). Two months later, at the end of my field study, the parents received a letter from the paediatrician informing them that a second, very rare mutation, had been detected in Lea's DNA and concluding that 'strictly speaking' the child has 'atypical cystic fibrosis'. The letter specifies that only two cases of this second mutation have ever been described worldwide: one was almost asymptomatic and involved a man who just had a form of infertility, and the other was symptomatic and involved a female child with chronic pancreatitis. Nearly three months later, the geneticist informed me that Catherine was two and a half months pregnant and had just undergone a prenatal diagnosis to check the genetic status of the foetus regarding these two mutations. He went on to explain: 'I was careful. There were no signs in Lea but we cannot make any guarantees for the future' (Biologist-Geneticist 1, 20.2.06). A week later, we learnt that the foetus was healthy and the question of possibly terminating the pregnancy did not arise. Later, in our final conversation, Catherine explained:

> What was clearly stated [in the consultation], was that the decision was ours ...
> but that we were strongly advised to have the prenatal diagnosis. [The arguments
> were] that as we had the means to identify the foetus's genetic profile, it would
> be a pity not to do so, bearing in mind that there was a risk [of miscarriage
> due to the sample being taken] but that it was pretty low ... and the second
> argument was that I'm fairly young ... and if worst came to worst we could have
> considered another pregnancy (Catherine, 8.8.06).

Thirteen months had gone by since Lea was born. The whole process had begun with a high level of trypsin, the signification of which is unknown.

Situation 2: Bastien and Caroline are the parents of little Zoé, who is given a sweat test after a positive IRT test and the detection of one mutation, the famous so-called mild R117H mutation, during newborn screening. Fortunately, the result of the sweat test (8) is clearly negative and the baby is classified as not affected. Shortly after, Caroline and Bastien consult the geneticist to find out whether the mutation is on the maternal or paternal side, with a view to warning their respective brothers and sisters, should they wish to have children. The consultation takes place like any other CF consultation. A few months later, Bastien receives a letter from the geneticist stating:

> The molecular testing conducted on your DNA ... shows that you are a carrier of
> the R117H mutation (associated with alleles 7T, 7T of intron 8) ... . We advise
> you to inform your brother that there is a 1 in 2 risk that he is also a carrier of
> this mutation so that he can seek the advice of geneticist if he so wishes ... . On
> the basis of this information ... the risk of you and your partner having a child
> with cystic fibrosis can be estimated to be in the order of 1 in 640, which is close
> to the risk in the general population.

The method for calculating the risk of CF is the same as for any other mutation of the CFTR gene, independently of the fact that this mutation, associated with the 7T allele, most often leads simply to infertility as explained previously. The genetic profile is therefore clearly included in the 'cystic fibrosis' category. This information is taken up by the parents who obviously do not have the required knowledge to make the necessary subtle distinctions. According to the results, Zoé's mother tells me: 'The information is important, to know that this is in the family ... It's important for the collateral relatives who want to have children'. As I reread the letter, she confides: 'The 7T allele doesn't mean very much to me' (Caroline, 10.10.06).

These two examples support the results described previously and allow us further analyze the issues raised by borderline forms, at the intersection of newborn screening and prenatal diagnosis. While genetic counselling has been the subject of many social science publications related to the moral dilemmas raised by the use of new techniques (Ettore 2000, Rapp 1999, Remennick 2006, Williams 2006), it has been little studied at this particular intersection. The two situations described above indicate that, in this centre and at this time, when a mutation detected during newborn screening was little known or mostly associated with a benign form, or in some cases, a classic form, prenatal diagnosis was offered for subsequent pregnancies. The last part of this chapter will seek to confirm these practices regarding genetic counselling and also to understand the professionals' logic of action and moral frameworks in this regard.

The observation of genetic counselling consultations offers a more specific vision of how uncertainty is broached with the couples or women involved. Directly linked to this question, two further examples concern couples mid-pregnancy in families where someone is already affected with a mild form of CF. It should be underlined that these two examples concern initial genetic counselling consultations during a pregnancy and do not presume what would happen if the mutations were known and the foetuses carried them.

In the first case, the patient is the aunt of a child affected with a mild form of the disease and says: 'My niece has mild cystic fibrosis, in the sense that she's not very ill'. The geneticist anticipates an insufficiently serious image of the illness and insists on how difficult it is to predict its severity. He specifies: 'It is very difficult to correlate a damaged gene with the symptoms; it is very difficult to say: "It's not serious this time, it won't be next time"'. He does not yet know what mutations are involved in the niece's case and bases his risk calculation independently of their nature, concluding: 'You have a 1 in 240 chance that the baby is ill'. He does not allude to the fact that certain mutations are in principle considered to be milder than others, although these are only tendencies and there are exceptions (Woman 1, Geneticist 1, Observation 25.4.05).

In the second case, the female patient has a male cousin affected with a mild form of CF, while her partner, coincidentally, had a cousin who died of CF as a child. Given the woman's experience of the disease, she sees it as mild. She speaks of her cousin as follows: 'He lives fine with cystic fibrosis; he's just a bit more tired, I've never heard him mention physio; I've never seen him suffer; I've never seen him ill, he even did his military service'. She makes a distinction between her theoretical knowledge of the disease and her experience: 'I know physio can be demanding, but I never saw him suffer'; 'What I see doesn't correspond to what I know'. The man at her side has a much more severe image of the condition. He has experience of serious illnesses, as one of his cousins died of CF and another member of his family has a severe mental illness. Once again, the geneticist looks to inform them (above all the woman) about the existence of serious forms of the condition saying, on the subject of her cousin: 'That's a moderate form, there are much more severe forms'. He insists on the uncertainty concerning how serious another case could be adding: 'It's difficult to know if it will be severe or not severe'. He does not go into the details of the variable and complex nature of mutations, and he does not know the full nature of these at this stage. The psychologist who is also present in the consultation warns the woman more indirectly saying that she is not 'easily worried' (Woman 2, Geneticist 1, Psychologist 1, Observation 25.4.05).

The question of risk is at the heart of the information given to these couples in genetic counselling, as is customary (Lauritzen and Sachs 2001, Rapp 1999). Reassuring them consists in showing them that their level of risk is close to that of the general population and warning them consists in calculating the degree to which they differ from that. This risk calculation is linked to the statistical thinking that emerged in the eighteenth century, as we have seen, and which later allowed Mendel's law on heredity to be elaborated. The notion of an individual who is 'at risk' is now widespread in medicine, where risk has constituted a major category for several decades (Clarke et al. 2010). While applying the sociology of risk would be going too far, this should nonetheless be linked to the fact that risk evaluation extends to many fields, whether in terms of environmental or food-related disasters, etc. leading to the use of the term 'a society of risk' (Beck 1992).

Let us now look at the professionals' interpretive frameworks and the potential constraints they face. The interviews carried out with geneticists in the centre where the local study was conducted testify to the caution displayed regarding the serious nature of the disease. One of them summarized his position as follows:

> The child is going to be ill one way or another, even if they have a moderate form it's still not a standard life. And yes, afterwards, given that we can't guarantee to the parents that if we see something moderate, this will also mean a moderate phenotype, we offer them a voluntary termination (Geneticist 1, 15.9.05).

The 'semantic network' (Good 1994) in play is one of guarantees and risk reduction. Moreover, when asked whether the risk not of carrying a mutation but of the severity of the resulting illness is mentioned in genetic counselling, the respondent answered:

> At the moment, this isn't possible, we don't know the modifying genes [the genes likely to influence the activity of the CFTR gene], or rather we don't know enough about them ... So it's entirely possible to have a serious mutation and a moderately serious mutation, and to therefore expect a somewhat milder form, when, in actual fact, an extremely severe form will arise (Geneticist 1, 15.9.05).

Another geneticist working at the same centre explained:

> We often work on the hypothesis that a mutation that is not serious will cause
> serious symptoms. ... Twenty years ago we would maybe have said the opposite.
> Doctors want to avoid as much risk and uncertainty for people as possible ... .
> Also because people are less ready to accept uncertainty (Biologist-Geneticist
> 1, 2.9.05).

This testimony confirms the practice that consists in emphasizing the hypothesis
of severity and establishes a link between geneticists' practices and parents'
wishes. A third geneticist further confirmed this, taking the example of the R117H
mutation:

> When there's a mutation [in newborn screening], even the R117H, people are
> sent to genetic counselling ... . So there you go, you're in the system, whether
> it's justified or not, I don't know [he sighs]. I don't know ... The uncles, aunts,
> cousins, they'll all go and see ... (Geneticist 2, 7.9.05).

This geneticist established a strong link between newborn screening and
prenatal diagnosis. His point of view was sceptical, illustrating that, just like
paediatricians, geneticists are capable of reflexive thought and are not all
convinced by their own practices. Regarding the famous R117H mutation
associated with 7T, he explained:

> We are reassuring, but at the same time we do qualify this somewhat. And
> so fairly often, unfortunately, the parents choose a termination, when in the
> majority of cases it is likely that the child would have been little affected if at all
> ... . People are scared of finding themselves in the small fraction of percentages
> where there will be a typical form of cystic fibrosis (Geneticist 2, 7.9.05).

The highest hypothesis regarding severity is reinforced here because, according
to this respondent, the information given to the parents about even the slightest
possibility of disease results in pregnancy terminations. However, over the
course of my local study, I did not observe any cases in which a positive result
for a borderline form led to pregnancy termination. Geneticists express the
subtleties of the situation and explain that they reason on a case-by-case basis,
which corresponds to the traditional approach, or even to the norm, in genetic
counselling. They say that they adapt themselves to the situation of each family,
according to the number of pregnancies and prenatal diagnoses, to their level of
distress, etc. In doing so, they extract themselves from the static framework of
Mendel's theories and the associated risk calculation and place themselves rather
in the daily life and lived experience of the people in question. They sometimes
base themselves on this necessary flexibility when referring to the bioethical laws
that regulate these practices. In this regard, they underline the fact that French
laws are not adapted to the reality of situations, particularly the one that stipulates
that: 'Prenatal diagnosis refers to medical practices that aim to detect *in utero* a

particularly serious disorder in an embryo or foetus'.[3] They also sometimes link the evolution of these practices to the more general context in which an increasing numbers of legal proceedings are brought about by parents regarding a lack of information about the future handicaps facing their child. One of the geneticists indicated the dangers of this evolution:

> There's definitely a pitfall. It's [that] when we don't know, it's always easier to say: 'The child is affected' … than to say: 'We don't know, the child may be healthy'. Because if the pregnancy continues and in the end the child is affected, then we risk getting rapped on the knuckles by the parents. It's one of the major dangers of the increasing litigious nature of our society… . Because once we've taken a knock back two or three times, we won't take the risk again (Geneticist 2, 7.9.04).

This position was confirmed during a workshop that brought together around 150 legal experts and clinicians working in the field of prenatal diagnosis.[4] One of the obstetricians present explained: 'It's harder for us to take the risk of bringing into the world than to abort … . Someone who's not very brave, when there's a small risk, they'll carry out an abortion' (Obstetrician 1, Observation 16.3.06). It therefore seems that professional reasoning has to take into account this shift from the risk of illness that faces the child and parents to the risk of legal proceedings that faces geneticists if not enough information is provided. However, they must also take into consideration the opposite reasoning, which consists in protecting themselves against a possible complaint from the parents for an unnecessary termination on medical grounds.[5] This shows how, on the one hand, the law is relatively restrictive and out of step with practice (it limits the situations justifying prenatal diagnosis) and yet, on the other, it encourages less restriction (leading to terminations on medical grounds when professionals want to protect themselves against legal proceedings).

The last question that can be asked in view of these results is at what point do professionals consider a disease to be serious enough to justify prenatal diagnosis? In the centre studied here, infertility constituted a boundary in terms of what was acceptable for prenatal diagnosis and termination on medical grounds. Geneticists considered that this was not sufficiently serious to warrant the latter. This was confirmed by my observation of the following situation. A mutation had been detected in a baby during newborn screening. This mutation was found in the father, whereas the mother was a carrier of another type of gene (that geneticist call an 'allele') that could, in combination with the father's

---

3 Law n°2004-800 dated 6.8.04.

4 Twenty-second seminar of clinical genetics: 'Deciding to terminate a pregnancy on medical grounds', 16.3.06.

5 This very rare situation occurred for the first time in France in another hospital during my field study.

mutation, lead to infertility in a boy (and nothing in a girl). In the parents' medical file, the geneticists concluded: 'It does not seem legitimate to us to offer these parents prenatal diagnosis for atypical cystic fibrosis as this would be outside the legal framework of a "particularly serious disorder"'. The letter that the parents received did not, in fact, mention the mother's allele or the risk of infertility for a male child, thus excluding the possibility of any request for prenatal diagnosis during a future pregnancy. The geneticists probably wanted to protect themselves from a request that would seem to them not only illegal but also, and above all, unethical. The 'quality of life' of the future individual, to take up a term not used here but frequently present in biomedical discourse and beyond, was considered to be sufficiently preserved.

To summarize, all these interviews and observations come together to show that uncertainty is a very sensitive issue. Moreover, in this centre the only situations excluded from prenatal diagnosis were those where it could be affirmed that the genetic profile would *certainly* lead to a form of infertility, as the professionals considered that a termination on medical grounds was not justified in this case. CF and infertility were therefore separated where ethical justifications for prenatal diagnosis were concerned, insofar as genetics is able to provide any 'guarantee'. However, both conditions come together at a genetic intersection when the same mutation may be present and there is no certainty about how serious it will be. A positive test therefore does not entirely, or not only, raise the question of knowing what life is worth living, as it sometimes suggested in social science studies on the subject (Remennick 2006), but rather of knowing what risk of a life not worth living is acceptable. Genetic knowledge does not always transform the danger of being struck by a mysterious illness into a risk that can be 'calculated and controlled' as is sometimes said (Beck 2005), because the risk regarding severity cannot be calculated. By taking practices that work more on a case-by-case basis and establishing tendencies, this study shows us that a DNA change that can be calculated using the classic laws of genetics and that is below a certain level (for example 1 in 640 in Situation 2) is considered acceptable and 'normal'. Whereas, a modification that cannot be calculated with as much precision is considered unacceptable and 'abnormal'. The 'attitude of uncertainty' (the fact of highlighting uncertainty, indicating it to patients, etc.) displayed by geneticists can also be linked with an 'attitude of caution'. These results are an encouragement for further investigation to be carried out from the standpoint of the parents looking at practices relating to terminations on medical grounds. One instance that supports this remark is a short article published in *New Scientist* describing pregnancy terminations in the United States on the basis of non-pathogenic genetic polymorphism detected by commercial 'kits' and confused with CFTR gene mutations (Concar 2003).

This study does not presume upon future developments in newborn screening, nor upon practices in centres other than the one in which it was conducted. Two remarks do arise however. First, it is interesting to note that the centre is credited with a high level of scientific and medical legitimacy. Second, today a consensus conference bringing together European paediatricians corroborates the caution displayed by the French, and notes that the R117H mutation associated with 7T – with the emblematic nature that we have seen – leads in the long term to variable clinical situations involving necessary monitoring (Mayell et al. 2009). Like the French paediatricians, this group shows a certain anxiety regarding inappropriate exclusion from the CF category. However, on the other hand, the working group of geneticists from all the French CRCM currently recommends that no family investigations be carried out when one healthy heterozygote is identified for the R117H mutation (contrary to what was described in Situation 2 above), which indicates that the situation is still unstable (HAS 2009: 127).

To return to the study itself, it shows, first, how the idea of abnormality is extended with NSCF, proceeding from its concomitant use of three approaches: a technologization of medicine, a preventive policy geared towards the whole population and clinical practices aimed at the individual. First, the technologization of medicine redefines the disease on a mode that is above all biological. Genetics is not the only reason behind this, which is why I agree in part with Anne Kerr (2005) when she argues that the existence of borderline forms of CF, uncertainty and preventive measures do not only depend upon the developments of molecular genetics. However, I would add that the latter reinforces this tendency, if only through the fact that the use of the mutation 'kit' plays no small role, by facilitating things materially and allowing entire populations to be screened. Moreover, genetics is also the only factor that impacts on how the idea of abnormality spreads throughout a family, both present and future. As for the preventive approach on the level of the population, it combines a policy that is exercised over a population with the constant search in medicine for early diagnosis. At a time when other techniques are being developed, such as 'DNA chips' making mass genetic testing a possibility, a conjunction is occurring between globalizing procedures (population screening) and individually-based techniques (medical consultations and genetic counselling). Finally, the individual clinical approach includes the scientific criteria of abnormality and encourages paediatric monitoring and follow-up care, even of a moderate variety. The question therefore arises of knowing whether there is not a form of 'over-diagnosis' in the context of anxiety concerning health issues already mentioned. This seems to be the case for many of these borderline forms. Adele Clarke and her colleagues (2010) use the term 'technoscientific identities' to refer, as the name suggests, to identities created through technoscientific means, for instance the identity of 'heterozygote' or 'healthy carrier' constructed by genetics. Following on from the work I have described here, the question of the identities produced by these practices remains to be developed, this time from the standpoint of the families and children.

Second, this study shows how, by bringing borderline forms into view, newborn screening can lead to an expansion of this trend through prenatal diagnosis. More generally, obstetricians estimate that of the 5,000 pregnancy terminations carried out for medical reasons in France every year, for all kinds of pathologies, questions could be raised about 10% of cases in terms of how justified they are – either because the symptoms are, in principle, moderate but variable according to the individual, or because they will only appear at adulthood.[6] Of course, prenatal diagnoses for so-called mild mutations can occur occasionally independently from NSCF, but the latter does amplify the phenomenon. In one respect, the knowledge we have today allows us to screen at birth and then monitor and treat children seriously affected (we should not forget that if 14% of affected screened children have borderline forms, this means that the others have classic forms). Furthermore, this knowledge means that when an initial sick child has been identified at birth through screening, it is possible to avoid families with several sick children by then offering prenatal diagnosis for subsequent pregnancies. In another respect, to echo Georges Canguilhem, the question arises of the consequences of the medical knowledge of a given time drawing a dividing line between normal and abnormal (meaning that a foetus with a good chance of not being affected with CF is nonetheless considered undesirable). In this regard, two remarks should be made. The first concerns the researcher's position regarding their subject of study and the potential effects of this study. It would be naïve not to consider that there is a risk that this issue, highly charged with moral stakes, will be taken up by those opposed to the right to abortion. Indeed, this question of borderlines cases could be used to deny women any right to terminate pregnancy, which would definitely pose a serious problem to a feminist researcher such as myself. It is therefore necessary to make sure that the issues at stake have been clearly defined and that the investigator's own position is made clear. The second remark concerns the results of my study. Beyond the obvious differences between neonatal and prenatal approaches, it seems that common reasoning comes to light. Three salient points in common can be identified: the cautious attitude of the professionals in situations of uncertainty, the apparent importance of 'cases' where the disease progresses badly and the impossibility of evaluating the risk of severity. A shift can then be seen between the normal and the norm, with the extension of abnormality appearing in the extension of the possibility of selection, including for family members (cousins, etc.). Moreover, this raises the entire question of the link between newborn screening and prenatal diagnosis as medical approaches.

---

6 These data were collected during the previously mentioned meeting bringing together legal specialists and specialists in prenatal diagnosis (Observation 16.3.06).

Chapter 5
Living with the Disease

Numerous results from this study have shown that links exist between neonatal and prenatal approaches. One such link, of a technical nature, relates to the tools allowing mutations to be identified both in screened babies and in foetuses. In theory, and all other considerations aside, this facilitates a shift from one to the other. Tracking the famous borderline forms brought a further link to light, this time based on departures from the norm: identifying these forms at birth can lead to prenatal diagnoses being carried out in cases that are, in principle, mild. A third intersection can be seen in the actions of the professionals in West Brittany who, as we have seen, combined NSCF with screening for heterozygote adults in the early 1990s, with a view to prenatal diagnosis in cases where there was a risk of disease. The fourth link rests on one of the Breton professionals' justifications for NSCF: newborn screening allows prenatal diagnosis to be offered during a second pregnancy before symptoms have appeared in the first child. It should be noted, though, that the last two points at least are contested by the AFDPHE as contravening its ethical principles. Nonetheless, all in all, four points emerge where the two approaches, on either side of birth, seem to mutually reinforce each other; in other words, it is as if a treatment-related approach encourages prenatal diagnosis, and visa versa. We can therefore draw the hypothesis that a broader issue lies beneath these links, which can also transform into tensions. And this question is connected to conceptions of what I suggest calling a 'quality life', which I shall analyze here in the context of CF. First, however, a few general points should be specified.

The historical movement that brought life and its optimization into political strategies, as described at the beginning of this book, is related to the notion of well-being. In fact, this notion is currently the subject of a wide rhetoric as can be evidenced by any number of advertising billboards (for instance, the well-being that a particular brand of mineral water is supposed to afford...). This rhetoric is linked to, and fuelled by, a rising number of scientific studies that look to measure well-being throughout life and to compare this between different countries (notably Blanchflower and Oswald 2008). The increasingly prevalent concept of 'quality of life' should be understood in this same spirit. For Alain Leplège (2004), the notion of well-being resembles the concept of quality of life and is close to 'happiness' as understood by many moralists and philosophers stretching back to Aristotle. Instruments measuring qualify of life therefore exist because of the idea that empirical distinctions can be made between policies in order to identify those that provide the greatest increase in general and collective well-being.

From a socio-historical point of view, the introduction of measures of activities of daily living (ADL) into health questionnaires at the beginning of the 1960s lead to focus shifting away from the immediate manifestations of the pathology (Armstrong et al. 2007). These were linked to disruptions in social activities, in parallel with the widened definition of health developed by the WHO mentioned in introduction ('a state of complete physical, mental and social well-being'). The instrument for measuring quality of life was built on these grounds, based mainly on four kinds of parameters: symptoms, mental health, ADL and social activities. It reflects a shift away from the traditional pathological referent: it is no longer a question of improving health or reducing suffering, but rather of understanding patients' experience and giving as much weight to post-disease effects, such as difficulty in going out, as to corporal lesions (Armstrong et al. 2007). According to their proponents, these measures of quality of life present the advantage of combining a quantitative approach, seen as objective (criteria about health, standard of living, family support, etc.) with a subjective perspective (the patient's self-evaluation, the evaluation of health professionals, etc.). They are characterized by the fact that the concept was taken on board by clinicians and their stated aim to take the patient's point of view into account. Moreover, as has been made clear, these indicators combine biological life (symptoms) with certain aspects of social life (meeting up with friends, etc.) and how they are taken into account in clinical practice remains to be analyzed.

This quest to not only optimize life but also measure its quality as precisely as possible, could potentially reinforce value judgments about lives. These judgments already emerge in all the biomedical techniques that make it necessary to evaluate 'quality of life' in order to make an informed decision about future action. The debates about choices in terms of euthanasia, neonatal resuscitation, amniocentesis and prenatal diagnosis can testify to this. This explains why sociologists and anthropologists highlight the fact that, behind prenatal diagnosis, for example, lies the question of what kind of life is worth living (Landsman 2003, Press and Browner 1997). I have already shown that, given the uncertainty surrounding prognosis, it is more a question of the 'risk' of living a life not worth living, but let us set this aside here. A significant example of the growing influence of biomedicine in this regard can be seen in *in vitro* fertilization and pre-implantation diagnosis in Great Britain. These practices were subject to the law of human fertilization and embryology, which stipulated that the well-being of future children had to be assessed beforehand by the medical unit, using medical and social criteria (Ehrich et al. 2006). The study carried out by Ehrich and colleagues shows, at the very least, a partial shift from solutions for handicaps based on the social (social well-being) towards those based on genetics (genetic well-being). And it has the value of pointing out the value judgments that are made about future living beings and specifying the criteria on which these judgments are based. Meanwhile, some ethicists are concerned about moves to generalize prenatal diagnosis on the grounds that they would mean that immensely talented individuals, such as Mozart or Einstein, would be deemed 'unfit to live' today.[1] From another perspective, as Nikolas Rose (2005) has stated '[the] attempts to eliminate such single gene disorders [do not] indicate that those born with such conditions are deemed "lives less worthy of life", less worthy of our care and sustenance'. In other words, the issue of making value judgments about potential or actual lives has different implications depending on whether it concerns life *before* or *after* birth. And naturally all these questions are charged with moral stakes, values and affects. This is why it seems useful to call upon an analytical framework that helps set preconceptions aside. Extending Mitchell Dean's (1999) analysis of 'ethical government', such a framework could include several dimensions: ethical substance (*what* we act upon), ethical work (*how* we govern this substance), ethical subjects (*who* we are when governed this way) and ethical practices (what this government *aims* to achieve). To summarize, taken together these elements can offer a way of reframing the question of well-being and quality of life within a general perspective of optimizing or evaluating life. They also allow certain points of intersection to be identified between this movement and prenatal practices, in terms of the value judgments made about potential or actual lives within ethical government.

Broaching this question of life and its quality and value naturally entails looking more closely at patients' daily life. A significant body of social science literature has arisen on the subject of living with a chronic illness. From as early as the 1970s, Anselm Strauss (1975) contributed to developing studies on the daily lives of patients affected with such conditions, including a dimension that was not strictly medical but also social (and sometimes psychological) in his approach to these diseases. He showed the specificity of such conditions in comparison with acute illnesses: their length (by definition); the uncertainty that they generate in terms of long-term life projects; the extent to which they intrude upon patients' and families' lives; the diversity of services and actors that they call upon, etc. In France, for instance, Isabelle Baszanger (1986) played a role in developing this kind of sociology. She showed in particular the negotiations and interactions that take place between the different actors involved, as well as how rules of social life are organized during the illness and how this organization changes. More recently, numerous studies have focused on patients' and/or families' experiences, the meaning they give to the disease and how it transforms their identity (in particular Johansson et al. 1999, Richardson, Nio Ong and Sim 2007, Young et al. 2002). However, here I shall focus less on the question of identity than on how the physical body is managed in relation to social life. In this line of thinking, sociologists have studied how the body can be integrated into the sociological dimension of the experience of chronic illness. In particular, biological facts can become social when other people respond to patients from the point of view of their bodily impairment (Kelly and Field 1996). This means that the biological does not only depend upon social factors, it can also create the social.

---

1   Cf. the article entitled 'La France au risque de l'eugénisme', *Le Monde*, 4-5.2.07.

While some pay attention to the body, others want to bring the disease itself back into the sociology of health. Indeed, other authors (Timmermans and Hans 2008) focus mainly on the disease and its symptoms and impairments, as well as its relationship with social life. In their view, sociology was initially too closely aligned with doctors in the 1950s, but since then, in attempting to take its distance, it has neglected the physiological side to disease (its severity, its symptoms, etc.) in its research subjects. They add that in order to understand health inequalities, for example, it is important to identify the ways in which the social is incorporated into the biological. Moreover, the authors of the article also reproach social science researchers their propensity to flatten out the differences between chronic diseases. Another study supports this idea indirectly by analyzing the experiences and discourse of patients suffering from genetic diseases in comparison with those suffering from non-genetic diseases (Peterson 2006). Due to the hereditary nature of genetic conditions, people affected as either patients or carriers mention their concerns about the lives of other family members, including future ones. This can raise issues linked to whether or not information about the disease is shared with these family members and concerns about the health or well-being of a future child can also emerge.

This introduction has already shown that the issues at stake here not only encompass but also exceed 'quality of life' in itself. In the case at hand, the link between NSCF and prenatal diagnosis means that the issue at stake includes the living being and existence itself. This is why I propose to exchange the concept of 'quality of life' for that of 'a quality life', which seems to be at the heart of related practices. In these final two chapters, I shall therefore come back to my field study in the hospital setting, looking at how the aim of preserving a quality life is pursued through NSCF. I will first look *at the efforts made to treat sick children in order to attain this aim of a quality life*. I will also question how patients, doctors and families see 'quality life' and how social and biological life are interlinked and/or co-produced. In order to answer these questions, I shall call upon the words and opinions of both clinicians and parents. In particular, I will highlight different aspects of disease and care provision, the ways in which life prospects are considered and how social life (going out, going to school, having fun, etc.) and biological life (looking after oneself, avoiding infections, etc.) are interlinked or co-produced. Far from any form of genetic essentialism, we will see both the processes through which patients stigmatize each other within the hospital space and the core of social inequalities in terms of health, which relates to living conditions.

Paediatric Semantic Networks

'It's a very time-consuming and difficult disease, with time-consuming and difficult treatment, on a daily basis, sometimes several times a day ... There are extremely difficult living conditions. The disease is present, you live with it all the time, all the time, there's no respite. It's definitely difficult' (Paediatrician 13, 24.2.05). This is how a young paediatrician, specialist in CF, described the condition in an interview. Most of her colleagues also described the extreme variability of the disease's severity, explained in the previous chapter. But what exactly are we talking about? To begin, we must reach a better understanding of the landscape of the illness. It involves teenagers whose condition suddenly worsens and young girls who can no longer cope with the two hours of daily care and the two months of intravenous treatment per year; it involves deaths and fears of death; it involves pregnant women in tears, but also cases of happy babies and healthy young people, who it is hard to imagine as CF sufferers. It is a question of better understanding not only the efforts made to treat sick children in order to achieve this aim of a quality life, but also the way in which the disease affects their lives. As this aim is obviously vast, I will limit the question by approaching it on the basis of the consultations I observed and the interviews I conducted. I will group together observations of young children screened with the disease and older teenagers, as the lives of the latter can shed light on the future lives of the former. According to anthropologist Brian Good, semantic networks are not simply adjacent words; they reveal deep-rooted associations (for instance, between obesity and self control today) that can afford a better understanding of disease. From a methodological point of view, in order to better understand these sick children's lives, I will therefore begin by outlining the 'semantic network' of the disease within paediatrics, in other words 'the "syndrome" of experiences, words, feelings and actions that run together' (Good 1994: 171).

Most of the paediatric observations I carried out involved consultations with a female paediatrician who played a very active role in the service in question. She treats around 100 patients all affected with CF and, like other professionals I encountered, combines research and clinical activities.

Germs, Weight and Treatment

The first point to be made concerns treatment and care provision, which doctors see as the elements that ensure the best life possible. Beginning with the slightest symptoms and moving towards treatment, a whole system of monitoring and care provision is put in place that Anselm Strauss calls an 'arc of work'. Dealing with a chronic disease also means looking after a body, both for the patient and their family. Among the *physical symptoms*, three interrelated areas can be identified: breathing, coughing and sputum; digestion and stools; and growth. When patients have a cough, paediatricians look to determine its frequency and type (loose or dry) and see if there are other associated signs (wheezing, sputum). Regarding stools, their frequency, consistency, colour and smell are evaluated. And in terms of growth, it is a question of measuring, weighing and drawing up growth curves. The 'objectivizing' form to such curves can correct some mothers' alarmist impressions, as they can be extremely concerned if their children have lost weight and satisfied if they have gained some. Given the extent of this sort of preoccupation, the paediatrician I observed took care to reassure mothers who were too worried so as to defuse any potential fixation on the question of food. Two key words emerge from this description of patients' general state: 'coughing' and 'losing/gaining weight'. *Beyond the signs and symptoms*, there is also more detailed monitoring through consultations (every month for the first six months, then twice a month) with a systematic bacteriological examination of sputum and outpatient visits every semester. Or at least this is the theoretical protocol in place. In practice, paediatricians and certain parents can choose for appointments to be less frequent, and we will see examples of this, or more frequent if the child's condition deteriorates. Sputum is 'examined' in both senses of the word, as both observation and test: the result leads to the verdict about whether the child has 'pseudo' (is infected by the pseudomonas germ) or not. The child can also have 'staph' (be infected with the staphylococcus germ) or other germs, but the first is undoubtedly the most feared. As for the detailed check-up in the outpatients' hospital, it provides a range of results, often at the cost of intrusive tests that can involve tubes in the nose or oesophagus, etc. As soon as newborns are diagnosed, 'physio' sessions begin (chest physiotherapy), *between monitoring and treatment*, on average twice a week in mild forms and in children who are well, but up to twice a day if they are congested. These 'physio' sessions can easily be overwhelming for the unaccustomed who suddenly find themselves faced with the efforts made to extract mucus from the infants' deepest airways. When they grow older, children and adolescents then face above all the repetitive and tedious nature of what are often daily sessions. Concerning treatment proper, when the medical situation is unsatisfactory, a plan of action is set in motion with wilful resolution prevailing ('We absolutely have to remove this germ', says the paediatrician). Should the situation become further complicated, the semantics at play can take on a combative or warlike nature ('We have to strike against pseudo' or keep 'armed vigilance', she adds). The arms in question are antibiotics, intravenous treatment courses, aerosols and ingested digestive enzymes. And the allies in this fight are a rich diet, good hygiene and certain life rules that avoid exposure to microbes. In cases of small children with fairly severe forms of the disease, for the parents this fight means two hours of daily treatment directly related to the condition. In an interview, Bruno, one of the rare fathers to have decided to stop working in order to devote himself to caring for his daughter, described repetitive days that are well structured and organized around the disease. This shows just how much the substantial treatment demands can lead to the complete reorganization of the life of the family carer. At the same time, paediatricians are aware that a quality life cannot be reduced simply to treatment, particularly because this is a chronic condition.

Dealing with a chronic disease on a daily basis does not only involve medical acts, it also calls upon all sorts of different actors involved with the illness and surrounding aspects – doctors or otherwise – in different spheres of social life. As Isabelle Baszanger (1986: 22) writes 'the patients must go beyond medically defined treatment work. They also have to deal with the consequences that the disease has on how they organize their lives [and] their relationships with others'. Given that the disease is a long-term condition, it cannot be considered as suspending the accomplishment of normal social roles. One of the issues at stake is, where possible, to maintain social insertion, as it is important to keep a balance between biological life (hygiene, treatment) and social life (games, going out, etc.). So how do paediatricians broach these aspects, which are not strictly medical, with the families? The following examples taken from consultations can give an idea of the balance in question, particularly when mothers ask the paediatrician for details about the kinds of leisure activities sick children can engage in without running the risk of worsening their condition:

> The mother of a sick child protests because she was not invited to the hospital's Christmas party:
> '[Irritated] Last year, there was the Christmas tree, this year, nothing...' (Mother 3).
> 'This year, the children in hospital were invited to the Christmas tree. [We can't mix] those with pseudo and the others. You wouldn't want [your child] to go home laden with presents, but with pseudo as well?' (Paediatrician 11, Observation 22.12.04).

> A mother asks the paediatrician:
> 'Should I take [Tom] out?' (Michèle).
> 'The weather's nice' (Paediatrician 11).
> 'I know, but I keep thinking he got sick twice when he went outside' (Michèle).
> 'He mustn't be in an environment with people who are coughing. He has to go to the park. I don't think I ever told you shouldn't take him out' (Paediatrician 11, Observation 16.3.05).

> A mother asks if she should remove a plastic swimming pool in the garden where her sick son plays. The paediatrician replies:
> 'I don't think you need to remove it, you should disinfect it … . Municipal pools aren't good'.
> 'And water jets in the garden, that's not a problem is it? I wondered about that with the pseudo he caught' (Isabelle).
> 'Pseudomonas is everywhere, he [Jules] can't be kept in a bubble' (Paediatrician 11, Observation 29.3.06).

This expression of children not being able to be in 'a bubble' came up several times during consultations and interviews. The mothers want to weigh up the benefits of leisure activities against the perceived risks that they entail. In these examples, the first mother is looking to negotiate – or even demanding – a moment of social interaction, while the others, with young children, are looking more for information. The balance between normalizing life ('He [the child] is normal' said the paediatrician at another moment) and 'abnormalizing' life due to the disease can be difficult to achieve (Strauss 1975: 58). More generally, there can be a conflict between, on the one hand, preserving children from infection and other risks and, on the other, enabling them to have a quality life that allows, or would allow, them to enter into the category of normality (attending the Christmas party, going to the park, playing in the pool). In this way, parents are strongly advised against sending their children to a crèche, due to the risk of infection, but encouraged to send them to school later (appointments between health professionals and school heads in order to ensure good integration are frequent).

This tension between safeguarding against infections and maintaining a quality life also emerges in health care centre summits bringing together several hundred professionals and some patient families (Observations 19.3.04). In one such setting, a paediatrician and lung specialist listed among medical aims 'reconciling close monitoring and quality of life ... , so that we have children in front of us and not cystic fibrosis cases' and 'bringing into line hygiene measures and maintaining quality of life'. The father of a sick child, one of the heads of a patient organization, also underlined: 'Our joint battle has one single aim which is to improve quality of treatment while maintaining quality of life'. The idea expressed here is that it is necessary to reconcile treatment and quality of life in order to achieve, I would add, a quality life. However, the balance in question can become harder to attain when play and treatment both carry potential dangers and benefits. In a workshop during this same conference, a discussion began about toys in hospital waiting rooms. It showed that, depending on the environment, toys can provide children with a quality life (at home) or can be a danger (in the hospital, as a source of germs). And during one consultation I observed, the paediatrician removed a hospital toy from the room remarking that it was a 'vehicle for germs'. This does not, however, prevent certain children diagnosed through screening from playing with them in the waiting room. In the same way, treatment can be seen both as a constraint weighing on children's lives and something beneficial providing them with better health, and therefore ultimately a better life. As a paediatrician and lung specialist said in another workshop during the same conference: 'We increased treatment; this could have been to the detriment of the children's quality of life and is relatively rare' and 'Basic proper hygiene leads to quality of life, quality of treatment underpins a better quality of life'. In this perspective, the tension between treatment and quality of life disappears because treatment *affords* quality of life.

In short, how can this complex situation be summarized? Doctors and parents are led to make sometimes cruel decisions between biological life (safeguarding health) and social life (seeing other children, playing). However these choices are not limited to a binary form because biological life can have a negative impact on social life (two hours of daily treatment can limit activities) but also a positive one (treatment enables children to feel better and therefore to enjoy these activities). In the same way, social life can have a negative impact on biological life (going to the swimming pool carries a risk of infection) but also a positive one (playing in water can be a way of maintaining *joie de vivre*). If the two are intertwined in this way, this is in part because social activities are taken into account in the notion of 'quality of life' as outlined in the introduction, and in part because these social activities in turn have effects on CF. We can therefore see the dilemmas and paradoxes that this entails. For instance, one mother's autobiographical book recounts her fear in face of the first chest physiotherapy sessions that she witnessed and the author adds: 'These children are manhandled and this violence is necessary for their survival! What a sad paradox!' (Laurent-Seguin 1999: 92). And this paradox could no doubt be taken further to say that 'these children are manhandled and this violence is necessary for them to have a quality life'.

Prospects of Life and Death

Considering the lives of children suffering from CF also unfortunately means sometimes considering death. In this regard, my local study illustrates the extent to which:

> the hospital is not only the site of the construction and treatment of the medicalized body, but the site of moral drama – of human suffering and fear, of the confrontation with illness and death on the part of both the sick and those charged with their care, and of efforts to contain and manage the drama (Good 1994: 85).

A certain inherent selective bias should be underlined, however, insofar as that patients whose condition has worsened are more often seen in hospital than the others.

In the case of young children diagnosed through screening, given that they have only been alive for a short period, the life referred to in my interviews or observations was above all the child's future life. The main issue at stake was the life prospects of these children. A study carried out in the United States in the context of NSCF showed that for many mothers who have just learnt about the illness, the hardest thing to hear are the statistics concerning their child's possible future, in other words life expectancy data and the description of the disease's natural history (Grob 2008, 2011). In the context of the study carried out here, examples from interviews can show how parents consider the future of their young child, diagnosed through screening. In these first cases, the disease had already proved quite severe:

> I was told: 'He's not going to die, he'll become a fine young man'. I believe it without believing it, but anyway... I believe it for the moment. But then it depends on the evolution of the disease, it's always the same. Because you can stay positive, I'm positive about Jules, but still, you can't delude yourself either (Isabelle, 19.5.05).

> For the moment, you don't have the impression that she's sick, but I know that one day we'll wake up in the morning and she'll start coughing and bringing

> up phlegm. We're not under any illusions. ... At the moment, the disease
> in her lungs is busy doing its work, there's nothing to be done. Every day
> her pancreas dies a little more. ... We don't try to hide from the reality, tell
> ourselves it'll get better. It's a disease that progresses (Bruno, 10.5.05).

In other cases, when there are almost no symptoms or only mild ones, logically
projections into the future are more positive. One mother described the disease
in an interview more as something that other children suffer from:

> I'm really lucky... that she doesn't have anything wrong with her lungs,
> nothing with her pancreas. ... I see other children, they're not as lucky. ...
> There are [parents] who found out about the illness at age two, and then the
> children are very very sick, they wear masks, they have oxygen, they have
> sterile rooms. ... It's hard (Jeanne, 30.6.05).

In such cases, the illness remains in part outside the family realm, without
preventing the mother from being on the alert. All in all, whether they are dealing
with a form that is, in principle, on the severe or the mild end of the spectrum,
these parents of young children (between eight months and two years) are well-
informed about the most classic and serious 'trajectories' of the condition, either
by the information provided by professionals or thanks to exchanges with other
parents, as well as by information obtained elsewhere (Internet, etc.). The term
'trajectory', which is applied in particular to chronic diseases, refers here not
only to the course of the illness but also to the organization of work necessary
over that course and the impact it has on those involved (Strauss 1985). Parents
take a somewhat similar view to doctors of all these events that are part of the
future life of the patient. The future 'emplotment' that they envisage does not,
at any rate, contradict the one provided by doctors, unlike what can be observed
with other conditions (Landsman 2003). Families encounter other older patients,
if only in hospital waiting rooms. And as the years go by, the problems of these
young patients often become more complicated.

As the illness evolves, the patient's medical state becomes a vital issue, in
the literal sense of the word, which interferes increasingly with social life (going
to school, going on holiday, etc.). During my observations, for instance, one
young girl with bad respiratory function had to undergo an endoscopy produced
by fibroscope under general anaesthetic, followed by a two-week course of
intravenous treatment, while another young boy had painful digestive problems,
often missed school and had to undergo a coloscopy and substantial enemas, etc.
Courses of treatment and hospital stays become more frequent as lung infections
become more chronic. The price to pay to avoid deterioration as much as possible
is clear: more and more treatment, more and more time devoted to care, etc.
Patients sometimes cry when told they will have to undergo another course of
intravenous treatment or another serious procedure. Consultations are therefore
often emotionally charged, as is often the case in medicine, and particularly

when they concern a disease that is often severe. This illustrates once more that Western medicine does not (always) correspond to the cold, distant and formal caricatured image that is sometimes suggested (Good 1994).

However, the picture is not always as morbid. On the contrary, other pre-teens are in good health and it is difficult to imagine that they are in fact ill. For instance, a brother and sister, Solenn and Adrien, are two adolescents with very few symptoms and who therefore only have six monthly appointments. Solenn was diagnosed at the age of 13 due to a respiratory disease. At the end of the consultation, the paediatrician measured her respiratory function and concluded: 'I think we only need to see each other once every six months ... . She's perfectly well, avoid taking her to the hospital too often, there are germs there' (Paediatrician 11, Observation 15.6.05). Moreover, quite often brother and sisters with the same mutations will have very different symptoms, as illustrated by the example of Gilles and Camille:

> Gilles was diagnosed from symptoms at the age of 7. Today he is severely affected and the paediatrician is beginning to consider a lung transplant. Just after her brother's diagnosis, his sister Camille presented the same classic mutations. However, she is a young girl of 17 who has so far had very few symptoms and considers herself normal. Concerns are rising, however, due to the signs of a first infection, and the paediatrician therefore says to her: 'You have a long life ahead of you, you have to retain your ability to play sport' (Paediatrician 11). She explains the possibility of genetic testing when she wants children and adds: 'I've seen lots of adults in your position, I even had a granddad of 70 [Camille smiles]. ... You have a normal life, the aim is to keep it that way' (Paediatrician 11, Observation 2.2.05).

Here we have two opposing cases in terms of life prospects: a lung transplant for the brother, carried out after severe deterioration of respiratory function, and a long life with children for the sister, provided she receives good care. This example encapsulates the hopes and fears of the illness. And we can see all the uncertainty regarding the consequences of mutations surfacing in concrete terms of life and illness, because while uncertainty is common in medicine, it is all the more so when the condition extends over time. The difficulty of making long-term plans, and of organizing or reorganizing one's life, makes the burden of the illness even greater.

As conditions deteriorate, these uncertainties and consequences can begin to be expressed in terms of death. For instance, one day the paediatrician treated the emergency case of a young girl who died the next day. She said later to the nurse: 'She saw herself go, she said: "I'm going to die"'. Another day, the paediatrician discussed a patient with the nurse and said: 'If we don't do anything, she's going to die'. Certain parents and teenagers are well aware of the danger. One adolescent cried during a consultation as she remembered children she had known who were no longer alive. Another teenager's mother said that her daughter was afraid of death. In these moments, everyone – patient, parent and doctor alike – comes close to the inevitably tragic side to medicine: the fact that everyone is mortal (Fox 2000). This dramatic perspective is necessary to better understand the disease, the treatment efforts deployed to ensure the best life possible, and the lives of those who literally live with the condition.

Two points are worth underlining as this section draws to a close. First, the difference with genetic consultations is clear in terms of the semantic networks surrounding the illness. In genetics, these networks concern above all geographical origin, the risk of transmission and biological links. In what is said by parents and doctors within paediatric consultations, the disease remains something that can be passed on genetically, but the potential danger lies in infection. Nutrition, weight and height, but above all the risk of infection, are the major issues at stake. Both discourse and distress seem to crystallize around germs not genes. Depending on the space in question, the illness is either purely genetic in essence (in the genetics service) or becomes a hybrid entity in which germs play a role that is as important as genes, given that the latter do not offer any therapeutic possibilities (in the paediatrics service). In other words, the semantic network of the disease changes before and after birth. Second, in paediatrics, the semantic network of the illness is schematically organized around two areas: biological life ('gaining/losing weight', 'coughing', 'pseudo', 'physio', 'life/death') and social/psychological life ('playing', 'quality of life', 'bubble', 'worried') where each term can be linked to others in the same group ('cough' with 'pseudo', 'playing' with 'bubble', etc.). Of course, there is strong crossover between the two groups ('playing' and 'pseudo', 'quality of life' and 'physio', 'death' and 'worried', etc.). Certain terms, like 'life/death' and 'quality of life' can shift from one group to another depending on the circumstances, or else belong to both. This is because in professionals' conception of things, while maintaining a quality life belongs mainly to the register of the biological life that they look after, it does also involve other aspects such as going out, playing, going to school, etc. Their vision of things is therefore not strictly biological, it also incorporates into clinical practices the changes brought about by the instruments for measuring quality of life, as outlined in introduction. At the same time, the link with intra-corporal lesions remains stronger than the changes described by David Armstrong and colleagues (2007), who define quality of life so broadly that it is sometimes measured on the basis of 'free-floating symptoms' free of 'any link' with lesions. This can be explained by the nature of the disease in question, that could not be more inscribed in the body.

Social Life and Biological Life

Let us now move on to look in detail at two conditions for a quality life for sick children: the first relates to infections encountered in hospital, which emerged as an important issue within my field study, and the second, less immediately apparent, relates to social inequalities. Both issues provide food for thought about the links between biological and social lives, albeit in very different ways.

The Threat of the 'Other'

I have already analyzed the central role of germs in establishing evidence of the benefits of NSCF, including as an unpredicted side effect. In the same vein, we have just seen the ambiguous status of toys that are mainly seen as beneficial, but can also present a danger in the hospital setting as germ carriers. More generally, hospital visits are both indispensable and not without disadvantages. More so than the toys, it is the other patients who present a potential source of danger. Although this is a classic problem for contagious diseases – which CF is obviously not – the situation is quite particular in this case, given that the danger arises within the very establishment that provides early treatment (courses of antibiotic treatment for infections) for the dangers that it can also transmit. How do health professionals and parents deal with this paradoxical situation and how are social relationships reorganized within this context?

Like all hospitals that date back to the nineteenth and early twentieth century, the hospital in which I carried out my field study has separate wards in order to reduce the spread of infectious diseases. Indeed, from this period onwards, such diseases were the main preoccupation of paediatricians and administrators alike, who had discovered that hospitals did not cure as much as they should. Today, given that CF sufferers die most often from cycles of infection-inflammation that eventually destroy their lungs, the risk of infection is a major issue in daily practices, including within the hospital itself. More specifically, on the one hand, health professionals make efforts and implement strategies to reduce cross-infection and, on the other hand, they encounter organizational and structural constraints inherent to the hospital setting and the disease itself. Among the strategies in question, for example, paediatricians schedule consultations without 'pseudo' before those with 'pseudo', so in cleaner rooms and atmospheres. This therefore creates two initial groups of patients: those with and those without 'pseudo', who must be kept separate. But a whole series of problems makes this overall principle difficult to apply in practice. The following observation illustrates in more detail what these potential issues can encompass:

> In the morning, the paediatrician is held back upstairs due to a serious emergency. During this time, Kevin, a child diagnosed through screening, who had an appointment at 8 a.m., arrives with his family at 9.45 a.m. Then the paediatrician arrives and consultations begin with Marie, who is around 10 years old, and her mother. Marie is colonized with 'staph' but does not have 'pseudo'. During the appointment, the paediatrician says to a nurse: 'Can you check that Céline [a child diagnosed through screening] is not in contact with the others. That waiting room really is a disaster ... . These consultations are badly organized, explain to [Céline's father] that the children without "pseudo" go first' (Paediatrician 11).

Céline's appointment was at 9 a.m., but she therefore goes in later, as she has 'pseudo'. Marie's consultation ends. The paediatrician asks the physiotherapist to tell the parents of Julie, another child screened as sick, to go and get a coffee and not mix with the others. Then Kevin's consultation takes place, during which the paediatrician asks his parents: 'Next come, come on time, otherwise there'll be a riot' (Paediatrician 11). Then comes Tom's turn; he also does not have 'pseudo'. His mother says in passing: 'I'll make an appointment in a month, because every time I come in at the last minute, it's not fair' (Michèle). Julie is next, a child diagnosed through screening who has had 'pseudo' but who, we learn today, is now free of it. Céline's consultation follows, a young girl who had a false negative screening result and who has now had 'pseudo' for several months. Finally, it's the turn of two older young girls, one colonized with 'pseudo' at a chronic stage, and the other with a germ undergoing isolation (Observation 16.3.05).

While, thankfully, every day of consultations does not combine as many problems, this particular one does highlight the organizational difficulties present. We can see in this example the accumulation of a number of elements: a medical emergency, a family arriving late, an appointment with 'pseudo' that has to be pushed back, a child who is thought to have 'pseudo' mixing with other children in the waiting room, a mother who comes in at the last minute, sometimes because her child is genuinely not well, and an interface between the 'pseudo' appointments (often older patients) and 'non-pseudo' appointments, which can lead to overlap. Other observations confirm these initial data, particularly concerning the interface between appointments with patients who do and do not have 'pseudo'. For instance, while in the waiting room, Mrs [X], the mother of little Julie, diagnosed through screening, went down to the floor below to get some paperwork. During her absence, a young girl of 16, infected with 'pseudo' and wearing a mask, took her place in the consultation. Another difficulty arises in that parents are not always free for the appointments that they are given as 'pseudo' or 'non-pseudo'. In this way, on one day, after a consultation with an older patient with a chronic infection, the paediatrician saw a 12 year-old patient. She began by throwing the window wide open and saying: 'I'm just opening the window, it's important'. During the consultation she explained to the physiotherapist: 'I'm seeing her at the end of my consultations, the mother knows about it, because of timetabling problems'. The mother worked and could not free herself up earlier. Sometimes the paediatrician will move to a different room between appointments.

In addition to these time-related difficulties, problems of space also arise. As the paediatrician said in one consultation: 'The waiting room is unsuitable'. This reflects the whole issue of space in the hospital, which arose from as early as the end of the eighteenth century. From this period onwards, research began to develop on the question of individualizing the space in which patients lived and breathed, including in waiting rooms. During my study, patient families were led to mix within the waiting room, usually sitting next to each other on a small bench. This physical proximity could go on for a certain amount of time, as waiting times could be long (from 30 minutes to two hours, or even longer). Furthermore, the patients of doctors [X] and [Y], whose cubicles were next to each other and who did not organize their appointments in the same way, also found themselves waiting on the same bench. This reveals the impact of architecture and spatial organization on health and social interactions. Unlike in the study carried out by Nick Fox (1997) on the physical barriers allowing a sterile regime to be established in surgical spaces, the temporal and spatial overlap identified here established a regime of proximity and possible contaminations. Infected patients are supposed to wear a mask, but while some do, the use of masks remains erratic. Teenagers in particular are sometimes reticent because they are fed up with the illness; they are aware that they are not completely 'normal' and they feel ostracized, too hot in summer, etc. The mask serves as a stigma of the disease, that is to say a discrediting object that prevents the adolescent from being considered as normal (Goffman 1963). And this is all the more the case given that the patients are not accustomed to stigmatizing situations because often their symptoms are not very apparent. Finally, another hindrance to effective separation of groups is linked to the fact that, at least during the first part of my field study, other doctors in the service, or in other services, treating CF patients sometimes used the same physiotherapy room – where much coughing and expectoration takes place – for different kinds of patients. This led the paediatrician to say to another health care worker:

> It makes me sick from an ethical point of view that our patients are seen in the same physio room.
> [She cites a colleague] is going to ask for two rooms (Health care worker).
> It's taken us two years to do it (Observation 1.2.05).

Here, this clinician calls upon the form taken by the 'ethical work' (how ethical government is exercised: seeing patients together in the same physio room) that seems to her to negate her work as a carer. Testifying to this desire to resolve the problem of the common physiotherapy room, a physiotherapist explained during one CRCM meeting that she had met with a manager, Mr [X], in order to see how to set up cubicles with and without pseudo, a suitable bin, systematic cleaning of the physio room after cyto-bacteriological examinations of sputum and a room for newly screened patients who are uncontaminated. All in all, despite the health care workers' best efforts, they remain at least in part constrained by the issues of space and organization within the hospital.

It should be noted that when the situation is observed in more detail, several groups are created rather than simply two. 'Pseudo' can take more or less chronic and dangerous forms (if the germ is encased in a little shell, generally in older patients, it becomes more and more resistant to antibiotics; if it becomes 'hypermutating' or 'multiresistant', it is resistant to everything). Consequently, health care workers created new sub-groups. Sports camps or support groups for teenagers are organized according to groups of germs and their resistance to antibiotics. During one consultation, the paediatrician suggested a ski programme to a young 17 year-old girl specifying: 'They have sensitive pseudo [like you]'. Likewise, during a CRCM meeting she said: 'The next teen group is Spseudo' [sensitive pseudo]. We'll see for Rpseudo [resistant pseudo] and staph [staphylococcus] later'. On the other hand, as the person making appointments explained to the paediatrician, the parents do not really know how to distinguish between chronic (resistant) forms of 'pseudo' and non-chronic (sensitive) forms; and indeed the secretary herself asked for clear written instructions. So what are the parents' points of view on this question?

Generally speaking, parents – or at least those who are the most aware about hospital-acquired infections – show concern about the issue of contamination within the hospital. They express more worry about this risk in interviews than they do with health care workers. For instance:

> We think of nothing else [microbes] because we know that most bugs, you catch them in the hospital. It's awful. I think about it. ... And we also think about the others, because, mainly at the beginning, we were sometimes given non-pseudo appointments, ... and in fact she had pseudo, so it was even dangerous for the others. ... We always make her wear the mask, but it's not healthy, it's not healthy for her, it's not healthy for the young kids with cystic fibrosis around her. ... Often they're running late, it's long (Bruno, 10.5.05).

Another displeased mother explained in an interview how her little girl was contaminated in the waiting room:

> I found myself next to a young girl [in the waiting room] ... , who was at least 18 and who was coughing, lots and lots. And that's what made me suddenly realise, I said to myself: she must have pseudo because every time we go, Mrs [X, paediatrician] asks us whether Julie coughs. And she was really coughing up her lungs, you could tell the mucus was coming loose and coming out. So then I went to get a mask for Julie, because at the beginning we didn't really know the principle of the mask, and this young girl didn't have a mask. ... Anyway, the fact remains that that day that young girl coughed up her lungs over Julie ... , we were sitting right next to each other on the little bench. When I saw that, I said to myself: take your daughter, go for a walk. And in the meantime another young girl had arrived, and so she was in contact with Julie ... , and the nurse said to her: 'Go and put your mask on, put your mask on'. The young girl said: 'I don't want to'. She told her off. ... So that was already two people with pseudo who were in front of Julie and weren't wearing their masks. Then [X, paediatrician] came out ... and she took me aside and said, 'Mrs [Z], I'd like you to go back there'... where the toys for the children are. She said to me: 'Go there, straightaway. ... I'll see you in another cubicle'. And she told her [the young girl] off. ... A month later, Mrs [X, paediatrician] called me and said 'Look, Mrs [Z], I'm sorry but we're Thursday today, tomorrow I want Julie

to come into the hospital for a course of antibiotic treatment because she has pseudo'. [She sighs]. Pfff ... (Corinne, 8.7.05).

This shows to what extent the risk of cross-infection is a source of tension between patients, and even between families and health care workers, sometimes revealing other social tensions. During an informal conversation, the paediatrician explained that the mother of Tom, a baby diagnosed through screening who had had an emergency course of treatment in hospital, claimed that her son had been infected while waiting for hours in the waiting room. According to the mother, this did not happen any which way but specifically when he was sitting next to a young child from a gypsy family who lived in a caravan and whose case will be outlined later. It should be specified that Tom's parents both work in the luxury goods business in one of the wealthiest areas of the Parisian region. The social gap between these two families emerges here in the shape of suspicion about contamination. In actual fact, among the cases I encountered during my field study, the two children screened with the disease who came from the most fragile social backgrounds were not infected and ran no risk of transmitting germs. However, their parents were the ones who spoke least about the problem of cross-infection and who were probably the least aware of the issue. At this stage, to summarize, we can see social groups emerging; groups of patients established not on the basis of their mutations or their genes but rather their germs. Moreover, these groups can give rise to tensions related to the dangers of infection, above all of a biological nature (germs) but sometimes linked to social factors (the socioeconomic disparity between families).

Other observations and interviews allow a more general perspective to be taken. During a workshop organized within the context of a care network summit, a discussion began between health care workers from different regions in France:

The speaker, a doctor, begins to read a slide: 'Things that are indispensable: Taking into account the bacteriological status of the patient when arranging an appointment'. He comments: 'It's not easy to stick to. What do you do with a child who isn't well when it's the day for the screened children [who are not infected yet]?'. He continues reading the slide: 'Avoid having germ-carrying patients in the waiting room' and mentions other measures relating to hand-washing and examination practices. A discussion begins in the room, with each participant describing the practices in their centre:
'We don't take [infectious] status into account'.
'We have a list with each child's germs. One day, it will be cepacia [name of a germ], the next, another germ. Emergency cases are seen either at the beginning or the end.
'Finally!'
'Is it manageable?'
'No'.
'At [X], the patients have very different days according to their status'.

'At [Y] we have days for children with or without pseudo. Children with cystic fibrosis never cross paths, we put an asthma case between the two'.
'We try and educate them about wearing a mask ...'.
'We leave masks at the reception desk. It's strongly advised. Sometimes they get put in pockets...'.
'There are some who are stubborn' (Observation 19.3.04).

Another paediatrician, incidentally more of a 'screener' than a 'clinician', explained how shocked he was to see patients stigmatizing each other on the basis of germ groups. During a patient organization meeting, the cystic fibrosis adolescents' group demanded that patients bring a bacteriological analysis to know whether or not they had the particularly dangerous cepacia germ. This paediatrician emphasized the risk of segregation between patients, here on their own behest and outside of the hospital system.

What we can see here is the current manifestation of a traditional idea within the hospital – the distribution of diseases and (formerly) of miasmas. On a small scale, a form of 'tertiary spatialization' is put in place, that is to say:

> all the gestures by which, in a given society, a disease is circumscribed, medically invested, isolated, divided up into closed, privileged regions, or distributed throughout cure centres, arranged in the most favourable way. ... [I]t brings into play a system of options that reveals the way in which a group, in order to protect itself, practises exclusions, establishes the forms of assistance, and reacts to poverty and to the fear of death (Foucault 2003: 17).

Here, however, this idea goes further still as it extends beyond the hospital framework and follows patients to the sports camps organized by the health care workers. Groups of children emerge according to the germs they carry. When teenagers participate in support groups or go on camps together, this distribution constitutes a new biosociality (Rabinow 1996), a form of sociality established on biological grounds as mentioned previously. However, unlike in the previous situations, this biosociality is not only genetic (CF) it is also built on infectious grounds (the associated germ). And it sometimes also influences the behaviour of patients and families among themselves. This therefore means that it carries less solidarity with it than in other cases, for example in Brittany with the 'Celtic' gene or within patient organizations. Here, the body is situated at the heart of social processes of segregation and stigmatization. In the end, where do parents lay the blame for these risks of infection? With teenagers who do not wear their masks, with doctors who have patients waiting together in the same room and sometimes with socially marginalized families. They do not mention the doctors' responsibility regarding the common physiotherapy room nor, on a public health level, the problem of excessive use of antibiotics that leads to resistant bacteria, although it is true that this is quite a specialist point. Like with infectious diseases as such, this responsibility brings tensions, when the 'other' represents a danger for

your own, or your child's, quality of life – or even life in general. The potentially
dangerous 'other' is therefore the 'older child' without a mask, and, in some cases,
the young child whose family is perceived as socially marginal. In comparison, in
the case of other infectious diseases like AIDS or the Ebola virus, the infectious
'other' is often a stranger or a member of a deviant group (this is less and less
the case for AIDS) (Washer and Joffe 2006). In the case at hand, the 'other' is
physically and socially closer, but is still blamed for spreading germs through
individual or social behaviour (spending time near babies without wearing a mask,
living in a caravan). Older children who fear being stigmatized due to their mask
will be stigmatized in the end for not wearing them. These children are seen as
a real danger and, what is more, as incapable of using their own moral sense of
responsibility. In this sense, the child is the figure of the stigmatized individual
as outlined by Arthur Kleinman and Rachel Hall-Clifford (2009), who suggest
rethinking stigma as an ordinary moral and emotional experience. Seen in this
way, stigma results either from the issues at stake within the local context, or
from what is perceived as a danger for agents' local moral experiences. However,
alongside this moral dimension, there is also an eminently political dimension.
In addition to this figure, there is the figure of the young gypsy, subject to power
relations within the small local world of the waiting room. To summarize, the lives
of patients suffering from CF involve being protected from these 'others' in both
a moral and political sense.

The Impact of Social Inequalities

The last point in this section concerns a less visible aspect to patients' lives. From
a social science perspective, the notion of quality life cannot be separated from
living conditions. In support of this idea, after having long been underestimated and
little known, studies increasingly attest to and demonstrate social inequalities in
health in France, particularly in terms of mortality according to socio-professional
categories (Kunst 1997). However, it should be noted that between perinatal
health, where such inequalities have been observed, and adulthood, the health
of young children remains understudied in France. And yet an epidemiological
study carried out in the United States has shown the relationship between chronic
infections and socioeconomic status in children aged between 6 and 16 (Dowd,
Zajacova and Aiello 2009). Family revenue, level of parental education and so-
called 'racial' origin correlated to the probability of infection in children, both by
microbes considered as linked to lack of hygiene and by widely spread microbes.
The authors of the study concluded that the differences in how exposed children
are to infection when very young could be one of the mechanisms through which
early social factors are incorporated and lead to more long term consequences in
the lives of future adults. Genetic diseases, which garner much attention around
the issues of prenatal diagnosis, have been subject to little study in terms of social
inequalities. It is possible that the 'naturalizing' aspect to approaching health from
the perspective of genes contributes to this. An older study nonetheless showed

the effects of social class and place of residence on the age of mortality in patients suffering from CF (Britton 1989).

During my field study, I observed diverse socioeconomic situations among the different patient families. Of the six families of children diagnosed through screening that I observed over time, one was of high socioeconomic status, three were of medium socioeconomic status and two were at the lower end of the scale. This heterogeneity is probably encouraged by the fact that screening is generalized across the whole population and patients are oriented towards specialist care centres at a very early stage. Does this mean that patients are all equal before the disease or that inequality is limited to genetic fatality? Certainly not. While all parameters other than social inequalities are fixed (by genes) or rendered more or less equal (by generalized screening and access to CRCM, and by the funding of CF treatment by the social security system), what doctors and biologists called the 'environment' and what I would call the 'core' of social inequalities, nonetheless remains, and NSCF offers a particularly suitable tool through which to examine this. I shall therefore look here at the way in which living conditions interfere with patients' lives and how this question is broached (or not) within the hospital. Without claiming to provide any exhaustive answer to these questions, I shall endeavour to bring shed light on them by using two specific examples. So let us now turn to the situation of two families living in very difficult social, economic and cultural conditions.

Josée is one and a half and was diagnosed at birth through screening. She suffers from CF but presents very few symptoms, she has never had a serious respiratory infection and her pancreas is working well. Her father Ali is 35 years old, of Algerian origin and works as a security guard, while her mother, Jeanne, is 25 and previously worked as a domestic help and then as a child minder. She stopped working when she found out about her daughter's condition.

The first consultation that I observed with the family began with a brief exchange about an outpatient check-up confirming the lack of any particular medical problem and went on to address the family's living condition in the following terms:

> Have you found bigger accommodation? (Paediatrician 11).
> No, we live in a studio, we don't have a shower inside, we make do... (Ali).
> [To Jeanne] Have you found work again? Or haven't you looked? (Paediatrician 11).
> I have looked, we need to find a solution for Josée, the crèche isn't an option' (Jeanne).
> [To Ali] You work nights, do you manage to sleep in the day? These aren't easy conditions (Paediatrician 11, Observation 2.3.05).

Here the paediatrician showed an interest in questions that go beyond the biomedical framework in the strictest sense of the word. As the consultation continued, I observed Josée because curiously she seemed more tired than ill. Her eyes were bright and puffy and she seemed somewhat lethargic. The mother mentioned this tiredness in another appointment when she explained that 'even if Josée sleeps 9 hours, she always seems tired'. An interview carried out at the family's home showed me that Jeanne, Ali and Josée lived together in one room of around 100 sq ft, within a working class area of the Parisian suburbs. When I arrived, I woke up Josée, who was sleeping on a small sofa while her mother watched television. During this interview, when her daughter began to cry a bit, Jeanne said to her: 'Josée, if you're tired, lie down'. The only place in the room where Josée could lie down was the sofa on which we were sitting, as the fittings and furnishings amounted to a small table, a few bags, a television, a computer, a shelf and a small washbasin. This washbasin was in addition to a shared shower on the landing. Given these circumstances, it became clear that Josée was very lucky to have developed a seemingly mild form of the disease especially in light of risk of infection linked to stagnant water for patients suffering with CF. As a doctor stated during a workshop about hygiene for patients aimed at professionals: 'The points on which we must not compromise are: the bathroom (sponges), the shower, stagnant water, floor cloths, liquid soap, the toilets and the kitchen' (Hospital doctor X, Observation 19.3.04). Moreover, Ali, who worked nights, had to rest on the sofa during the day in short stretches of a few hours. Over the past two years, he had made several housing applications for the French equivalent of Council housing, but none had been successful. Similarly, despite having a professional qualification in electronics and having run a small electronics company in Algeria, his job applications in the field had not proved fruitful. In the interview, he spoke of the racism he felt he encountered in his daily life, but when asked about whether he also felt this at the hospital, his reply was clear:

> On the medical side of things, I've never felt that, personally, no ... . It [health care] should be something that's global ... . A child, a person who's sick, they need treatment, whatever their colour or race. ... In the street ... yeah maybe you'll be looked at if you're white, black. But in hospitals, no, I've never felt that (Ali, 30.6.05).

In other words, for Ali, health care as a value transcends differences in origin in the eyes of health care workers. Although obviously no generalizations can be made on this basis, his opinion offers a better understanding of the context of the field study. Certain studies do contradict it, however. In the United States, in 'high discretion' medical cases that do not require emergency intervention, subtle differences in interactions with doctors are reported. These can lead in particular to variations in likelihood to recommend certain drugs depending on people's origin (Dovidio et al. 2008). One way or another, the case of Josée and her family offers an initial illustration of the impact of social inequalities on the life of a child suffering from CF (tiredness, living in close quarters, the problem of the communal shower, etc.). One final remark to be made concerns the value of carrying out interviews in the home setting, as it can highlight aspects of health care problems that are not immediately visible. For Josée, the issue is not access to treatment (it is funded by the social security system); rather it is her living conditions that affect her biological life. My second example adds an educational and cultural dimension to these questions.

Kevin is one and a half, was diagnosed through screening at birth and suffers from CF in a form that does not seem to be too severe. He lives in a caravan with his parents, Lila and Micha, who are both 18 years old and unemployed. Lila, the mother, can read but cannot write, and Micha, the father, is very withdrawn and has little involvement with the illness. Kevin's mother spoke in an interview about the members of her group as gypsies or Evangelical Christians, and his paternal grandmother, who can neither read nor write, described them as travellers or gypsies. At the beginning of the trajectory of the disease, Lila had difficulty in ensuring that Kevin was monitored and treated. An energetic young woman, she seems to have taken control of the situation and receives support from all the family. Often a small family group goes with the parents and baby to the hospital for appointments with the paediatrician, despite the problem of distance from the health care centre that faces the travellers. The two grandmothers, in particular, are very present. Lila would like to have access to a house in the winter due to the cold, particularly since Kevin's illness, but her freedom of movement is important to her. As she said in an interview: 'We get down if we stay in the same place all the time'. The family's whole way of living is in question and leads to negotiations concerning treatment. The first paediatric consultation that I observed with this family began as follows:

> The family has not attended an appointment with the paediatrician for four months. Lila explains that she is not well and mentions a recent pregnancy that she had to terminate. After a short exchange about this, the paediatrician specifies to me: 'They live in a caravan, you can imagine for physio'. And then she asks Micha if he is working, which is not the case, and if they are managing to live on their benefits. Lila answers that they do not receive the 'benefit specially for his illness', in other words benefits allocated in the case of chronic disease. Although the parents could have been eligible for more than a year, postal issues, complicated by changes in address (also affecting consultation reports) have impeded the process. The paediatrician telephones the social worker at the health care centre to inform her about this. And she comes back to the pregnancy termination and the foetus, bringing Lila to make the following remark:
> 'It's a shame you know, because she wasn't ill you know' [she did not have cystic fibrosis] (Lila).
> 'You need to talk about this. Are you sleeping? Do you cry?' (Paediatrician 11).
> 'Sometimes' (Lila).
> 'Would you like to see a psychiatrist?' (Paediatrician).
> 'No, if I talk about it, it's even more' (Lila) (Observation 19.1.05).

As this consultation began, a combination of medical, psychological and social issues thus arose. By not coming to consultations for several months, the parents were clearly out of step with the therapeutic protocol of screening, leading the paediatrician to insist repeatedly on the need to come regularly in the future. For her part, Lila spoke in interview about the difficulty of reconciling an itinerant mode of living and regular treatment: 'We was three months without coming, I was pleased 'cos we can move' (Lila, 5.10.05). During this consultation, the paediatrician alluded to 'physio' problems, because physiotherapists in general refuse to go out to caravans and the parents have to take Kevin to their office every day. From her perspective as a health professional, she disapproves of caravan living, as expressed in another consultation: 'He [Kevin] doesn't have his own room, that's the problem... . If you didn't live in the caravan, you'd shut the door'. Moreover, although she takes the social and financial problem linked to benefits into account, she can obviously not resolve it herself. During another consultation, somewhat irritated, she replied to Lila that the social worker was in the office next door and that it was her job to deal with this. What transpires in this excerpt is the gap between the means available in terms of psychological care provision and those available in terms of social aid, and I will come back to this. The consultation continued with Kevin's care proper:

After an exchange concerning an allergy to an antibiotic, Lila asks what she should do with some paperwork that she has received. The paediatrician explains that there are examinations to be carried out and that the documents have to be sent back to the CAF. Then she asks if Kevin is eating well because he has lost a little weight, but she reassures the mother who is worried about this and tells her not to fixate on the question of weight. She also asks if Kevin coughs, checks whether Kevin has been taking the medication to help with digestion, that he does not like taking, and asks about stool frequency. The father notes:
'He's really difficult' (Micha).
'You have to set boundaries. No means no' (Paediatrician 11).
'For sleeping, it's a problem, we have to put him in the [our] bed until 2 [in the morning]' (Lila).
'... Parents sleep in one bed, children in another. Otherwise, you're going to have huge problems with this child. ... You have to set limits for him. It's going to be a huge problem, he's sick, he won't want to be treated. He'll make your lives impossible – he has a chronic illness, all children refuse treatment – if you don't manage to impose daily constraints. ... I do know that for you the child is a little emperor, it's cultural' (Paediatrician 11, Observation 19.1.05).

The paediatrician tries to take culture into account, or rather the somewhat generalized knowledge she has about her patients' culture ('for you, the child is a little emperor', or at another moment 'For you, the grandmother's role is very important'). The rest of the consultation shows that, unlike other families, the parents are encouraged to put their child in a day nursery as the health care workers consider that the need to play with other children is more important than the risk of infection. Given that the child is in good health overall, a quality life in his case means removing him from in front of the television and getting him to play and go out. However his mother, obsessed with the question of his weight, thinks that he might lose weight if he plays outside. More generally, most of the consultation was geared towards educating the young parents, as it were, about educating their child. It is true that while Kevin was sometimes agitated in consultations, as the months went by he seemed to watch less television, play more and be calmer. This raises the implicit question of the relationship between health and education, which is even more obvious within paediatrics than in other specialities. The paediatrician established a link between the two through the issue of refusal of treatment ('it's going to be a huge problem, he won't want to be treated') and this is illustrated by the difficulty encountered in administering his digestion medicine. She is well acquainted with the problems linked to refusal of treatment as children grow older. Similarly, in another consultation, she explained that Kevin should not be given too much sugar or too many sweets (Lila puts five sugars in his bottle) if only to protect his teeth. Nevertheless, the link between health and lifestyle is sometimes more ambiguous and it is the parents' youth that accentuates this confusion. A certain shift between quality life and lifestyle can be observed. And in fact Lila explained in an interview that she had trouble accepting medical interference in her conception of education:

> I think that everyone raises children their way. ... I'd gave Kevin sweets, I was told: 'No,... you mustn't give him sweets, you have to give him bread instead'. If Kevin wants to eat sweets, well I think that ... . Ok, so you have to do physio, all right. And yeah, he should eat fatty foods, lots of salt, lots of vitamins, I mean yeah ok, all of that it's true, but ... if Kevin wants to stick his tongue out ... and even if Kevin wants to leave the telly on. We don't live like you and so you don't live like us. ... Some people'll put their children to sleep at eight o'clock and others it's ten o'clock ... . It's that too, I think it's too much (Lila, 5.10.05).

Here Lila outlines what, in her opinion, falls under the rubric of health (doing physio, eating fatty foods, vitamins, etc.) and what falls under education (eating sweets, watching television, sticking his tongue out, etc.) and clearly separates the two.

As for Mariana, one of the grandmothers, she makes it a point of honour to explain how she follows the doctor's instructions meticulously, contrary to the preconceptions she assumes – probably accurately – that the health care workers harbour. However, she also said in an interview: 'When we go see the doctor I tell you, sometimes, he says stuff to us in medical term, and then honest I tell you I don't understand. I tell you sometimes we don't understand the word, speak to us straight up, honest' (Mariana, 5.10.05).

Likewise, in an interview Lila made it a point of honour to describe how she cleans the caravan, from top to bottom every morning and the nurse and paediatrician confirmed this. However, the fact remains that the family tends to be tempted to travel far from the town centre and that it is cold in the caravan during winter. Moreover, the parents and grandparents do not have the educational resources to follow all the ins and outs of medical treatment. And, as expected, studies have shown that a low level of literacy is directly or indirectly linked with unfavourable consequences in terms of health (Nutbeam 2008). From a Bourdieusian perspective (Bourdieu 1984), Kevin's family enjoys reduced cultural capital, if we take this to mean the knowledge that can be called upon to face the disease. On the other hand, his family capital (affective or material support in face of the illness) is solid, constituting a form of capital linked to culture and tradition. In short, the family's itinerant lifestyle, the lack of creature comforts, the parents' minimal medical knowledge and various other factors will all have a negative impact on Kevin's life as a patient.

These examples feed into the new attention that is now paid to social inequalities in health and present two interesting features. First, unlike in other studies that rely on identifying socioprofessional categories without any mention of origin (Leclerc et al. 2000), they link socioeconomic, educational and housing concerns with the origin of the individuals in question. Ali's night job and a certain professional downgrade due to having left Algeria contribute to Josée chronic fatigue. The question of housing, which should be linked to the substantial level of poor housing in France, is also crucial in both families. These elements reinforce the idea that the structural and political context of the social world of chronic diseases is crucial for a quality life, and all the more so in a context of rising social inequality (Leclerc et al. 2000). Second, these examples shed a different light on the stakes of medical genetics from those usually identified. What is of interest here is not how the disease is produced (it is genetic) nor its consequences in terms of mortality (the children are very young), but the intermediary process concerning the current and future lives of these children. On the one hand, biomedical technology provides equal access to diagnosis through screening, but on the other the treatment rationale reaches its limits when it comes up against people's living conditions. And yet public health discourse tends to focus on unequal access to health care, neglecting hygiene, living conditions, etc. (Aïach and Cèbe 1994). This kind of analysis can counterbalance such a restrictive notion. Finally, my last remark relates to the social and the mental, broadly speaking. In the paediatric and genetics services in which I carried out my study, no less than five psychiatrists and psychologists were employed whereas only one part-time social worker was present. My intention is in no way to undermine the contribution of the former, given how difficult the disease can be in certain cases, but rather to point out this imbalance and attempt to analyze it. For Patrice Pinell (2004b), paediatrics is the sector of somatic medicine that is most open to different 'psychological' approaches. For my part, I would add that here it is as if material conditions were not as important in life as psychological ones. Is mental life more important in providing a quality life than economical and social life? Robert Castel (1991) has analyzed how the medical influence in terms of mental and psychological health has extended within society. In parallel, other authors have underlined the disintegration, or even death, of the social, particularly in Anglo-Saxon countries following attacks on the welfare state (Rose 1996). The phenomenon is therefore more general and extends beyond what can be observed within the paediatric space. In any case, the limitations of societal understanding of the impact of living conditions on patients' lives should be underlined.

This study in a screening and health care centre has allowed us 'to investigate how local medical worlds – including those of biomedicine – formulate and respond to illness, comprehend aspects of reality, produce distinctive forms of medical knowledge and shape a crucial dimension of medical experience' (Good 1994: 177). The following elements, presented above, were drawn from the space of consultations to offer ways of analyzing patients' lives: the need to preserve biological life, without completely forgetting social relationships; the creation of social groups on genetic and infectious grounds; the way the 'other' sick person is kept at bay; and the considerable attention paid to mental life, unlike that paid to living conditions.

This part of my study therefore offers a different perspective on the results developed thus far throughout this book. The emotions aroused by the differences in life expectancy and deaths of patients were discussed in the context of how evidence was constructed, but here they take on a sadly more concrete resonance. And the clinicians' arguments in favour of screening ('you don't know what it's like to see people come in with kids age 4, 5 [that are not being monitored/ treated]'), analyzed previously in terms of government oriented towards patients, are also based on what was seen in these observations. The cases examined here also further illustrate the uncertainty and variability of the disease, in terms of biological criteria, sometimes within the same family. And yet the arguments put forward by NSCF's greatest sceptics also find support here. The risks of infection at the hospital, which were not really anticipated in the first discussions about screening, prove to be a very real issue. And they give rise to tensions due to cross-infection, thus leading us far away from the 'biosociality' of the patient organizations. Moreover, other invisible, or less visible, issues come to light, such as health inequalities not in terms of access to care but rather in terms of living conditions. Far from simply being counterpoints to the previous data, these observations offer a more nuanced perspective on this research and reveal aspects that were not sufficiently brought out during interviews. And they do this by giving a less theoretical existence to the illness and by approaching more closely the daily lives of health professionals often confronted with sensitive situations. My observations also clarify the difficulties facing clinicians in their work as well as their 'point of view' in the literal sense. The contribution made here, albeit imperfect and partial, is that of a more accurate understanding of the stakes and effects of screening. Now we shall turn to another dimension to patients' lives, related to time, and to the link between newborn screening and prenatal diagnosis.

Chapter 6

Maintaining a
Quality Life

So far, I have examined different dimensions to the efforts deployed to treat children screened with CF. I shall now turn to another aspect of what I previously suggested calling the aim of a 'quality life'. On the one hand, we have a morally consensual policy, focused on the suffering child, and on the other, more controversial practices, focused on foetal selection. This chapter will analyze how the relationship between the two is dealt with in the field.

The conjunction between the lives of sick people and the issue of prenatal diagnosis makes it possible to bring together two social science research traditions. The first concerns reproductive health or what is at stake in genetic techniques, while the second concerns the experience of illness and policies for handicapped persons, with variants in the latter regarding treatment for the sick and the social integration of handicapped persons as such. A small number of studies have attempted to combine these questions, either in terms of the 'disability rights' critique of prenatal diagnosis and possible responses to that critique (Parens and Asch 2000), tension between the biomedical potential to both screen out imperfect lives and to enable people with significant disabilities to survive and flourish (Rapp and Ginsburg 2001, 2003), later reproductive choices of parents with a handicapped child (Kelly 2009), comparative social history of the areas in which perinatal medicine intervenes and social policies around disability (Ville 2011), or the question of whether newborn screening for and prenatal diagnosis of metabolic diseases are converging or diverging (Buchbinder and Timmermans 2011). The idea informing many of these texts is that there is tension between including handicapped persons in society and excluding disease-affected foetuses, or at least that the two actions reflect contradictory viewpoints. Moreover, most of these authors do not seem to wish to directly address *the question of how prenatal diagnosis connects with the lives of sick people understood as subjects of treatment*; in any case they have not developed methodological means for addressing that question. My analysis here was designed to focus on just that question and to determine what it can tell us about the value of life.

Beyond different professional practices, we will see how these two approaches, before and after birth, are either interlinked or opposed and how they can converge overall. We will also see how the idea of early treatment, and the question of timeframe more broadly, bring this link into play. Finally, the conclusion to this chapter will suggest a way of characterizing these practices.

Gaining Time and Passing Time

As we have seen previously, one of the overriding arguments in favour of deciding upon NSCF related to the idea of early treatment and therefore to the notion of timeframe. However, the timeframe in question was that of the doctors. Here, within the context of actual practice, the timeframe we will see is just as much that of the parents as of the doctors. It is a question of showing how the question of a quality life for CF patients presupposes that the medical timeframe be taken into account. More specifically, I will show the role played by timeframe in the conditions for diagnosis, in telling parents about the disease and in alerting parents to its possibility (in cases of false positives).[1]

Reading through the various quotations in this book, the reader will perhaps already have noticed that 'quality of life' was mentioned as a theme in most of the documents justifying NSCF and *early* care provision. An example of this can be seen in this excerpt from the leaflet given to parents in the maternity unit: 'With early and rigorous care, the frequency of clinical manifestations can be substantially reduced. This enables the patient to have a better quality of life, even though there is no specific treatment which can cure the disease' (AFDPHE 2001b). This phrase was taken up again in the press release concerning the announcement of NSCF being launched by the AFDPHE and the Cnamts: 'It is important to screen [for CF] as early as possible, to improve the quality of life of the children who are screened with the disease and increase their life expectancy'. Many other examples could also be given.

As for the parents of children screened as sick, when I asked them about their opinion on newborn screening in interviews, they were unanimously strongly in favour. These parents did not express the desire, described by Rachel Grob (2008) regarding NSCF in the United States, for screening to be delayed by two or three months in order to preserve the early moments of bonding with the baby. Given that what they have to say overlaps with examples that I have already given, I will simply offer a summary here. In short, the most frequent argument in favour of screening regards time gained. Sometimes the parents bring this argument up again by comparing their situation with the situation faced by parents they have met whose children were diagnosed much later, although they do not know what the future holds for their own (screened) child at the same age. The second main argument relates to avoiding suffering and medical complications, while the third refers to understanding the situation. These themes recall those seen and analyzed previously – during the field study about consent in maternity units (knowing, receiving care early on) and among the Breton clinicians' arguments for screening in the 1980s (screening early, directing children towards suitable centres, avoiding serial misdiagnosis). For parents and health care workers alike, maintaining a quality life therefore means above all 'knowing' and receiving care at an *early*

---

1   I will not look at the timeframe of treatment here, as this would fall under observations in the home.

stage. However, if we look more closely, we can see that two different practices are combined here – screening itself and care provision. This is unsurprising given how closely they are linked in France, which is not the case in other countries. Nonetheless, I shall try to separate them somewhat artificially so as to better understand what they entail.

Understanding the effect of newborn screening alone, independently from care provision in specialist centres, is a complicated matter. It is difficult to know what would have happened to children who screened positive, and more generally what their lives would have been like, had screening not existed. However, an example taken from my field study can offer a way of better understanding the value of screening itself.

With three children already at home, Jules' mother decided to leave her job as a leader in a centre for children's extra-curricular activities before he was born. Her husband is unemployed and used to run a small shop. From the very beginning in the maternity unit, the health care workers realized that Jules was gaining little weight. But the mother left the maternity unit in the normal fashion, insisting on going home to look after her other children. The town paediatrician, whom she consulted shortly after, assured her that she could go on holiday with little Jules. Jules was tired, not gaining weight, bringing up his milk and generally not very well, but his mother was not the anxious type and did not realize any of this. When the screening results showed the suspicion of illness, the health care centre tried to contact the family to call them in for a sweat test, but the mother, away on holiday, could not be reached. The paediatrician finally managed to get in contact and the child was taken into hospital at the age of two months, already undernourished and anaemic. After two and a half months in hospital, Jules had gained weight and was much better. At this time, the paediatrician said of him: 'We saw him completely transform'. Screening was useful in this case because of the combination of several factors: a child with health problems right from birth, a mother and paediatrician who were not particularly anxious, and the holiday away. It was because of screening that Jules was called back and given the appropriate diet before his health deteriorated further. For Jules, the benefits of screening *in itself* are clear. The fact that diagnosis took place so quickly has allowed him to live the best life possible so far. However, for most children diagnosed through screening, more than screening itself, it is the early and appropriate care provided that constitutes one of the conditions for a quality life. So let us shift our focus to this question of care provision.

Based on the consultations I observed, the parents of children screened with the disease had positive, even laudatory, opinions about the care provided, particularly regarding the paediatrician (it should be noted that this field study did not concern treatment provided during hospital stays for courses of antibiotics or when children's conditions worsened). Parents highlighted the paediatrician's level of involvement and the time she spent with them and their child, sometimes setting her apart from other, more conflictual, relationships with different health care workers, interns, etc. For example, during the following interview:

> I like her [Doctor X] a lot. ... [When the illness was confirmed], she said to her
> nurses: 'Listen, cancel everything I have upstairs, I'm going to spend a lot of
> time with the parents, we have to talk'. ... She really took her time with us, she
> explained lots of things to us over and over. She really looked after us for a while
> (Corinne, 8.7.05).

Pushing this a little to the extreme, one could say that the paediatrician's
involvement in the quality life of her patients extends to include her own life.
The parents do not hesitate to phone her early in the morning or in the evening
for emergencies, which can sometimes lead to tensions in consultations:

> One mother protests during a consultation:
> 'Last time, ... you saw her in a real rush, your meeting was more important than
> [my child]' (Isabelle).
> 'I have appointments until 9 p.m., I was here at 6 a.m., I'm a human being'
> (Paediatrician 11).
> Finally, shortly after, the mother apologizes. The paediatrician replies:
> 'I'm too available. I had a phone call at 7 in the morning [from the mother of
> a sick child], I'm seen as an object, it's unbearable for me' (Paediatrician 11,
> Observation 16.2.05).

Another paediatrician explained in an interview that looking after patients
with this disease is a time-consuming and difficult task: they require time for
treatment, discussion and explanations. This recalls the remark made by one
of the Breton paediatricians, who said that health care workers 'put [their]
heart and soul' into treating CF sufferers. However, we should not draw too
idealized a picture either. One of the parents gave a more nuanced opinion when
he said the hospital turned into a 'factory'. While care provision is considered
to be good, particularly at the beginning, the affluence of patients restricts the
amount of time that can be spent with each one. Nonetheless, the fact remains
that what these parents praise (and sometimes demand) in these interviews is
the early care provided but also the availability of the carers, the time they
spend explaining, listening and treating. In short, the waiting time for diagnosis
and care provision should be short, but the time devoted to care should be
sufficiently long for them not to feel as if they are in 'a factory' or being seen 'in
a rush'. Two timeframes collide here: the short timeframe in which diagnosis
and care provision occur, and the longer timeframe devoted to explanations.
These two timeframes are also at the heart of the procedure for breaking the
news of the NSCF diagnosis.

Breaking the News

When a serious illness is announced, the people concerned often suffer a shift
leading to 'the unmaking of the world' (Scarry 1985). Health care workers consider

that the moment at which parents are told about the CF diagnosis is one that they remember the most throughout the whole trajectory of the disease. The issue in question is of course extremely serious, because it means telling parents their child will have the life of a sick person and, moreover, a life that will probably be curtailed. A questionnaire study carried out by psychologists and doctors has shown that during the consultation in which they are told, more than 80% of parents think: 'My child won't live as long as the others' (Gueganton, Rault and De Braekeleer 2004). It is therefore definitely the child's future, in terms of both length and quality, that is at stake. Consequently, how are these life prospects announced and what role do timeframes play in how the news is broken?

Paediatricians are well aware of the specific nature of giving a diagnosis after newborn screening. As they explain in interviews, the diagnosis does not come in response to parents actively seeking a doctor's opinion to answer the question: 'What is wrong with my child?' More often than not, these parents are happy and busy with their newborn, or at least far from thinking about illness. In this situation, they have not been called upon as subjects, except through the consent they gave in the maternity units and we have already seen that this remains partial. This is linked to how soon diagnosis is made after screening in NSCF (the child is only one and a half months old) and the fact that the baby often has no symptoms. One of the usual stages in the trajectory of an illness, the 'pre-diagnosis' stage to paraphrase Anselm Strauss, disappears. Under these conditions, learning about the illness can only be even more brutal, a real 'bombshell' as one of the paediatricians put it. The parents use similar words on the subject, employing expressions such as 'a huge blow', and the shock is exacerbated by the discrepancy with the child's seemingly good state of health. During one consultation, a mother said: 'It's hard to take in news like this, when he's well'. In other words, the experience of apparent good health clashes with the illness that is being announced. The child's identity changes and the results of screening mark the end of the experience of being the parents of 'normal' children and the beginning of a life as parents of sick children (Grob 2008). As with other kinds of screening (Kaufert 2000), a certain innocence is lost and the people involved are made aware that their child's body will be different to how they imagined it.

On another hand, while the parents are often completely out of step with any diagnosis made, on the day of the consultation every effort is made to make the news less hard to bear and to prepare them for the care programme that will follow. The procedure for giving this news is the result of reflection on the part of the health care workers and is almost a protocol. We should remember here the words of the father in Brittany who was particularly shocked by the way in which he was told about his child's illness years before: a doctor had told him in a corridor that his son had a 'defect' and the disease was the cystic fibrosis of the pancreas [former name of CF]. Things have changed substantially since then as evidenced by the interviews I carried out with the parents of children diagnosed through screening, who recounted the day of the positive sweat test and the moment they were told about the disease:

> We were seen by doctor [X] who first of all asked us questions, talked about
> our families, our jobs, our genotypes, but we didn't know where she was going
> with this. And then after an hour, an hour and a half, she explained that it was an
> imbalance in the pancreas. We had tests done, including sweat and blood tests,
> ... she explained us what it was, how we should already have hygiene rules,
> what we were going to do about medication, milk. ... She led us very gently,
> very intelligently, with a lot of sensitivity, to cystic fibrosis. ... We arrived at
> 11.30 a.m., it was 5 in the afternoon when we left (Michèle, 26.11.04).

The information given is controlled and the different people involved (paediatrician,
nurse, psychologist) are all present. However, this subtle and well-oiled procedure
can also fail when, for one reason or another, the news is not given by the CRCM.
Of the six families of children screened with the disease that I encountered during
my field study, three families did not go through this linear process in which the
disease is diagnosed and then announced.

The first family who received the news in a different way were Kevin, Lila and
Micha. As the parents did not have a fixed address, the letter was sent to them in
Marseille, in the South of France, through an association. And one day, a doctor
from the association telephoned Lila advising her to take Kevin to the nearest
hospital, while reassuring her that it was not serious. The family therefore went
to a small hospital in the North of France and met with a doctor. This is how Lila
described what happened next in an interview:

> So in the end, I seen a doctor from that hospital. 'No, no, no' he says, 'We
> can't tell you [what is wrong with Kevin]. I says 'Why?' [He said:] 'It's too
> serious. We can't even tell you what it is, what it comes from'. I says: 'Mister, I
> don't understand nothing, I says what is it, this illness?' [He said:] 'No no no, I
> won't tell you'... . So I don't even know what's attacking at him, I didn't know
> nothing. They didn't want to tell me. ... They said: 'Go to the hospital in [X]
> [large town]'. So I was like a whole week without knowing what it was, without
> knowing what's attacking at him. So it was like... really really scared (Lila,
> 5.10.05).

So in one small hospital, a doctor can tell a mother who has just given birth that
her child is suffering from an illness that is too serious for him to tell her what
it is. The mother waits for an appointment at the nearest CRCM in order to get
the information about the disease. For her, the timeframe of the verdict about the
child's future life is therefore much longer. This situation is both rare, because it
concerns a family of travellers, and informative, because it sheds light on how
unprepared and even tactless some health care workers can be in this respect.
Nevertheless, the situation remains close to that of other screened children insofar
as the screening protocol in itself worked and was only disrupted by issues related
to addresses and the post. Conversely, the other two families who did not hear the
news through the planned route were in situations where screening did not work

or did not apply. These examples reveal the problems that can arise when there is no protocol for giving this news, which was the norm before screening existed.

The second family was a case of a false negative screening result. These cases are few and far between – they represent around 3% of patients screened – but they are interesting in that they can shed light on symptom-based diagnosis. Bruno and Annick are the parents of little Céline. Bruno left his job as an office worker when Céline was diagnosed and Annick is an executive assistant. Despite a few abnormal signs during pregnancy (a black mark on the intestine), the baby was born without problems. Newborn screening was carried out in the usual routine fashion and the parents heard nothing back about it. But as soon as Céline left the maternity unit, she did not gain enough weight. After what the doctors believed was a milk allergy, she went into hospital for three weeks. Once home again, despite large bottles, she was still not gaining enough weight and her stools were oily and odorous. Alerted by someone from *Protection Maternelle et Infantile* (Mother and Infant Protection),[2] the parents took her to casualty. She went into hospital for four weeks, in an establishment that did not specialize in the disease, and was fed for three days by a gastric tube in her nose, which was understandably a real ordeal for the parents. A series of tests were carried out and they did include CF, although the health professionals were sceptical on this count because of the negative screening result. And yet two sweat tests proved positive and a sample was sent to a specialized centre for confirmation. Bruno explained in an interview how vague the information given to the parents was at this time:

> There was a young intern there, who didn't really know what to say because honestly he didn't really know anything about it. Even the nurses didn't know anything about it, they had never had any cases. ... So no one talked to us about it. The only one who knew anything about it, and even then, with hindsight, I know she ... made technical mistakes in telling us certain things about the disease that aren't true – [was Professor [Y]]. So even Professor [Y] wasn't a specialist in cystic fibrosis, there's no getting away from it (Bruno, 10.5.05).

Beyond the lack of information, the health care workers' lack of tact was also mentioned through the following anecdote:

> One day, we knew absolutely nothing, but straightaway the Professor [Y] asked for a physio to come by. ... We were talking, [the physio] says to us: '... Don't worry ... people who have cystic fibrosis, I treat some, young adults, and they don't regret the life they've had at all'... So we said: 'Sorry, what do you mean, young adults and they don't regret the life they've had?'... She said to us: 'What you have to know is that people who suffer from cystic fibrosis do have a much shorter life expectancy'. Well, I just can't tell you what effect that had on us. ...

2　The PMI, as the names suggests, is a system in place to protect mother and child, created in France at the end of the Second World War.

> So then we had a really big shock… . Of course, we would have found things
> out later, but maybe a different way, or maybe there is no way, I don't know. At
> any rate, it was rough (Bruno, 10.5.05).

Shortly after, the parents were seen at the CRCM, the diagnosis was confirmed and
the treatment protocol was put in place. A month later, a 'pseudo' infection was
found during an examination. The CRCM paediatrician ascribed this particularly
persistent infection to the stay in the non-specialist hospital. Nonetheless, Céline
was developing correctly, gaining weight and seemed, at least for the time being, to
be out of the woods. This example illustrates both a screening error (a false negative)
and, implicitly, the value of the procedure for telling parents about the disease that
is linked to screening, even though, as Bruno said, this is obviously always difficult
news to take in. Without functional screening, the wait for diagnosis takes longer
and then the news is broken in far too brief a manner: this is precisely the opposite of
what health care workers recommend. When formulated in terms of life prospects,
the information being given is dismal and particularly abrupt.

My study revealed another example in which screening did not play its role in
how the news about a life of illness was broken to the parents. This case concerned
a young girl who had an intestinal obstruction and nearly died in the days following
her birth (in roughly 10% of patients, CF leads to an intestinal obstruction at birth,
that doctors call 'meconium ileus'). I shall not go into the details of her case here,
for reasons of brevity. To summarize, this baby, whose first weeks of life were so
turbulent and filled with serious treatment, slipped by the screening process due
to more urgent medical interventions. In such a dramatic situation, the news was
broken in different stages (during the turmoil of treatment in a corridor in the
middle of the night, then by information given another evening, and then abruptly
on the day of the consultation). The timeframe was short, in the first instance. The
explanations came later, when the diagnosis was confirmed and the paediatrician
specializing in CF was brought into the treatment plan.

Two comments can be made as this section draws to a close. In the context of
traditional sociology of chronic disease, waiting for a consensus on the cause of a
health problem can be a long and progressive process, in which the patient plays
an active role by largely directing the doctor's diagnostic work (Baszanger 1986).
There are even strategies of delay in which the doctors puts off diagnosis with a
view to reducing the risk of misdiagnosis, waiting until giving the bad news and
making it easier both to communicate with the family and for them to adapt. In the
case of NSCF, this slow process is usually disrupted. There is no real 'negotiated
order' between doctor and families because there is no moment at which the
patients (or in this case, the parents) 'feel that their participation in diagnosis is
essential' (Baszanger 1986). Conversely, the timeframe in which the news is given
is diluted to make what is being said about life prospects more bearable for the
parents. During my field study, however, in three out of six cases, the screening
process did not play its usual role and the child's life prospects were presented in
a particularly brutal fashion. Finally, the last comment to be made here concerns

the effects of this compressed timeframe on the identity of the child screened as ill. Rachel Grob (2008) presented a study carried out on the basis of interviews in the United States on the experiences of parents of children suffering from CF who were screened at birth, in comparison with those of parents of children diagnosed from symptoms. The study shows in particular that screening orients the parents' role around the disease and changes the early relationship between parents and child, by placing the illness at the centre of their bond with the child. I should add that there is not yet enough hindsight to know what will happen later; it remains possible that such differences will fade away over time. At any rate, it would seem that during the initial months, the parent-child relationship is not built in the same way if the diagnosis is established at birth or if it is established later. And this remark will become important for the next stages of my study.

Outside the Illness, Looking in

Having looked at the moment at which the news is broken, this part of the chapter will now focus on the period during which parents are alerted to a potential problem. This concerns families who stay in screening 'limbo' but remain outside the illness itself. From a more factual perspective, we see this situation when families are initially alarmed by being called in for a sweat test and then reassured. In such cases, parents are alerted to an 'intangible threat of possible future calamity' (Rose 1985: 35). As with being told about the diagnosis, the issue at stake is substantial: the results determine whether or not these tiny children will enter into a life of sickness. In this section, I shall examine how the threat facing a quality life is approached, rather than the actual news being broken, and I will look at the impact of timeframe on this, particularly in terms of the issue of 'worrying' versus 'reassuring'. Three main points will be broached: the tight management of time, the parents' worry and the medical space in which this diagnostic test takes place.

On a quantitative level, between 2002 and 2004, the sweat tests resulting from NSCF concerned more than 1,000 families per year. And yet 85% of these tests were negative and this illustrates one of the disadvantages of these treatment efforts (that is, the initial false positives that occur). Due to the changes in thresholds and in the screening flow chart that we saw at the beginning of the field study, this number was substantially lowered from 2005 onwards, leading to few false positives in the end. On a practical level, I have already outlined the stages of screening: the IRT assay, the search for mutations, potentially a second IRT assay and the sweat test, which is the diagnostic test. As we saw, screening is often forgotten about by parents in maternity units, due to its routine nature among numerous other practices. When the parents are contacted again because a second IRT assay is necessary and/or because they need to have a sweat test carried out, the least we can say is that this does not go unnoticed. I observed six sweat tests in order to compare these with the six families whose children were screened positive (therefore studying 12 families in all). Out of these six sweat tests, two followed on from new IRT assays and four were carried out after a mutation had been detected (the reason for specifying this will become clear later).

First, health care workers manage time very tightly between the call back and the result of the sweat test – during what we could therefore call the period of alert. It is a question of not keeping parents in this difficult limbo, filled with worry (and often anxiety, even terror), uncertainty and the only partly reassuring words of the professionals. Initially, all these parents are called back urgently to the hospital for a sweat test, either the same day or, more often, the next day. They therefore receive a phone call from the paediatrician out of the blue. And these paediatricians find themselves in an ambiguous position: on the one hand, they are calling the parents to come in urgently for a 'trypsin test', and on the other, they want to be reassuring. They try to avoid mentioning the term CF, unless the parents are very insistent. The letter that the parents also receive on top of the phone call is along the same lines. On the one hand, it is stamped 'Urgent', which is not insignificant for the parents, and, on the other, it shows the same verbal discretion in avoiding the term 'cystic fibrosis'. This is because during this period of alert, every word takes on great resonance given what is at stake. While historically the clinic has called upon the metaphor of the 'alphabetical structure' of disease, in other words while a disease could be assimilated to a name composed of the 'letters' that were the different symptoms (Foucault 2003), here it is a question of not saying the name of the disease, because it has not yet assembled its 'alphabet'. These verbal precautions are not always enough, however. Indeed, out of the six families I studied, three identified the disease in question, either by finding specific information about the paediatrician's work on the Internet, or because the letter was signed by a paediatrician in the 'cystic fibrosis' category of the headed notepaper. And in fact, after the end of my study, the health professionals decided to no longer send this letter and simply use the telephone call to ask parents to come in, once again due to problems of timeframe: the parents either received the letter too late (after the sweat test) or too soon (several days before). Above and beyond the various more or less successful tactics used by health care workers to reduce the anxiety generated, let us look at how the parents experience this.

The short time between the child being born and the sweat test obviously leads to a certain element of surprise, already mentioned in relation to when the news is broken. Here is an example of a mother's point of view, taken from an interview:

> It's one of those things that you just don't expect at all, to get a phone call like that out of nowhere, in middle of everything else, it's really destabilizing. Bearing in mind that the appointment was the next day, I think, … it's really abrupt, to be told that (Catherine, 21.9.05).

Most testimonies make an explicit or implicit link between the routine nature of screening in the maternity unit and the fact that they are not informed about these possible further tests. And the field study that I discussed previously, carried out in the maternity units, confirmed this lack of information.

Second, parental concern and anxiety is predictably the main and common factor in this experience. More specifically, two types emerge in these examples – immediate worry and what we could call secondary or delayed worry. This interview excerpt illustrates the first type:

> [Professor X] told us [on the telephone] that other tests had to be done, that it was important. And so he offered us an appointment … . And when we said it was a bit tight, if we could push it back, he said to us: 'No no no, it's better to come now', in a very nice, calm, reassuring tone (Perrine).
> Saying above all that it wasn't serious (Luc).
> Yes, but that we had to come. So in our heads, … you can't change the appointment, so it has to be really serious … . The world fell apart in a few seconds. … It didn't mean Nicolas was ill, I know he told us that, but we had to come now. I think it was the whole now, urgent, thing that made us more anxious (Perrine, 15.7.05).

There is no doubt about the effect ('more anxious', etc.) wherein the urgency of the matter is very important, despite the paediatrician's precautions. This worry can also sometimes last even longer. Some of the things the biochemist carrying out the sweat test had to say also illustrated the issue of tight time management during the period of concern. While performing the test, she often alluded to the babies' weight, which she linked to the technical possibility of the test. In doing so, she explained that she had seen many cases where the three-week-old baby was too small for a proper sample to be taken. In these cases, the families are called back later and left in complete uncertainty. We can see here one of the limitations placed on reducing time: the aim is to act as quickly as possible so as not to leave parents with uncertainty, but the baby is sometimes so small that the sweat test is not possible and the family does end up left in a state of anxiety for longer. Moreover, when the biochemist finished the test, she would anticipate the result – at this point every minute counts – and relieve the parents of some of their fear by telling them that the result was 'reassuring', even if she took care to specify that the paediatrician would need to confirm this. In most cases (usually the same day or later if the baby is too small), the parents' relief came during the second consultation with the paediatrician following up on the sweat test. The paediatrician then used words aiming to lift any possible ambiguity: the level of categorical refutation is as high as the fears that preceded it. For instance, in the following observations:

> Forget about me, … it's over, over (Paediatrician 14, Observation 31.05.05).
> Everything is normal, this formally excludes cystic fibrosis … . You can go home with your minds at ease … she doesn't have cystic fibrosis, it's absolutely certain (Paediatrician 14, Observation 12.7.05).

Here the paediatrician seeks to push the family out of his sphere of intervention, because it is associated with CF. He also looks to erase any persistent worry, that we could call secondary. In three cases (including the two mothers of children without mutations), this attitude worked efficiently, because all the mothers' doubts and fears had lifted at the end of the day, as they explained in interviews. When the child does not have a mutation and has a normal sweat test, the paediatricians completely reassure the parents and the situation is simple. When the child has a mutation (and is a so-called heterozygote) and a normal sweat test paediatricians also reassure parents but the situation is slightly more complicated. First, the parents receive a letter of conclusions and its phrasing might seem somewhat strange, as it reads: 'The sweat test has detected a chloride level of [X]mEq/l, which is perfectly normal. In principle, your child therefore does not have cystic fibrosis'. In the increasingly litigious context already mentioned, this legally cautious expression 'in principle' can be explained by the fact that the risk of disease is extremely low, but not nil. This expression can raise doubts once again, as it could seem to mean 'at first glance', as shown in the following interview:

> I received a letter that he said: 'In principle, your child does not have cystic fibrosis'. So then I jumped up again and called him [the paediatrician] saying 'But why do you say "in principle"? You said she didn't have cystic fibrosis'. He said: 'No no, she won't have cystic fibrosis'. 'So why do you put in principle?' And he said to me: 'No no, she 100% won't have cystic fibrosis' (Laurence, 22.9.05).

Another element responsible for confusing the issue lies in the fact that the idea of being a heterozygote can leave its mark on parents, no matter how clear or affirmative the doctors are. In two of the three families I studied with a heterozygote child, this notion instilled doubt as evidenced by this interview with a mother:

> It's silly, but if he has a little cold, something like that, we still think about it. … Even though we know there's nothing wrong with him, that there won't ever be anything wrong with him, it's still imprinted in our flesh. … Maybe with time I won't think about it anymore, but it's true that right now I'm bound to think about it. And it's not for long, it's three seconds: and what if they got it wrong? … But with me, it's more like something irrational, because I trust what he said to us. But I can't help it (Perrine, 15.7.05).

In these two cases, the mothers take on board and rationalize the information provided by the doctors, but cannot get rid of their doubts. It should be noted that these disruptions do not change the parents' positive opinion of screening, which we saw was unanimous in maternity units. Methodologically speaking, it would be worth carrying out such a study over a longer timeframe, when greater hindsight is possible ('maybe with time I won't think about it anymore'). More generally, a Canadian study has shown that half the people who see a genetic counsellor remain unclear about what it means to be a heterozygote (Mischler et al. 1998). If these results were confirmed by a larger number of families, they would support the questions raised by one of the organizers of newborn screening. She has substantial experience of the problem, both as a former geneticist and as the founder of a support and information group for families. She explained in an interview:

> The real problem is all these parents who panicked for no reason because they were given a result that was suspect, which then proved to be normal. When you tell people something, it stays in their minds. ... They don't forget, it takes absolutely ages. ... As soon as you call a child somewhere because they are suspect ..., it stays in their minds. When you have a heterozygote test, all the heterozygotes, even if their sweat is normal, the parents [say]: 'But are you completely sure?' (Geneticist-Paediatrician 1, 31.1.03).

A third point to mention, which links in with the following section, concerns the medical space in which the sweat test is carried out. Temporally speaking, it takes place just after birth and thus logically combines the approaches and semantic networks of genetics with those of paediatrics. For example, during a consultation prior to the sweat test, the paediatrician begins by looking for small signs or family symptoms in the parents (such as asthma)[3] or the newborn (such as a salty taste when kissing the baby). At this point, the paediatrician is mainly situated in the space of paediatrics or, at least, of the clinic. However, at other moments of the consultations, he changes register. When a mutation has been identified, he explains briefly the risks of transmission as in the following observation: 'She is a carrier, she has one normal gene. One person in 25 within the population is a carrier. ... Maybe she and her partner will consider doing a test when she wants children' (Paediatrician 14, Observation 6.9.05).

And if a mutation is detected in a child, the parents are encouraged to consult a geneticist and they are reminded of this in the letter sent to them after the sweat test. In short, when the sweat test results are reassuring (that is, negative), it is genetics that provides the way out. We can even push this further and say that paediatricians do everything in their power, at the end of consultations, to leave the space of paediatrics. The aim is to calm parents down by assuring them that their children do not need treatment because *they are not ill*. There should be no doubt left in their minds (although this is not always the case, as we have seen). What is interesting here, and I will come back to this in more detail later, is that by identifying the baby as a heterozygote, the paediatrician makes an initial link with prenatal diagnosis.

To summarize, these results show the effect of this threat that looms over a quality life for a while before disappearing. Although delays are always possible

---

3 Heterozygotes with CFTR gene mutations are sometimes prone to developing asthma.

(parents on holiday, lack of sweat, etc.), time is generally reduced as much as possible between birth, potential call-backs, the sweat test and the conclusion. This short timeframe exacerbates the effect of shock and surprise, and further illustrates the effect it can have when the result is positive. Moreover, in the case of CF the combination between 'worrying' and 'reassuring' leads to a mode of communication in which every word is carefully considered, perhaps even more so than in usual clinical medicine. These ambiguities (acting quickly without causing too much worry, giving information but not too much) lie at the intersection of many aims, which are sometimes contradictory: informing people of a disease as early as possible, but without worrying them too much and without worrying too many of them. This protocol and flow chart were conceived and adjusted (with the lowering of thresholds) precisely to reduce anxiety as much as possible. This should be linked with the fact that the worry generated in parents of a child without CF was one of the main arguments levied by the long-standing opponents of NSCF who, much more than the clinicians, geared their mode of government towards the population as a whole. Finally, this part of the study allows us to go back in time, from sick children to birth, following the doctors' rationale of intervening earlier and earlier – a rationale that families also follow. It suggests a link between NSCF and prenatal diagnosis when a heterozygote child is identified and we move from the space of paediatrics and genetics to the space of pure genetics. After having shown how time intervenes in screening practices to pursue this aim of a quality life, let us now look at this issue of the actual link between neonatal and prenatal approaches.

The Impact of Newborn Screening on Prenatal Diagnosis

Genetics is omnipresent in prenatal situations and also important at birth due to its role as a diagnostic tool. However, its limitations are apparent in terms of prognosis and its role recedes over the course of care provision. My observations of paediatric consultations showed that it was relatively rare for the nature of mutations to be mentioned or for genetic techniques and knowledge to be called upon. This can be explained by the absence of correlation between mutations and symptoms, as well as the absence, in the short-term, of therapeutic prospects derived from genetics. However, as we have seen, the notion of transmission remains present in this paediatric space, particularly in the shape of prenatal diagnosis. The aim of this section is to try to understand how the logic of care and of foetal selection combine in the field and are part of the same movement towards maintaining health.

Searching for Good Health and Refusing Ill Health

The reader will recall that one of the arguments for NSCF put forward by the Breton paediatricians and biologists was to avoid families with several children suffering from CF. In this respect, screening allows prenatal diagnosis to be offered in the case of a second pregnancy, or to a related couple, before the first child has begun to show symptoms. Likewise, during my hospital field study, when parents of a sick child wanted to have another baby, the CRCM paediatrician encouraged them to see a geneticist with a view to a possible prenatal diagnosis as attested by the following interview excerpt: 'I told [X (paediatrician)] that I was pregnant and she got an appointment for me right away with the geneticist' (Isabelle, 19.5.05). During my study, three mothers of children screened as sick underwent prenatal diagnosis in the year following newborn screening (the foetuses were all unaffected). With their experience of the illness, which I will come back to later, none of these mothers I encountered envisaged giving birth to another sick child (only one of them expressed hesitations about pregnancy termination for religious reasons). In particular, one of them said in an interview: 'I wouldn't put them through that [I wouldn't put my child through that illness]' (Isabelle, 29.3.05). This shows that the questions regarding the value of a life in which treatment looms so large can arise, given the frequently serious and difficult nature of the disease, as described in the previous chapter. In short, these mothers reflect the fact that, in France, more than 80% of women terminate their pregnancies when CF is detected in the foetus (Agence de la biomédicine 2010).

These practices give rise to little debate among professionals, given how difficult caring for a sick child can be, for both patients and families. Traditionally, the question is problematized in terms of the risk of giving birth to another sick child – a risk that is considered to be high because, for a recessive disease like CF, it is of 25%. For example, one geneticist said in an interview: 'I tell people: you have a high risk of having a pathological pregnancy' (Biologist-Geneticist 1, 2.9.05.). This therefore constitutes a first point of intersection between the neonatal and the prenatal.[4]

Another point of intersection relates to heterozygotes. We have already seen earlier that newborn screening identifies a small percentage (400 to 500 newborns per year) of the population of heterozygous neonates that are born every year. This means that children screened at birth as heterozygous can later request a genetic test when they want to have their own children. Likewise, relatives (uncles, aunts, cousins, etc.) are encouraged to consult a geneticist so as to be able to benefit from prenatal diagnosis should they have an 'at-risk' pregnancy. In this way, a paediatrician said the following during a consultation after a sweat test: 'You should inform your brothers and sisters [that you are a heterozygote and they could be too], you shouldn't adopt the ostrich policy' (Paediatrician 14, Observation 5.4.05). The fact that some heterozygous individuals are identified through newborn screening, albeit in limited numbers, thus induces the possibility of new prenatal diagnoses being carried out in the more or less long-term.

The mothers I interviewed expressed a positive view of these practices relating to heterozygote screening. One of them in particular said: 'It's true that

---

4   This result was also observed in a study concerning newborn screening for metabolic diseases in the United States (Buchbinder and Timmermans 2011).

I find that afterwards you feel uneasy, but it's good to know' (Laurence, 22.9.05). Contrary to the previous case of a second pregnancy following the birth of a first child with the illness, here, for the most part, the families do not have any experience of a child suffering from CF. They do know enough about the illness, however, to consider that information regarding heterozygosity is interesting.

For certain doctors, this practice is seen as positive, as it could allow an increasing number of heterozygotes to be identified in the general population, making more prenatal diagnoses possible and leading, in the end, to the eradication of the disease (this was one of the arguments put forward in the history of screening in Brittany). The following interview excerpt illustrates this:

> If it's well designed, a maximum number of heterozygotes will be identified, so in the end ..., prenatal screening will be offered. ... So we could say to ourselves: treatment for this disease is actually still ... relatively ineffective, so this will be a means ... of eradicating the disease, as it were. ... I think it's a good thing for people ... to be aware of the possible risk of having a child who would be sick (Biologist-Geneticist 1, 28.1.05).

However, most clinicians have a negative perception of identifying heterozygotes, for several reasons. First, the aims of their actions, and indeed the very meaning they ascribe to them, are at stake. Detecting heterozygous individuals is not the same thing as identifying sick people for the purpose of treating them; instead it means detecting a genetic characteristic that may lead to a prenatal test. This shift is likely to cloud the actual aim of the action, as defined by the AFDPHE (diagnosing and providing care to sick children) and to shift health care workers into a sphere that, in their eyes, is darker and detached from its initial target: 'Diagnosing heterozygotes ... is a necessary related consequence that cannot be neglected, but it's a problem. Let's just say it raises questions' (Paediatrician 15, 26.9.05).

Second, they may question how far their own practices are actually or potentially going. As they see it, identifying heterozygous individuals at birth and informing parents could lead to an increasing number being identified and some fear that as the information gets passed from relative to relative, this may lead to mass screening for heterozygotes or 'eugenics': 'We're following a fairly incredible line of logic here, where newborn screening for cystic fibrosis actually amounts to undisclosed mass [prenatal] screening' (Geneticist 3, 29.1.05). These actors therefore raise questions that, although phrased differently, can be linked to the notion of 'flexible eugenics' (Taussig et al. 2005), in other words a form of eugenics arising from the tension between the tendency to normalize foetuses through genetics and the sum of parents' individual choices.

Third, the unexpected consequences of the actions in question can also raise concerns for professionals, linked to the fact that these practices can identify heterozygote children with a mutation classified as mild in principle, who are then likely to ask for genetic counselling as adults. This brings us back to the debate surrounding the issue of the mutations involved in borderline forms of the disease. To summarize, three elements define the ethical concern about professionals' collective practices concerning heterozygotes: the sphere of intervention (acting in the therapeutic domain), the quantitative aspects (keeping genetic counselling to an individual mode) and the qualitative aspects (limiting it to forms of diseases for which it is justified). More than moral subjects, in this case we should refer rather to a 'configuration' of moral subjects, with 'configuration' taken to designate individuals belonging to a community and who are both individually and collectively responsible for actions (Elias 1978).

All these moral questions mean that professionals are showing a great deal of interest in a new technique for NSCF that is currently being studied. This technique, based solely on biochemistry, does not involve DNA testing. It would therefore avoid identifying heterozygotes and potentially reduce the cases in which borderline forms of the disease were identified. We can see here a desire for 'de-genetizication' on the part of paediatricians and the national screening officials, with the wish to modify ethical government by focusing on the suffering child and abandoning the more controversial practices. This remains to be confirmed by the future developments of this technique.

More fundamentally, another aspect through which newborn screening interacts with prenatal diagnosis is linked to the fact that it changes people's thinking on the latter. More specifically, it changes how people see mass screening of pregnant women. At several points in the local field study, doctors explained that after their child was screened positive at birth, certain parents asked why this test was not carried out during pregnancy. In order to fully understand this, it is important to know that in France there is no legal time limit on pregnancy termination for medical reasons, which can be carried out up to term. Thus, in the following interview:

> People get up in arms about the fact that a child is born today with cystic fibrosis: 'How it is possible, doctor, that it wasn't seen to?' ... . In their minds, they confuse newborn screening and eradication. They don't understand why, if there is screening, children are born with cystic fibrosis. ... 'How come, doctor, with all your hype... around genetics, how come we're not able to eradicate the damn illness? ... Is it possible technically?' 'Yes, it's possible' 'Why wasn't that done to me?' ... So here, through this newborn screening for cystic fibrosis, we're giving credit to, we're transmitting, an ideology of much earlier and much broader screening. We're legitimizing an approach of mass screening. ... Given that screening exists, why not prevent the first child from being affected (Geneticist 3, 29.1.05).

This situation does not seem to be specific to the centre where the field study was carried out because, during a national meeting of paediatricians and geneticists involved in CF care provision, a geneticist from the South West of France explained that among couples with one child screened sick, many ask: 'Why wasn't the test done before?' Likewise, in an interview a Breton biologist attested to the fact that a certain number of couples who have given birth to an affected child say: 'But why weren't we told before?' According to the professionals, the link between prenatal and newborn screening is therefore established by parents on different modes: the similarity between the techniques used for both types of screening ('is it possible technically?'), a shift backward in time ('why wasn't the test done before?') or a combination of these two elements. These testimonies are enlightening when it comes to answering the questions outlined in introduction, but they remain reported discourse. Let us now look directly at what the parents themselves have to say.

Of the six families of sick children diagnosed through screening that I observed over time during my study, four brought up the sorts of questions reported by clinicians. A methodological point that should be underlined is that these always came up *spontaneously*, with no prior allusions on my part to prenatal screening. For example, just after her son was screened positive after birth, one mother explained from the very beginning of an interview:

> We lost a lot of time, the parents' choice of bringing a child into the world with cystic fibrosis or not was taken away. ... It's good to do it at birth, ... but it's a shame not to do it before. ... It's true that today I don't regret having my son, but if I'd been able to know before, it's true, at a time when I could have had an abortion legally in France, I think I would have taken that option, yes. You don't want to bring a child into the world today ... who's going to become an adult who will already have a much heavier burden to bear than another. You can live from [with] it, yes, but you're taking away evolution, freedom, from people. ... It's really a huge blow. ... Then, everyone makes their own choice ... . Today [my baby] is here, I love him, he's my child, he's beautiful, he's not even ill, he's not in crisis. ... Having a sick child is quite something (Michèle, 26.11.04).

Another mother of a child screened as sick said in an interview:

> *With newborn screening, the diagnosis didn't take too long? (Me).*
> Yes. I think that's great, I really do. To be honest if on top of that they could do ... just a blood test when a woman's pregnant. ... To look at him... he seems fine, but you know, it's not always easy. If I had to do it over again, let me reassure you, I'd still have this one [she looks at her son]. He's still a great little guy ... . But yes, it's true that it's not easy for him and also for us. ... It's a bit difficult, yes. And it's true that it's always ... you never know. ... It means living from one day to the next all the time (Isabelle, 19.5.05).

When fathers were present during the interviews or observations, they sometimes expressed the same wish, for example:

What do you think about screening for cystic fibrosis at birth? (Me).

There's nothing better. ... It's essential. I don't know why it wasn't done before [slight laughter]. [...] It's good that it's done, but shouldn't it be done before? (Patrick).

Before birth you mean? (Me).

Before birth... . No, it's good, but could it be done better, yes, maybe (Patrick, 19.5.05).

In a less straightforward manner, during an informal discussion with the father and grandmother of another child screened as sick, they said:

I don't know if it would have been possible to take a sample [during pregnancy] (Grandmother 1).

At worst, they'd have said: 'It's cystic fibrosis', I don't know... (Bruno).

It's always pretty much been running through our heads (Grandmother 1).

[Later, he says again, spontaneously] If we'd been told: 'Your child has cystic fibrosis...'... I don't know (Bruno, 22.12.04).

During another informal discussion, his wife said more directly: 'We wondered why they didn't screen all mothers before birth' (Annick, 10.5.05). Likewise, when the question of a possible prenatal diagnosis for a second child was raised in interviews, another father called for generalized screening on all pregnant women:

Personally, I prefer a prenatal test for everyone. ... Why should a child have to be born sick for it to be offered to parents? ... If they was concerned with the child not being born ill, it would be better, it's more a way of avoiding the disease more (Ali).

Anyway, people prefer to have children in good health (Jeanne).

... As soon as she's pregnant, he [the doctor] should offer parents ... to know if they've got the mutation, if there's a chance their child will have the disease. ... When you have a sick child, you have to look after them their whole life. For the social worker, for the parents... . It avoids less of [sic] a load for parents and for medical treatment (Ali, 30.6.05).

Finally, one of the six mothers of a child who screened negative mentioned her questions on this subject just before an interview. In this excerpt, she repeats them:

Before we started, you said to me: 'Why doesn't screening happen before birth?' (Me).

Yes... Whereas now it's true you can't even know it. It's true that you find yourself with a handicapped child, which is already not easy, and then the child isn't happy. You don't have a child for them to be ill, do you? Even if cystic fibrosis isn't a big deal for some people, for me it's huge. A child who can't run, who's out of breath straightaway, it would have been really painful for me... .

> It would be good, I think, if we tried to see if we couldn't detect some diseases before, when the amniocentesis is done (Sylvie, 27.9.05).

First, for a substantial proportion of families (roughly half of families with a child who was screened sick or well), these different excerpts corroborate what the doctors summarized previously. Moreover, we can see the question of time arising once again ('we lost a lot of time', etc.). It is very much as if the concern for early detection that infuses the entire newborn screening process had been extended backward into the prenatal period. And from the moment at which generalized screening is promoted, the issue arises about the kind of life, or future life, the child will have, and how to evaluate this ('an adult who will already have a much heavier burden to carry than another', 'it's very particular kind of life, it's a bit difficult', 'it's not always easy', 'the child isn't happy', etc.). Of course, this question clashes with the love and attachment that the parents feel towards their child ('I don't regret having my son', 'Today [my baby] is here, I love him, he's my child', 'If I had to do it over again, I'd still have this one', 'I don't know…'). And in the last case, where the father cannot bring himself to say something that he probably sees as negating the very existence of his daughter, whom he cares for so attentively, in the end it is his wife who actually says it. The child's value is sometimes reasserted at the same time ('He's still a great little guy'). Finally, the parents sometimes link the difficulties facing sick children and their parents with the family's socio-economic environment, on the one hand, and the country's social policies, on the other. Before analyzing these results, however, let us turn to the positions held by the professionals themselves.

Where the paediatricians and geneticists are concerned, none of those I encountered during my hospital field study openly advocated generalized screening for CF during pregnancy (or before), unlike what was seen in Brittany. One of the geneticists nonetheless expressed a more ambiguous position in an interview, which was also confirmed by a consultation I observed:

> It's true that, given the substantial amount of money spent on this newborn screening, it could have been worth asking whether it would not actually be better to screen before pregnancy? Bearing in mind that if we do that, we are leaning towards a system not of eugenics, but … it's true that there would be a slightly disturbing side to saying 'All the children who could potentially be born with cystic fibrosis won't be born'. [Later in the interview, spontaneously] The only question we can ask is: 'Why wait until a child is affected to offer prenatal diagnosis?' (Geneticist 1, 3.3.05).

The same geneticist said in passing during a genetic counselling appointment: 'We screen at birth. It would perhaps have been better to do it pre-natally, but that's how it is' (Geneticist 1, Observation 11.5.05).

Does this mean that newborn screening can also change professionals' thinking about prenatal screening? In part, no doubt, and further data on this subject will be presented below. However, this interview shows that the possible association between prenatal screening and eugenics (or a similar idea) controls any impulse to generalize such screening. The respondent in question was probably not familiar with the details of the history of eugenics, but he is immersed in an ethical government that cannot remove itself from that context. And this makes it difficult to defend prenatal screening, or even utter the idea, because of certain moral values.

The professionals therefore mention a form of prenatal screening that relies on a different method: the development of a technique for identifying mutations in the foetal cells present in the mother's blood at the very beginning of pregnancy. This method is currently used experimentally. It allows CFTR gene mutations to be identified by a simple blood test and pregnancy terminations to be offered very early on. It therefore links in with the issue of early intervention, as it aims to avoid late, and always traumatizing, pregnancy terminations as well as the risks of miscarriage linked to amniocentesis.

As Patricia Kaufert notes (2000: 176) 'The temptation, particularly for clinicians, is to continually push back the boundaries and "find" the disease at an earlier stage'. Consequently it is not surprising that a substantial proportion of parents of children screened with the disease express their desire to go back in time and their surprise at newborn screening, which they consider too late. However, the mothers that I interviewed found themselves in a paradoxical position because they were simultaneously involved in fighting the illness, loving the child who emblemized it and evaluating that child's life. Along the same lines, Gail Landsman (2003) has explained that mothers of mentally handicapped children find themselves caught up in a paradox, saying both that they love their children and that they would do anything to change them (that is, to remove the handicap). It is possible that the points of view held by mothers in the case of CF change as the child grows. As Gail Landsman (2003) writes, mothers who have just received the diagnosis of their child's handicap speak rather about 'developmental delay' (implying that it will be possible to catch up) whereas later they refer openly to 'handicap' (without this notion of catching up). She adds that when mothers understand that their child will probably never become what is considered as 'normal', most reconsider the meaning and value of normality and develop a critique of any discourse that would diminish their child's value.

Furthermore, the reasoning reproduced by the mothers I encountered in the field study is age-old amongst French doctors: in their thinking, there was often no hiatus between action preceding and action following birth. As early as the seventeenth century, a discipline called '*callipédie*' (the art of bearing beautiful children) was devised to handle problems relating not only to pregnancy and birth but also early child-raising (Carol 1995). In the late nineteenth century, medical disciplines such as paediatric nursing and venereology gave paediatricians medical experience that gradually led them to look into the question of forebears in their attempts to explain and combat certain pathologies (Carol 1995). Although the aims are different, there is therefore a body of historical evidence suggesting a tendency to follow a path backward in time, some aspects of which can be linked to the fact that French eugenics was influenced by the hygienists (Gaudillière 2006). In this way, today NSCF – in combination with different prenatal diagnostic practices – has contributed to changing thinking about generalized prenatal screening. Another episode can confirm this.

On the National Level

The last aspect to this study concerns the national level rather than the space of the screening and health care centre. It is important to know that, like in North Finistère, several experimental programmes for generalized screening of heterozygotes with a view to prenatal screening were carried out from the 1990s onwards, in particular in Great Britain and the United States. Today, prenatal screening for CF is widely available in the United States even if it comes up against technical difficulties. In 2002, a pilot programme for generalized prenatal screening of CF was put forward to the *Comité Consultatif National d'Ethique* (CCNE – the National Consultative Ethics Committee for Health and Life Sciences) in France. This committee is mainly composed of doctors and biologists asked to give 'opinions' on ethical questions of a medical or biomedical nature. This pilot problem was designed by a molecular geneticist, who had been working on CF for many years. His work encompassed teaching, research and medical analysis, bringing him into contact with families with cases of CF. His idea consisted in carrying out screening for the mutation most frequently involved in CF, the famous ΔF508 mutation, in all pregnant women. The aim was to identify the heterozygous women, after obtaining their consent, in order to offer a mutation test to the future fathers in question, and then a possible prenatal test on the foetus in so-called at risk pregnancies (when both parents are heterozygotes). In an interview, he explained how this idea came about as follows:

> Why did that [the idea of offering prenatal screening] form in 2001? It was because of the implementation of newborn screening. … While we were doing newborn screening, I said to myself: 'But what is the point of this newborn screening?'. … You know, the number of children you see in the laboratory who are screened as neonates, and you say to yourself: 'We didn't give that child's parents the chance to make a choice', it's disturbing (Molecular geneticist 1, 14.10.05).

Here, the idea of screening before birth follows on from newborn screening and is linked to it. The geneticist calls into question the efficiency of this newborn screening because, in his view, it only saves a few months in terms of diagnosis and does not really change much in therapeutic terms. In the interview, he justified his proposal as follows: 'I promise you, a kid with cystic fibrosis is no joke … . Even if life expectancy increases, but life expectancy increases while being… It's no joke' (Molecular geneticist 1, 14.10.05). It should be noted that in the proposal for this pilot programme (2002), it was no longer a question of the patients' lives but rather of their *survival* after NSCF: 'The aim of newborn diagnosis of cystic fibrosis is to improve the children's survival, which is currently more than problematic' (Proposition d'une étude pilote 2002).

In short, it was definitely a question of evaluating life because the improvement of treatment did not, in his view, lead to a quality life for the sick children. Finally, this geneticist considered prenatal diagnosis to be an alternative solution to NSCF. For the geneticists and biologists in the Finistère, as we have seen, screening before and after birth were not considered to be antagonistic. This geneticist, however, puts forward the opposite viewpoint: if newborn screening is efficient, and the children are well treated, prenatal diagnosis is not justified; conversely, if newborn screening proves insufficient, prenatal screening will be developed further.

On this point – and this point alone – his point of view resembles that of the AFDPHE officials. Offering prenatal screening when newborn screening had just been set up seemed paradoxical to them. Hélène Ravenel, a pillar of the association, took this idea even further. During an informal discussion, she spoke of the fact that 'newborn screening should kill prenatal screening'. When I asked her what she meant by this during an interview, she replied:

> If parents take the decision to have a pregnancy termination for medical reasons, … it means that there isn't a good quality of life… . If we were right to set up newborn screening, I'll be satisfied if in ten years' time prenatal diagnosis for cystic fibrosis no longer exists (21.7.04).

This point of view is based on the premise that the more care provision for a disease progresses, the less parents request prenatal diagnosis. This seems to be confirmed in the case of phenylketonuria, which is now treated by following the requisite diet. As Bernard Robin put it in an interview, there is no prenatal diagnosis for phenylketonuria because 'you don't diagnose to kill a foetus when you know how to cure it'. But generally speaking, the situation is more complex. As one geneticist said, other parameters aside from the more or less treatable nature of a disease come into play in the development of prenatal tests:

> *In general, when life expectancy increases, does this mean the number of requests for prenatal decrease? (Me).*
> No, it's more complicated than that. Actually, prenatal requests are linked to several things. They are linked to parents' anxiety, which is created by knowledge… the knowledge brought to them by the doctors surrounding them and also the knowledge they can get from the Internet (Geneticist 1, 3.3.05).

The fact remains that the long-standing AFDPHE officials who, as we saw previously, had been fiercely hostile towards the prenatal CF screening offered to all couples in North Finistère at the beginning of the 1990s, also opposed the 2002 prenatal screening proposal. The arguments put forward in opposition to the proposal were summarized in a text written when one of these officials was interviewed by the CCNE when it examined the proposal. These arguments were of several types: medical (the disease is not sufficiently serious to justify this action when newborn screening exists to ensure care provision); technical (the test offered intervenes at a late stage, the number of predicted false positives and false negatives according to the suggested protocol is too great); economic (the screening and associated information and consultations are too expensive); and moral (on the one hand, eliminating future sick people in order to eradicate an illness poses an ethical problem, on the other hand, for technical reasons that are too long to go into here, certain at risk couples would be detected without the possibility for prenatal diagnosis). These different arguments cross over to a large extent with those put forward by the CCNE, who refused this proposal for generalized prenatal screening for CF in 2004, and they also give technical, organizational, medical, economic and ethical dimensions to the issue (CCNE 2004). All in all, this episode shows that newborn screening can also change certain professionals' thinking about screening during pregnancy and that this sometimes involves evaluating patients' lives. And, indeed, we also saw that this was the case in Brittany. However, technical and organizational aspects aside, the ethical dimension seems to be a real obstacle to generalization. In other words, the 'regime of entrenchment' (Koch and Stemerding 1994) of NSCF, which makes the advent of generalized screening before birth easier, is curbed by a problem of moral acceptability. Let us therefore try and understand this issue in a little more depth.

One of the main AFDPHE officials explained the ethical argument in an interview: 'Hitler eliminated everyone who wasn't tall with blue eyes, and who was also Jewish. Right, so here, I'll eliminate any child who will have cystic fibrosis' (Paediatrician-Geneticist 1, 17.11.05). The comparison with the policies of Hitlerian eugenics gives a controversial aspect to the position and emphasizes its moral dimension. This therefore tends to flatten out the differences between particularly authoritarian policies and something that is a norm: Hitler's policies, in one case, genetic testing in the other. It also flattens out the differences between 'ethical substances' (Dean 1999), in other words the substance upon which ethics works: children or adults in one case; foetuses in the other. One way or the other, the issue at the heart of the debate is what means should be used in order to achieve the aim of a quality life: treatment versus eradication. In order to fully understand this position, it is necessary to take a look at the AFDPHE's practices and moral foundations.

First of all, we should remember that the association officials are not opposed to prenatal diagnosis on principle: within their own professional activities, they have carried out many such diagnoses and developed certain such tests. Although they were not (are not) in favour of abortion (except for medical reasons) – which was the case for many people in France in the 1970s – they were not against pregnancy terminations for medical reasons, having themselves been confronted with difficult family situations, and it is also probable that their views have evolved along with society. As an example, let us look at how Bernard Robin described his past experience in prenatal screening of chromosomal anomalies in an interview:

> The risk of recurrence meant providing genetic counselling, meant listening, and also meant making possible prevention available to the parents. ... (Paediatrician-Geneticist 1).
> *So the idea linking your two areas of work [paediatrics and genetics] was in fact the idea of prevention? (Me).*
> Yes, that's it. That's it, I had a family with a sick kid, the parents were saying: 'But if we have another what's going to happen?' ... . It just followed on from that, I suppose, on it's own (Paediatrician-Geneticist 1).
> *That's also the idea that we can see in the aims of the AFDPHE, at the beginning. Perinatal prevention? (Me).*
> Yes, the AFDPHE did both. It was part of a prevention programme that began with phenylketonuria and hyperthyroidism. And then it was led to, because ... they were paediatricians, but they were geneticists as well, they were in the same situation as me. They had all diagnosed, they all did genetic counselling (Paediatrician-Geneticist 1, 17.11.05).

Through this testimony, we can see how the notion of prevention, which was at the heart of the founding activity of the AFDPHE, builds a bridge between newborn screening and prenatal diagnosis. As the association officials wrote in the 1980s: 'Genetic counselling, prenatal diagnosis and newborn screening are the foundations of perinatal prevention for a certain number of handicaps in children'. This will come as no surprise to the reader who is familiar with the notions of primary prevention (avoiding the causes of disease, here the development of the sick foetus), secondary prevention (preventing the physical consequences of the disease) and tertiary prevention (avoiding social handicap and complications) that are mentioned in public health studies (Armstrong 2012). The aim of the association was originally perinatal prevention, until prenatal diagnoses shifted to the remit of the Cnamts, during the 1990s, and thus left the sphere of the association. The different preventative approaches were organized around two disciplines, paediatrics and genetics, which were interwoven in the professional career paths of the promoters of the association. One of them estimated that until genetics became an autonomous independent specialism, 80-90% of geneticists were paediatricians. But for the AFDPHE officials, bridging the gap between neonatal and prenatal approaches was subject to certain conditions, because the principle of legitimacy for prenatal diagnosis was that of so-called at-risk pregnancies: when families already had a sick child or when ultrasound or biochemical signs indicated the risk of disease. It should also be noted that prenatal screening for Down's Syndrome, which is currently being extended to all women in France (Vassy 2006), does not subscribe to this principle. While the comparison with prenatal screening for Down's Syndrome would be going a little too far, it should be noted that it does not immediately entail DNA analysis. This can perhaps explain in part why it has not been contested in the same way as prenatal screening for CF in France. It seems that prenatal techniques extended to whole populations and with immediate recourse to genetic analysis are linked to the notion of eugenics and this notion creates a veritable barrier.

Beyond the AFDPHE, national statistics for France confirm that these principles are indeed practised. Approximately 560 prenatal foetal tests in connection with CF were carried out in France in 2009, leading to approximately 50 pregnancy terminations for medical reasons (Agence de la biomédicine 2010); 180 sick babies were born. In Brittany, a study shows a significant drop of approximately 40% in the incidence of CF, linked to prenatal diagnoses (all techniques included) (Scotet et al. 2012). In short, prenatal diagnosis is considered to be legitimate – by the AFDPHE and beyond – when a certain proportion of affected children are allowed to be born. The limitation that professionals place on 'ethical practice' is linked to the problem of genetic practices being extended with a view to eradication. However, highlighting the role of the *individual* identified as being at-risk remains acceptable. While the majority of health care workers may be of this opinion, it is nevertheless not unanimous. Indeed, on the other hand, the logic of prevention continues, as we saw above with the example of one geneticist's proposal for generalized prenatal screening. After having moved back in time to birth, in order to intervene as early as possible, finally some parents and professionals move beyond the threshold of birth and reach back to the foetus. Once this threshold has been crossed, the earliest possible intervention during pregnancy is also advocated. More broadly, it is particularly interesting to note that the decrease in incidence of CF linked with NSCF is not specific to France, as it has also been observed in regions of Great Britain and Australia (Scotet et al. 2012).

The hypothesis outlined in introduction was based on the idea that the issue of a quality life is at work in this link between screening before and after birth. As Giorgio Agamben (1998: 131) wrote in *Homo Sacer*: 'One of the essential characteristics of modern biopolitics (which will continue to increase in our century) is its constant need to redefine the threshold in life that distinguishes and separates what is inside from what is outside'. Birth certainly strikes people as a threshold separating the sick child from the foetus. Though this seems obvious today, the anthropology of law shows that this threshold has changed (Cayla and Thomas 2002). Historically, the Declaration of Human Rights of 1789 in France held that the mere fact of *being born* carried with it certain rights. As Agamben (1998: 127) put it:

> Declarations of rights represent the originary figure of the inscription of natural life in the juridico-political order of the nation-state. The same bare life that in the ancien régime was politically neutral and belonged to God as creaturely life … now fully enters into the structure of the state and even becomes the earthly foundation of the state's legitimacy and sovereignty.

In short, birth, life and rights have coincided ever since that period, and this strengthens the threshold effect of birth.

However, my study shows that there is tension surrounding this birth. The first part of this tension comes from the fact that the threshold of birth is becoming less pronounced, for several reasons: the temporal link (that can be drawn between the foetus of eight and a half months and the one month-old newborn), the similarity between techniques used (when looking for mutations in children or foetuses), the notion of prevention (as applied both to prenatal and postnatal situations) and, more fundamentally, the right to good health (called upon in both cases). For these different reasons, and despite the fact that prenatal and neonatal approaches are enacted by different types of specialists using different intervention modes with different effects, it is not really tenable to separate them entirely. What my study shows here is that we are not dealing with mere parallel advances in two different practices, but with a causal link between the two. Against the widespread understanding that social inclusion of handicapped persons is antagonistic to the exclusion of 'sick' foetuses, the quest for good health and the elimination of poor health do not seem to neutralize each other or even to combine but rather to bolster each other: the more attentive we are to including sick persons, the more likely we are to exclude foetuses. This process is no doubt inherent to health and biopolitical practices as, to paraphrase Anne Carol (1995) it reflects a desire for 'absolute prevention'. In this context, the Breton professionals in particular defended an ethical position in emphasizing their experience with treating sick patients and their desire to reduce suffering by promoting the eradication of the disease. The second aspect to this tension lies in the positions taken by other ethical subjects. This desire for disease prevention was curbed by the positions taken by the AFDPHE officials (who took care to clearly separate NSCF from prenatal diagnosis) and by the questions raised by paediatricians and geneticists during the hospital field study (who called into question their own practices): in both cases, there is reflection about a way to 'de-geneticize' practice. The recognition of ethical obligations can be encouraged by professional deontology (the role of the doctor is to treat patients), the code adopted (one of the criteria for the legitimacy of newborn screening is that it must be beneficial to the child being screened) and/or law (French law restricts genetic tests). Some would also add questions or accusations relating to 'eugenics'. I will not use that term myself in this context because, following Nikolas Rose (2007), I see today's policies and practices as sufficiently complex and new to deserve their own vocabulary. What my field study suggests is that the tension seems to be shifting towards a move backward in time. The future will tell whether or not this observation is well-founded.

Conclusion

Policies of screening for genetic conditions on whole populations are developing rapidly. And the use of so-called 'new generation' sequencing allowing searches for more than 400 diseases (Bell et al. 2011), as well as the new genetic tests available on the Internet, show that genome profiling is no longer purely fictional (Goldenberg and Sharp 2012). It is therefore important to understand the stakes of these changes and what they can tell us about broader societal issues.

In this book, I grounded my analysis in Foucault's theoretical tools, using the concept of 'field of experience' that links together scientific, political and moral issues. The screening policy I analyzed stems from the medical genetics of the early twenty-first century and constitutes a field of experience in which these three types of issue are present and linked by interrelated questions. Knowledge (genetics, statistics about incidence or life expectancy, etc.) contributes to the rise of new practices that have political effects (directing patients towards centres, producing different subjects, drawing benefits from financial and human support) and raise moral questions (diagnosing borderline forms, identifying heterozygotes, etc.). The political dimension, in turn, affects knowledge (screening produces knowledge about CF, etc.) and moral questions (about acting in keeping with the law on consent, etc.). And moral values also act upon scientific practices (not carrying out a 'randomized controlled trial', envisaging screening without DNA testing, etc.) and political practices (considering generalized prenatal screening as unacceptable, etc.). This shows the extent to which each of the three dimensions is linked to the other two or slots into the interstitial spaces they create. Understanding how they are connected can allow a more accurate interpretation of the actors' motivations, particularly regarding their convictions, their social positions and/ or their doubts. And it also enables a better understanding of the signification of a screening programme positioned at the interface of science, medicine and politics. This interweaving of different spaces shows that we are definitely looking at a 'field' (in the sense defined in the introduction) and justifies the decision to avoid placing emphasis on one particular dimension to the detriment of the others. Nonetheless, I did attempt to separate these different facets to the issue with a view to clarity and I shall do so once again here.

Due to the specific characteristics of genetics as a form of knowledge (it tends to essentialize features, it is part of what is often seen as 'progress' and it can affect everyone), it highlights social processes that could, at first glance, seem to be far removed from its remit. In this sense, it can prove of interest to researchers or individuals who are not directly concerned by its practices. My study threw into light an initial tension existing between the social construction of a problem and genetic essentialism. As we have seen, health questions generally tend to be based on 'constructed reality', but when looking at genes it is even more important to emphasize the social dimension to how these questions are problematized. In the 1980s and 1990s in Brittany, the idea people had of CF was of course partly grounded in the reality of the disease, and how it was inscribed in the body, but it was also partly the result of the actors' mobilization. This fact therefore allows us to set aside conceptions seeing genes as the essence of a person and the truth of a disease. And the fact that CF has a determining genetic origin, and that social construction could seem, at first glance, to have a very minimal role to play, makes this all the more striking. Such essentializing conceptions of genetics were rife at this time, and although they may seem outdated today given the greater inclusion of environmental factors in genetic research (Lock 2010, Niewöhner 2011), they have not entirely disappeared, particularly in people's common understanding. The second tension revealed by my research exists between a new technical approach (using the tools of molecular biology to screen for a genetic disease) and a simple, older approach (preventing cross-infection in hospitals through measures of hygiene). This brings questions about the risks of hospital-acquired infections to the fore, which were subject to little consideration in the lead-up to screening. The technically oriented approaches of biomedicine were carried forward by their own momentum and sometimes seemed to forget the more ordinary dimensions to health. This underscores the actual importance of the seemingly trivial aspects to health that carry little professional prestige. Finally, genetics reveals the core issue of social inequalities in health. In this case, the parameters of the disease seem, on the one hand, to be dictated by genes, and on the other, to be made equal by generalized screening at birth and access to well-organized care programmes. In other cases, the problem of access to health care can obfuscate the various other social factors at work. Here, the processes through which the disease can worsen due to social inequalities in housing, education and living conditions appear all the more clearly.

Another dimension to the scientific issues at stake relates to the statements considered as 'true' in biomedical discourse today: how they are constituted, what rules they must obey and how they circulate in situations of uncertainty. I highlighted several regimes of scientific rationality, embodied by the 'mavericks', the 'screeners' and the 'clinicians'. Each of these groups of actors revealed more particularly a different aspect to the question: self-evidence, doubt, and evidence itself. The social role of self-evidence retained my attention in particular as it appeared at several moments of the study (the launch of NSCF in the Finistère region, the support for the newspaper's 'cause', the funding provided by a *Conseil général*, the mothers seen in maternity units, etc.). The mechanisms of self-evidence provide material for research that can take a critical perspective of potential relevance in all number of fields. Moreover, the question of how evidence is produced, disseminated and received has particular resonance in societies that give such an important role to expertise and scientific criteria. Given the substantial role played by 'evidence-based medicine' in the medical sphere today, it seemed appropriate to question this current on its own ground, in other words that of evidence itself. This allowed me to show criteria for scientificity both close to, and conversely far from, evidence-based medicine, while also highlighting the importance of contingent details and the social role of emotions in the construction of evidence. More fundamentally, and beyond the specific case of CF, studying this screening programme from a historical perspective offered an example of the relationships established between reason and action. I highlighted in particular the connections between, on the one hand, elements of knowledge (the genetic approach, measures of incidence of CF, calculations of life expectancy), and, on the other, rather than power strategies, the stakes and effects of power (the problematization of genetic diseases and, within these diseases, of CF, the means made available to the large centres, etc.).

Besides this important connection, the political stakes lie mainly in how a number of factors are interrelated: power relations and legitimacy; types of domination; conceptions of the individual and the collective; and spaces of freedom. In order to make such a statement, it is necessary to unpick the different power relations at work between medical, associative and institutional actors, as well as the forms of legitimacy on which they are grounded (such as the reliability of the professional association, the experience of the clinicians and the patients'/parents' lived experience of the disease itself). Analysis of these relationships shows above all the preponderant influence of the professionals, including within the patient organization, and more specifically of the 'clinicians' who, on a national level, base their legitimacy on that of the AFDPHE 'screeners'. The mechanism at work is perhaps not of dominance, but at the very least of hierarchy. This illustrates the limitations that exist with regard to calling professional expertise into question in favour of the population or of patients – something that does exist in other cases and has been described by other authors (Lascoumes 2005). In the same spirit, borrowing the term used by Adriana Petryna (2002) about the people exposed to the Chernobyl radiation, Nikolas Rose (2007) speaks of a certain 'biological citizenship' that accounts for citizen-led projects linked to their biological existence as human beings. If we take the term 'citizen' to refer to the notion of people who are fully engaged in public action and/or whose rights are recognized, it would perhaps be more appropriate in this case to talk about 'biological subjects' because, as we have seen, the term 'subject' enables the idea of a possible inversion with objectivation. A further ambiguity inherent to subjectivation in matters of genetics lies with how consent is obtained in maternity units: the subjects are convinced by screening, but in practice their remit remains limited. In short, clinicians are the actual 'subjects' in the fullest sense of the term and this is why they are able to assert their conception of government (in the sense outlined in the introduction to the book). This conception is directed more towards the individual and marked more by patient 'cases' than by the population as a whole. This leads to an effect of fragmentation that also recalls the influence exerted on ministerial leaders by pressure groups, both on the part of clinicians and associative actors, when the supposed differences in life expectancy for CF patients were announced.

There is incidentally no doubt that these political leaders are convinced of NSCF's strong social legitimacy. The policy is grounded in various spaces of freedom, through the requirement for written consent, as well as in the almost unanimous approval of parents in maternity units and in the clinicians' agreement in principle to follow the protocols for screening and care provision. Moreover, the policy meets with the approval of the patient organization, even if the complex nature of the organization's role, and its various medical and non-medical actors, has been demonstrated. In short, these spaces of freedom reactivate the legitimacy of screening in a bottom-up movement stemming from the maternity units. It should also be underlined that the issue of the link between power and freedom clearly extends far beyond the field of genetics and biomedicine. This link is present in all number of fields today ranging from the 'choice' of working on Sundays to the 'choice' of retiring late, to take a couple of examples from recent current affairs. And this fragmented conception of 'government' is neither specific to France nor to medicine. The issue at stake in many policies can be seen to be negotiating the balance between what is considered as good for a population overall and what is considered suitable for the individual. These remarks illustrate the fact that a newborn screening programme for a rare illness can give rise to reflections that are of relevance much further afield.

My work also integrated the moral dimension by dealing with how actors take up certain positions and question their own actions, within a framework of rules and values. These professionals develop collective thinking about their own practices that result in these practices evolving, for example regarding procedures for breaking the news of the illness or the decision to change the screening thresholds. They all invoke 'ethics', as this notion is almost a prerequisite in biomedical discourse today, among other areas. And in doing so, they come together to create a configuration of ethical subjects defending various positions either alternately or together: an ethics of conviction (judging it to be unethical not to launch a screening programme that can benefit children), an ethics of avoiding suffering (considering that screening for heterozygotes avoids suffering for patients and families), an ethics of care (believing newborn screening should be solely geared towards providing care for patients), an ethics of the acceptable limits of genetic counselling (viewing infertility as the limit for prenatal diagnosis), and an ethics of doubt (questioning whether they themselves are involved in an uncontrolled expansion of practices and wondering how borderline forms should be considered). It becomes clear therefore that, in the end, in these different cases, 'ethical practices' (Dean 1999) are also a question of compassion and of avoiding suffering, sentiments that are echoed in the values of solidarity that were put forward in particular in the mobilization of the population in Brittany. Above and beyond these shared values and stated principles, however, the means – or the 'ethical work' – through which suffering should be avoided are varied and sometimes opposed. This diversity can even give rise to controversy when the differences are erased between adults and foetuses as 'ethical substances'. Related to this question, at several times in my study it became clear that screening at birth was interlaced with screening before birth. This raises the question of the link between treatment practices and the logic of foetus selection. More fundamentally, this link also brings up questions regarding what I suggested calling a 'quality life' for sick people and how to achieve this, within a much wider movement towards optimizing life. The hospital is informative in this regard because it is a space in which we can observe these criteria for 'quality of life' being put into practice, targeting biological life but without completely neglecting social life, or the sick children's overall life prospects, in the process. Moreover, during the interviews I conducted certain value judgments about the lives of very young children rose to the surface or were made explicit. We have seen that while birth continues to be a threshold, as the point at which certain rights are conferred upon the individual, this boundary is nonetheless sometimes eroded and the effects of this erosion can be contradictory. Clinicians find themselves contributing to the shift from looking to maintain good health (through treatment) to looking to eradicate bad health (through foetal selection). These two aspects converge and mutually reinforce one another giving rise to ethical questions for some professionals. I therefore attempted to show not how practices in care provision and prenatal diagnosis have advanced in parallel, but rather the causal link between the two. Understanding this also contributes to better grasping, on the one hand, the political and moral space of genetics – which I will return to later – and, on the other, the developments of biomedicine.

These different results need to be considered within the context of the concern with health mentioned in my introduction. Biology and the techno-sciences have taken this huge sector of modern anxiety on board and new techniques have therefore been developed that seek to predict the future. At the same time, this future potentially marked by disease seems more and more unbearable and worrying. In wealthy countries, the old saying that prevention is better than cure now goes hand-in-hand with a desire for prevention to be extended to more and more diseases. This theme is a key part of a historical process that, according to Michel Foucault (2001b: 727), is part of 'a certain displacement, or at least broadening, of objective: it is no longer a question of eradicating the disease when it appears, but of preventing it; better still, as far as possible, of preventing any disease whatsoever'. In my introduction, I emphasized the need to consider the differences in health priorities between different social worlds, so I will not fully align myself with a point of view expressed in such generalizing terms. However, this general context remains useful in better understanding the transformations of biomedicine. Care provision for CF over the last 20 years has brought longer life expectancy to children suffering from a disease that used to prove fatal at a young age in most cases. Newborn screening itself avoids serial misdiagnosis, contributes to the restructuring of health care and avoids families with several sick children. However, here it is interesting to note that beyond its medical effects, it also highlights certain boundary areas of the biomedicalization process. These areas are first of all linked to temporality. One of the characteristics of this screening is that it is informed at all levels by the idea of early intervention, because whether before or after birth, the idea is to establish a diagnosis as early as possible. This means that clinicians have to try and reconcile contradictory aims when it comes to alerting the parents of 'suspect' children, who often have few or no symptoms, without worrying them too much and without providing too little or too much information. Another boundary area of biomedicalization is linked to this last point and concerns the people to whom its influence extends. We have seen that this screening programme contributed to producing abnormality because children who would previously have been considered normal now fell into this category. It also contributes to the anxiety of parents and professionals, leading – today at any rate – to clinical over-diagnosis and demands for 'guarantees' concerning foetuses. At the same time, this brings professionals to call their own practices into question. These two dimensions – the timeframes in question and the extension of the groups of people concerned – both seem to contribute actively to processes of biomedicalization. While all screening programmes cannot be lumped together – some are beneficial while others are not – this tendency towards early screening for diseases that are difficult to interpret and include an increasing number of borderline forms, and/or forms with sometimes limited treatment possibilities, can be seen in many other contexts today (various kinds of newborn screening in the United States, as we have seen, but also screening for Alzheimer's, prostate cancer, etc.) and this also gives rise to debate.

On another level, this study gives food for thought on the matter of research approaches in the social sciences. It seems timely at this point to plead in favour of an approach that is interdisciplinary, that pays attention to social dynamics and that is bolstered by observations. Interdisciplinarity is increasingly encouraged in research practice today. I hope that I have shown that it can be useful and functional not only within research teams but also at the level of the individual researcher. In the same spirit of breaking down disciplinary boundaries, I also made use of different social science approaches, in particular political anthropology, the sociology and anthropology of science, medical anthropology and the sociology of health. It seemed appropriate to call upon a sufficiently wide panel of social science approaches so as to explain both practices and interactions between actors, as well as the structural constraints to which they are subject. Taking these constraints into consideration seemed all the more appropriate in a political and social context that seeks to impose increasingly individualizing and cognitivist conceptions of the world. My second point concerns social dynamics. My research here attempted to offer an account less of the stable aspects to society and more of its transformations, whether through processes constituting a policy, changes seen in scientific knowledge, the dynamics of evidence or the transformation of norms. It seemed that this offered a fairer view of actors whose points of view sometimes changed, or who were perhaps in control of an issue only for it to slip away from them further down the line. It also seemed to correspond better to the rapid developments occurring in genetics and in the contemporary world more widely (linked to the Internet, to transport systems, etc.). Finally, my last remark pertains to the observations I carried out. This study showed the importance of spending time with patients in consultations, in order to better understand the disease, and with families, in order to consider the question of life and death. And it also underscored the value in observing the brevity of interactions between mothers and health care workers in maternity units so as to understand consent beyond its somewhat theoretical legal framework. The social sciences seem to be subject to increasingly strict conditions of access to the field, due to ethical constraints and the standardizing of rules for publication, and this could well encourage shorter one-off field studies. And yet it seems to me that everyone – researchers and non-researchers alike – stand to lose a lot if observation studies are limited in this way.

Finally, I would like to put forward two suggestions for further discussion. The first relates to the link between the biological, the social and the political. We saw that NSCF was, to a large extent, seen as a means through which to direct patients towards specialized centres. In other words, in this case, biological techniques are used for purposes of social organization. The specificity of NSCF lies above all in the fact that the way it functions establishes a link between the development of techniques (screening at birth, including with DNA tests) and the history of techniques of government (directing patients towards specialized centres). Does this mean that biological tools are more effective today than social or political tools for organizing health care provision? If other examples of this kind were to arise, they would be worth noting. Moreover, the relationship that NSCF creates between the biological, the social and the political also presents other aspects. This screening produces, or seeks to produce, social ties: we saw how a movement of solidarity was created in West Brittany, on grounds of regional and genetic identity (the Celtic genes 'we' share) as well as on compassionate grounds (the sick, suffering children, aside from the gene). We also saw how the patient organization sought to create a greatly extended community of people who could potentially transmit the disease through their genes, using a publicity insert in the media, taking the number of people concerned from 5,000 to 2 million. In this case, the patient organization sought to shift from Celtic or Breton bio-identity and the 'biosociality' of its members (Rabinow 1996) to a much wider bio-community of people carrying mutated genes. Extended networks of actors and patient organizations thus build or seek to build social ties on both biological grounds (the gene) and health grounds (the patients). Moreover, the spaces of both the hospital and leisure activities appear as a locus for tensions in social lives based on the patients' biological lives. Indeed, when young screened children find themselves alongside older children, this proximity raises issues of spatial organization and risks of cross-infection. While tensions can exist between patients or their families independently of screening, this can be exacerbated by the fact that NSCF concerns very young children. In this regard, Kaja Finkler (2005) carried out anthropological research questioning the nature of the ties established within families on the basis of genetics. She described situations in which genetics redefined family ties on biological grounds, a tendency that runs counter to the evolution of contemporary society which has seen an increase in the number of blended families and adoptions. In speaking about genetics, Finkler (2005: 1067) takes up the expression used previously by Bauman about a 'sociality' that 'does not require sociability'; in other words, social ties that do not require social relations. With NSCF, in the space of the waiting room, the disease creates, on the contrary, forms of relations based on physical proximity because in this context this genetic condition seems to be similar to an infectious disease. Overall, what rises to the forefront here is first, a technique of government functioning through a biological test when this could have been decided otherwise (as in other countries or for other diseases) and second, two forms of sociality: one that is grounded in genetics and solidarity (in Brittany and within the organization) and the other that can lead to both contamination and concern (in the waiting room). We can see here the different ways in which the biological produces the social and/or the political – through organization, solidarity or stigma – and therefore contributes to the foundations of social relations and/or political relations between individuals.

The second point of discussion concerns the political and moral space in which newborn screening programmes and prenatal diagnoses evolve. Defining this space offers a way of envisaging the future of this evolution with more precision. I mentioned in my introduction the increasing number of genetic tests and newborn screening programmes. Researchers in the United States and Great Britain in particular are questioning the possible use of new 'chip'-based techniques for the 'genetic profiling' of newborns, or in other words for studying their genomes (a 'chip' is a strip that is smaller than that of a microscope and on which several hundred thousand DNA fragments can be placed for analysis taken from one single sample). Researchers in the United States are arguing in favour of developing these chips in order to analyze the DNA of newborns, basing their views on 'the popularity and enthusiasm for newborn screening' as well as on a series of other arguments (Alexander and Van Dyck 2006: S351). According to them, this would avoid serial misdiagnosis, would help with reproductive decisions before symptoms appeared on a firstborn child, would afford the benefits of care provision even when no cure is available, and would allow children to partake in research programmes for innovative treatments. Some of these arguments are now familiar. Moreover, while overall industrial and market practices were little involved in the decision-making process for NSCF in France, they must of course be taken into account for the next stages in the process, particularly on an international level. Given these elements, and the results I have presented here, I suggest considering three periods in the political and moral space of genetics in Western countries. Historically, from the end of the nineteenth century onwards, the first period is that of eugenics, biopolitical figure *par excellence*. We should recall that eugenics aimed to improve the quality of the population by favouring 'the more suitable races' and that it linked science to a socio-political project (Gayon 1997). Designed with regard to populations, this project was intended as collective and, while it took on several different faces of more or less presentable natures according to political and social contexts, its harshest imaginable programmes were implemented under the Third Reich. Overall, it developed very little in France, as we have seen, where it translated mainly into pro-birth politics (Carol 1995). With the decline of the ideology of eugenics, a second period emerged within the political and moral space of genetics. As Jean Gayon (1997) explains, in this new configuration of biological knowledge and power, questions, concerns and hopes shifted extensively from populations to individuals. Against a backdrop of individual genetic counselling, voluntary participation and consent, this conception echoed, and continues to echo, a power in which the 'other' is recognized as a subject of action in a position to exercise freedom. Freedom was thus established as one of the main modes for the ethics of genetics, and this continues to be the case. Today, while these precepts remain strongly alive, screening on populations has created an unprecedented political and moral period, when compared with the previous configurations. CF offers a prime example of this. NSCF is both collective (the whole population is concerned) and individual (the patients and their families are seen individually). Moreover, it is relatively consensual from an ethical point of view because it is first and foremost aimed at sick children, even if, as we have seen, it does raise questions for professionals. Furthermore, while it is socially acceptable, compassionate and firmly grounded in care provision for suffering children, it does not offer sufficient therapeutic prospects to render prenatal diagnosis pointless. The prenatal diagnosis that it offers is very different from individual prenatal diagnoses, traditionally carried out on the basis of one sick person within a family, but also from generalized screening of adult heterozygotes, liable to cause controversy about actual or supposed eugenics. In short, NSCF is all at once collective, individual, compassionate, relatively ethically consensual and linked in part to prenatal diagnosis. This is where its ordinary nature resides, even if it raises much less ordinary questions. And this is why there is little risk in claiming that newborn screening and the related prenatal diagnoses will continue to develop. I would wager that if genetic tests continue to increase at the current rate, this new political and moral space will have to be taken into consideration in any future research looking at politics regarding the living being.

References

Agamben, G. 1998. *Homo Sacer: sovereign power and bare life*. Stanford: Stanford University Press [1995].

Alexander, D. and van Dyck, P.C. 2006. A vision of the future of newborn screening. *Pediatrics*, 117, S350-354.

Aïach, P. and Cèbe, D. 1994. Les inégalités sociales de santé. Une injustice inéluctable? *La Recherche*, 261, 100-109.

Akkad, A. et al. 2004. Informed consent for elective and emergency surgery: questionnaire study. *British Journal of Obstetrics and Gynaecology*, 111(10), 1133-1138.

Angell, M. 1997. The ethics of clinical research in the Third World. *New England Journal of Medicine*, 337(12), 847-849.

Armstrong, D. 1995. The rise of surveillance medicine. *Sociology of Health & Illness*, 17(3), 393-404.

Armstrong, D. 2002. Clinical autonomy, individual and collective: the problem of changing doctor's behaviour. *Social Science & Medicine*, 55(10), 1771-1777.

Armstrong, D. 2012. Screening: mapping medicine's temporal spaces. *Sociology of Health & Illness*, 34(2), 177-193.

Armstrong, D. et al. 2007. Health-related quality of life and the transformation of symptoms. *Sociology of Health & Illness*, 29(4), 570-583.

Armstrong, N. and Eborall, H. 2012. The sociology of medical screening: past, present and future. *Sociology of Health & Illness*, 34(2), 161-176.

Atkinson, P. 1984. Training for certainty. *Social Science & Medicine*, 19(9), 949-956.

Atkinson, P., Glasner, P. and Lock, M. 2009. *Handbook of genetics and society*. London, New York: Routledge.

Baszanger, I. 1986. Les maladies chroniques et leur ordre négocié. *Revue Française de Sociologie*, 27(1), 3-27.

Beck, S. 2005. Putting genetics to use. *The Cyprus Review*, 17(1), 59-78.

Beck, U. 1992. *Risk society. Towards a new modernity*. London: Sage Publications [1986].

Becker, H.S. 1963. *Outsiders: studies in the sociology of deviance*. New York, London: Collier Macmillan.

Becker, H.S. 1966. *Social problems: a modern approach*. New York: John Wiley.

Beecher, H.K. 1966. Ethics and clinical research. *New England Journal of Medicine*, 274(24), 1354-1360.

Bell, C.J. et al. 2011. Carrier testing for severe childhood recessive disorders by next generation sequencing. *Science Translational Medicine*, 3(65), 65ra4.

Berger, P. and Luckmann, T. 1966. *The construction of reality*. New York: Doubleday.

Biehl, J. 2005. Technologies of invisibility: politics of life and social inequality, in *Anthropologies of modernity. Foucault, governmentality and life politics*, edited by J.X. Inda. Malden, Oxford, Victoria: Blackwell, 248-271.

Bijker, W.E. 1995. Sociohistorical technoloy studies, in *Handbook of science and technology studies*, edited by S. Jasanoff et al. Thousand Oaks, London, New Delhi: SAGE, 229-256.

Bizeul, D. 2007. Que faire des expériences d'enquête ? Apports et fragilité de l'observation directe. *Revue Française de Sociologie*, 57(1), 69-89.

Blanchflower, D.G. and Oswald, A. 2008. Is well-being U-shaped over the life cycle? *Social Science & Medicine*, 66(8), 1733-1749.

Blume, S. and Tump, J. 2010. Evidence and policymaking: the introduction of MMR vaccine in the Netherlands. *Social Science and Medicine,* 71(6), 1049-1055.

Blumer, H. 1971. Social problems as collective behaviour. *Social problems*, 18, 298-306.

Bonnet, D. et al. 1998. Les associations de malades: entre le marché, la science et la médecine. *Sciences Sociales et Santé*, 16(3), 5-16.

Borraz, O. and Loncle-Moriceau, P. 2000. Les politiques locales de lutte contre le sida. *Revue Française de Sociologie*, 41(1), 36-60.

Boudon, R. 1992. Connaissance, in *Traité de Sociologie*, edited by R. Boudon. Paris: PUF, 491-531.

Boulton, M. and Parker, M. 2007. Informed consent in a changing environment. *Social Science & Medicine*, 65(11), 2187-2198.

Bourdieu, P. 1984. *Distinction: a social critique of the judgment of taste*. Cambridge: Harvard University Press.

Bourdieu, P. 2004. *Science of science and reflexivity*. Chicago: University of Chicago Press.

Bowker, G.C. and Star, S.L. 2000. *Sorting things out. Classification and its consequence*. Cambridge, London: The MIT Press.

Buchbinder, M. and Timmermans, S. 2011. Medical technologies and the dream of the perfect newborn. *Medical Anthropology,* 30(1), 56-80.

Brenneis, D. 2006. Reforming promise, in *Documents: artifacts of modern knowledge*, edited by A. Riles. Ann Arbor: University of Michigan Press, 41-70.

Britton, J.R. 1989. Effects of social class, sex, and region of residence on age at death from cystic fibrosis. *British Medical Journal*, 298(6672), 483-487.

Cambrosio, A. et al. 2006. Regulatory objectivity and the generation and management of evidence in medicine. *Social Science & Medicine*, 63(1), 189-199.

Cambrosio, A. et al. 2009. Biomedical conventions and regulatory objectivity. *Social Studies of Science*, 39(5), 651-664.

Cambrosio, A., Young, A. and Lock, M. 2000. Introduction, in *Living and working with the new medical technologies. Intersections of inquiry*, edited by M. Lock, A. Young and A. Cambrosio. Cambridge: Cambridge University Press, 1-16.

Canguilhem, G. 1978. *On the normal and the pathological*. Dordrecht, Boston, London: D. Reidel Publishing Company [1966].

Cardon, D. et al. 1998. Mais qui fait bouger le compteur du Téléthon ? Une construction télévisuelle de la solidarité. *Sciences Sociales et Santé*, 16(3), 17-40.

Carol, A. 1995. *Histoire de l'eugénisme en France. Les médecins et la procréation XIXᵉ-XXᵉ siècle*. Paris: Seuil.

Castel, R. 1991. From dangerousness to risk, in *The Foucault effect: studies in governmentality*, edited by G. Burchell, C. Gordon and P. Miller. Chicago: Chicago University Press, 281-298.

Cayla, O. and Thomas, Y. 2002. *Du droit de ne pas naître. A propos de l'affaire Perruche*. Paris: Gallimard.

Chagnollaud, D. 1999. *Science politique. Eléments de sociologie politique*. Paris: Dalloz.

Charon, J.-M. 1996. *La presse quotidienne*. Paris: La Découverte.

Chopplet, M. 2001. La double hélice d'une utopie, in *L'utopie de la santé parfaite*, edited by L. Sfez. Paris: PUF, 335-361.

Clarke, A.E. et al. (eds.) 2010. *Biomedicalization: technoscience, health, and illness in the U.S.* Durham: Duke University Press.

Claustres, M. et al. 2000. Spectrum of CFTR mutations in cystic fibrosis and in congenital absence of the vas deferens in France. *Human Mutation*, 16, 143-156.

Commaille, J. 2006. Sociologie de l'action publique, in *Dictionnaire des politiques publiques*, edited by L. Boussaguet, S. Jacquot and P. Ravinet. Paris: Les Presses de Sciences Po, 415-423.

Concar, D. 2003. Test blunders risk needless abortions. *New Scientist*, 178(2393), 4-6.

Conrad, P. and Gabe, J. 1999. Sociological perspectives on the new genetics: an overview. *Sociology of Health & Illness*, 21(5), 505-516.

Corcuff, P. 1995. *Les nouvelles sociologies*. Paris: Nathan.

Corrigan, O. 2003. Empty ethics: the problem with informed consent. *Sociology of Health and Illness*, 25(3), 768-792.

Dalgalarrondo, S. and Urfalino, P. 2000. Choix tragique, controverse et décision publique. Le cas du tirage au sort des malades du sida. *Revue Française de Sociologie*, 41(1), 119-157.

Dean, M. 1999. *Governmentality: power and rule in modern society.* London, Thousand Oaks, New Delhi: SAGE.

Desrosières, A. 1998. *The politics of large numbers: a history of statistical reasoning.* Cambridge, London: Harvard University Press [1993].

De Vries, R. and Lemmens, T. 2005. The social and cultural shaping of medical evidence: case studies from pharmaceutical research and obstetric science. *Social Science & Medicine,* 62(11), 2694-2706.

Dixon-Woods, M. et al. 2007. Beyond 'misunderstanding': written information and decisions about taking part in a genetic epidemiology study. *Social Science & Medicine,* 65(11), 2212-2222.

Dobrow, M.J. et al. 2006. The impact of context on evidence utilisation: a framework for expert groups developing health policy recommendations. *Social Science & Medicine,* 63(7), 1811-1824.

Dodier, N. and Barbot, J. 2000. Le temps de tensions épistémiques. Le développement des essais thérapeutiques dans le cadre du sida. *Revue Française de Sociologie,* 41(1), 79-118.

Dovidio, J.F. et al. 2008. Disparities and distrust: the implications of psychosocial processes for understanding racial disparities in health and health care. *Social Science & Medicine,* 67(3), 478-486.

Dowd, J.B., Zajacova, A. and Aiello, A. 2009. Early origins of health disparities: burden of infection, health, and socioeconomic status in U.S. children. *Social Science & Medicine,* 68(4), 699-707.

Ducournau, P. 2007. The viewpoint of DNA donors on the consent procedure. *New Genetics and Society,* 26(1), 105-116.

Ducournau, P. and Beaudevin, C. 2011. Of deterritorialization, healthism and biosocialities: the companies' marketing and users' experiences of online genetics. *Journal of Science Communication,* 10(3), 1-10.

Ehrich, K. et al. 2006. Social welfare, genetic welfare? Boundary-work in the IVF/ PDG clinic. *Social Science & Medicine,* 63(5), 1213-1224.

Elias, N. 1978. *What is sociology?* London: Hutchinson [1970].

Elias, N. 1987. *Involvement and detachment.* Oxford: Basil Blackwell [1983].

Elias, N. 1991. *The society of individuals.* Oxford, Cambridge: Blackwell [1987].

Elias, N. 1992. *Time: an essay.* Oxford, Cambridge: Blackwell [1984].

Ettore, E. 2000. Reproductive genetics, gender and the body: 'Please doctor, may I have a normal baby?' *Sociology,* 34(3), 403-420.

Evidence-Based Medicine Working Group. 1992. Evidence-based medicine. A new approach to teaching the practice of medicine. *Journal of the American Medical Association,* 268(17), 2420-2425.

Farley, J. and Geison, G.L. 1974. Science, politics, and spontaneous generation in nineteenth century France: the Pasteur Pouchet debate. *Bulletin of the History of Medicine,* 48, 161-198.

Farrell, M.H. and Farrell, P.M. 2003. Newborn screening for cystic fibrosis: ensuring more good than harm. *The Journal of Paediatrics,* 143, 707-712.

Farrell P.M. et al. 1997. Nutritional benefits of neonatal screening for cystic fibrosis. *New England Journal of Medicine,* 337(14), 963-969.

Farrell, P.M. et al. 2001. Early diagnosis of cystic fibrosis through neonatal screening prevents severe malnutrition and improves long-term growth. *Pediatrics,* 107(1), 1-13.

Farrell, P.M. et al. 2005. Evidence on improved outcomes with early diagnosis of cystic fibrosis through neonatal screening: enough is enough! *The Journal of Paediatrics*, 147(3), S30-36.

Fassin, D. 1996. *L'espace politique de la santé. Essai de généalogie.* Paris: PUF.

Fassin, D. 1998. Politique des corps et gouvernement des villes. La production locale de la santé publique, in *Les figures urbaines de la santé publique. Enquête sur des expériences locales,* edited by D. Fassin. Paris: La Découverte, 7-46.

Fassin, D. 1999. L'indicible et l'impensé: la 'question immigrée' dans les politiques du sida. *Sciences Sociales et Santé,* 17(4), 5-35.

Fassin, D. 2004. Public health as culture. The social construction of the childhood lead poisoning epidemic in France. *British Medical Bulletin,* 69, 167-177.

Fassin, D. 2007. *When bodies remember. Experiences and politic of AIDS in post-apartheid South Africa.* Berkeley, Los Angeles, London: University of California Press.

Fassin, D. 2009. Another politics of life is possible. *Theory, Culture & Society,* 26 (5), 44-60.

Fassin, D. and Bourdelais, P. (eds.) 2005. *Les constructions de l'intolérable. Etudes d'anthropologie et d'histoire sur les frontières de l'espace moral.* Paris: La Découverte.

Fassin, D. and Memmi, D. (eds.) 2004. *Le gouvernement des corps.* Paris: Editions de l'Ecole des hautes études en sciences sociales.

Featherstone, K. et al. 2005. Dysmorphology and the spectacle of the clinic. *Sociology of Health & Illness,* 27(5), 551-574.

Feuer, L.S. 1974. *Einstein and the conflict of generations in science.* New York: Basic Books.

Finkler, K. 2005. Family, kinship, memory and temporality in the age of the new genetics. *Social Science & Medicine,* 61, 1059-1071.

Foucault, M. 1980. *Power/Knowledge. Selected interviews and other writings 1972-1977 by Michel Foucault,* edited by C. Gordon. New York: Pantheon Books [1976].

Foucault, M. 1985. *The history of sexuality. The use of pleasure.* New York: Random House [1984].

Foucault, M. 1988. The political technology of individuals, in *Technology of the self. A seminar with Michel Foucault,* edited by P.H. Hutton, H. Gutman and L.H. Martin. Amherst: University of Massachusetts Press, 145-162.

Foucault, M. 1989. *Foucault live (Interviews, 1966-84),* edited by S. Lotringer. New York: Semiotext(e).

Foucault, M. 1998. *The history of sexuality. The will to knowledge.* London: Penguin [1976].

Foucault, M. 2001a. *Dits et écrits I, 1954-1975.* Paris: Gallimard [1994].

Foucault, M. 2001b. *Dits et écrits II, 1976-1988.* Paris: Gallimard [1994].

Foucault, M. 2003. *The birth of the clinic.* London: Routledge [1963].

Foucault, M. et al. 2001. *Power. The essential works of Michel Foucault, vol. 3.* New York: The New Press.

Fox, N.J. 1997. Space, sterility and surgery: circuits of hygiene in the operating theatre. *Social Science & Medicine*, 45(5), 649-657.

Fox, R.C. 1957. Training for uncertainty, in *The student physician*, edited by R.K. Merton, G. Reader and P.L. Kendall. Cambridge: Harvard University Press, 207-241.

Fox, R.C. 2000. Medical uncertainty revisited, in *The handbook of social studies in health and medicine,* edited by G.L. Albrecht, R. Fitzpatrick and S.C. Scrimshaw. London, Thousand Oaks, New Delhi: SAGE, 259-276.

Fox Keller, E. 2000. *The century of the gene.* Cambridge: Harvard University Press.

Frattini, M.-O. and Naiditch, M. 2004. Mucoviscidose, spécialisation en médecine et dépistage néonatal systématique. *Sciences Sociales et Santé*, 22(4), 61-71.

Fullwiley, D. 1998. Race, biologie et maladie: la difficile organisation des patients atteints de drépanocytose aux Etats-Unis. *Sciences Sociales et Santé*, 16(3), 129-157.

Gaudillière, J.-P. 2006. *La médecine et les sciences XIXᵉ-XXᵉ siècles.* Paris: La Découverte.

Gayon, J. 1997. Eugenics: an historical and philosophical schema. *Ludus Vitalis*, 5(8), 81-99.

Getz, L. and Kirkengen, A.L. 2003. Ultrasound screening in pregnancy: advancing technology, soft markers for fetal chromosomal aberrations, and unacknowledged ethical dilemmas. *Social Science & Medicine*, 56(10), 2045-2057.

Gilly, R., Barbier, Y. and Garcia, I. 1987. Le dépistage néonatal de la mucoviscidose. *Archives Françaises de Pédiatrie*, 44, 731-734.

Goffman, E. 1963. *Stigma.* Englewood Cliffs: Prentice-Hall.

Goldenberg, A.J. and Sharp, R. 2012. The ethical hazards and programmatic challenges of genomic newborn screening. *Journal of the American Medical Association*, 307(5), 461-462.

Good, B. 1994. *Medicine, rationality and experience.* Cambridge: Cambridge University Press.

Green, J. 2000. Epistemology, evidence and experience: evidence based health care in the work of Accident Alliances. *Sociology of Health & Illness*, 22(4), 453-476.

Grimes, D.A. and Schulz, K.F. 2002. Uses and abuses of screening tests. *Lancet*, 359(9309), 881-884.

Grob, R. 2008. Is my sick child healthy? Is my healthy child sick? Changing parental experiences of cystic fibrosis in the age of expanded newborn screening. *Social Science & Medicine*, 67, 1056-1064.

Grob, R. 2011. *Testing baby. The transformation of newborn screening, parenting, and policymaking.* New Brunswick, London: Rutgers University Press.

Gros, F. 1996. *Michel Foucault.* Paris: PUF.

Grossman, E. and Saurugger, S. 2006. *Les groupes d'intérêt. Action collective et stratégie de représentation.* Paris: Armand Colin.

Hacking, I. 1999. *The social construction of what?* Cambridge: Harvard University Press.

Hacking, I. 2005. Seminar 'Façonner les gens', Collège de France, Paris, Available at: http://www.college-de-france.fr/default/EN/all/historique/ian_hacking.htm

Hacking, I. 2006. *The taming of chance.* Cambridge: Cambridge University Press [1990].

Hassenteufel, P. et al. 1998. L'émergence problématique d'une nouvelle santé publique. Forums d'action publique et coalitions de projets à Rennes et à Brest, in *Les figures urbaines de la santé publique. Enquête sur des expériences locales,* edited by D. Fassin. Paris: La Découverte, 84-109.

Heath, D., Rapp, R. and Taussig, K.-S. 2004. Genetic citizenship, in *A companion to the anthropology of politics,* edited by D. Nugent and J. Vincent. Malden, Oxford, Victoria: Blackwell Publishing, 152-167.

Hedgecoe, A.M. 2003. Expansion and uncertainty: cystic fibrosis, classification and genetics. *Sociology of Health & Illness,* 25(1), 50-70.

Hedgecoe, A.M. 2005. 'At the point at which you can do something about it, then it becomes more relevant': informed consent in the pharmacogenetic clinic. *Social Science and Medicine,* 61(6), 1201-1210.

Heinemann, T. and Lemke, T. 2013. Suspect families: DNA kinship testing in German immigration policy. *Sociology,* in press.

Hilgartner, S. and Bosk, C.L. 1988. The rise and fall of social problems: a public arenas model. *American Journal of Sociology,* 94(1), 53-78.

Hindmarsh, R. and Prainsack, B. (eds.) 2010. *Genetic suspects. Global governance of forensic DNA profiling and databasing.* Cambridge: Cambridge University Press.

Illich, I. 1974. *Medical nemesis.* London: Calder & Boyars.

Jacob, M.-A. 2007. Form-made persons: consent forms as consent's blind spot. *Political and Legal Anthropology Review,* 30(2), 249-268.

Jacob, M.-A. and Riles, A. 2007. The new bureaucracies of virtues: introduction. *Political and Legal Anthropology Review,* 30(2), 181-191.

Johansson, E.E. et al. 1999. The meanings of pain: an exploration of women's descriptions of symptoms. *Social Science & Medicine,* 48(12), 1791-1802.

Kaufert, P.A. 2000. Screening the body: the pap smear and the mammogram, in *Living and working with the new medical technologies. Intersections of inquiry,* edited by M. Lock, A. Young and A. Cambrosio. Cambridge: Cambridge University Press, 165-183.

Keating, P. and Cambrosio, A. 2000. 'Real compared to what?': diagnosis leukemias and lymphomas, in *Living and working with the new medical technologies. Intersections of inquiry,* edited by M. Lock, A. Young and A. Cambrosio. Cambridge: Cambridge University Press, 103-134.

Keating, P. and Cambrosio, A. 2009. Who's minding the data? Data Monitoring Committees in clinical cancer trials. *Sociology of Health and Illness,* 31(3), 325-342.

214 *The Birth of a Genetics Policy*

Kelly, S.E. 2009. Choosing not to choose: reproductive responses of parents of children with genetic conditions or impairments. *Sociology of Health & Illness*, 31(1), 81-97.

Kelly, M. et al. 2010. Evidence based public health: a review of the experience of the National Institute of Health and Clinical Excellence (NICE) of developing public health guidance in England. *Social Science and Medicine*, 71(6), 1056-1062.

Kelly, M.P. and Field, D. 1996. Medical sociology, chronic illness and the body. *Sociology of Health & Illness*, 18(2), 241-257.

Kerr, A. 2000. (Re)constructing genetic disease: the clinical continuum between cystic fibrosis and male infertility. *Social Studies of Science*, 30(6), 847-894.

Kerr, A. 2005. Understanding genetic disease in a socio-historical context: a case-study of cystic fibrosis. *Sociology of Health & Illness*, 27(7), 873-896.

Kerr, A. and Cunningham-Burley, S. 2000. On ambivalence and risk: reflexive modernity and the new human genetics. *Sociology*, 34(2), 283-304.

Khoshnood, B. et al. 2006. Advances in medical technology and creation of disparities: the case of Down syndrome. *American Journal of Public Health*, 96(12), 2139-2144.

Kingdon, J.W. 1984. *Agendas, alternatives, and public policies.* Boston, Toronto: Little, Brown and Company.

Kleinman, A. and Hall-Clifford, R. 2009. Stigma: a social, cultural and moral process. *Journal of Epidemiology & Community Health*, 63(6), 418-419.

Knaapen, L. et al. 2010. Pragmatic evidence and textual arrangements: a case study of French clinical cancer guidelines. *Social Science and Medicine*, 71(4), 685-692.

Koch, L. 2004. The meaning of eugenics: reflections on the government of genetic knowledge in the past and the present. *Science in Context*, 17(3), 315-331.

Koch, L. and Stemerding, D. 1994. The sociology of entrenchment: a cystic fibrosis test for everyone? *Social Science & Medicine*, 39(9), 1211-1220.

Koch, L. and Svendsen, M.N. 2005. Providing solutions-defining problems: the imperative of disease prevention in genetic counselling. *Social Science & Medicine*, 60(4), 823-832.

Kunitz, S. 1974. Some notes on physiologic conditions as social problems. *Social Science & Medicine*, 8, 207-211.

Kunst, A. 1997. *Cross-national comparisons of socio-economic differences in mortality*. Rotterdam: Erasmus University Press.

Lambert, H. 2006. Accounting for EBM: notions of evidence in medicine. *Social Science & Medicine*, 62(11), 2633-2645.

Landsman, G. 2003. Emplotting children's lives: developmental delay vs. disability. *Social Science & Medicine*, 56(9), 1947-1960.

Larédo, P. and Kahane, B. 1998. Politique de recherche et choix organisationnels de l'Association française de lutte contre la mucoviscidose. *Sciences Sociales et Santé*, 16(3), 97-127.

Lascoumes, P. (ed.) 2005. Expertise et action publique. *Problèmes politiques et sociaux, La Documentation Française*, 912.

Latour, B. 1987. *Science in action: how to follow scientists and engineers through society.* Cambridge: Harvard University Press.

Latour, B. and Woolgar, S. 1979. *Laboratory life. The construction of scientific facts*. Princeton: Princeton University Press.

Lauritzen, S.O. and Sachs, L. 2001. Normality, risk and the future: implicit communication of threat in health surveillance. *Sociology of Health & Illness*, 23(4), 497-516.

Leclerc, A. et al. 2000. *Les inégalités sociales de santé.* Paris: La Découverte.

Lemke, T. 2004. Disposition and determinism. Genetic diagnostics in risk society. *The Sociological Review*, 52(4), 550-566.

Leplège, A. 2004. Qualité de vie (Mesures de la), in *Dictionnaire de la pensée médicale*, edited by D. Lecourt. Paris: PUF, 939-940.

Lindee, S. 2005. *Moments of truth in genetic medicine.* Baltimore: Johns Hopkins University Press.

Lippman, A. 1992. Led (astray) by genetic maps: the cartography of the human genome and health care. *Social Science & Medicine*, 35(12), 1469-1476.

Lock, M. 2000. Accounting for disease and distress: morals of the normal and abnormal, in *The handbook of social studies in health and medicine*, edited by G.L. Albrecht, R. Fitzpatrick and S.C. Scrimshaw. London, Thousand Oaks, New Delhi: SAGE, 259-276.

Lock, M. 2010. Dementia entanglements in a postgenomic era. *Science, Technology & Human Values*, 36(5), 685-703.

Lock, M. and Nguyen, V.-K. 2010. *An anthropology of biomedicine.* Malden, Oxford: Wiley-Blackwell.

Mahadeva, R. et al. 1998. Clinical outcome in relation to care in centres specialising in cystic fibrosis: cross sectional study. *British Medical Journal*, 316, 1771-1775.

Markovic, M., Manderson, L. and Quinn, M. 2004. Embodied changes and the search for gynecological cancer diagnosis. *Medical Anthropology Quarterly*, 18(3), 376-396.

Marks, H. 1997. *The progress of experiment: science and therapeutic reform in the United States, 1900-1990.* Cambridge: Cambridge University Press.

Marshall, E. 2001. Fast technology drives new world of newborn screening. *Science*, 294(5550), 2272-2274.

Mayell, S.J. et al. 2009. A European consensus for the evaluation and management of infants with an equivocal diagnosis following newborn screening for cystic fibrosis. *Journal of Cystic Fibrosis*, 8, 71-78.

Mény, Y. and Thoenig, J.-C. 1989. *Politiques publiques.* Paris: PUF.

Mérelle, M.E. et al. 2001a. Newborn screening for cystic fibrosis (Cochrane Review). *The Cochrane Library*, 3, CD001402.

Mérelle, M.E. et al. 2001b. Influence of neonatal screening and centralized treatment on long-term clinical outcome and survival of CF patients. *European Respiratory Journal*, 18, 306-315.

Mérelle, M.E., Meerman, G.J. and Dankert-Roelse, J.E. 1999. The influence of treatment at a specialized centre on the course of the disease of patients with cystic fibrosis, in *Neonatal screening for cystic fibrosis*, edited by G. Travert. Caen: Presses Universitaires de Caen, 301-324.

Miller, F.A. et al. 2005. Ruling in and ruling out: implications of molecular genetic diagnosis for disease classification. *Social Science and Medicine*, 61(12), 2536-2545.

Mischler, E.H. et al. 1998. Cystic fibrosis newborn screening: impact on reproductive behavior and implications for genetic counselling. *Pediatrics*, 102, 44-52.

MMWR Recommendations and Reports. 1997. Newborn screening for cystic fibrosis: a paradigm for public health genetics policy development. 46 (RR-16), 1-24.

MMWR Recommendations and Reports. 2004. Newborn screening for cystic fibrosis: evaluation of benefits and risks and recommendations for state newborn screening programs. 53 (RR-13), 1-37.

Moreira, T. 2005. Diversity in clinical guidelines: the role of repertoires of evaluation. *Social Science & Medicine*, 60(9), 1975-1985.

Moreira, T. 2007. Entangled evidence: knowledge making in systematic reviews in healthcare. *Sociology of Health & Illness*, 29(2), 180-197.

Munck, A., Houssin, E. and Roussey, M. 2008. Le dépistage néonatal de la mucoviscidose: le point depuis sa généralisation en France. *Archives Françaises de Pédiatrie*, 15, 741-743.

Mykhalovskiy, E. and Weir, L. 2004. The problem of evidence-based medicine: directions for social science. *Social Science & Medicine*, 59(5), 1059-1069.

Nelkin, D. and Lindee, S. 1994. *The DNA mystique. The gene as a cultural icon.* New-York: W.H. Freeman and Company.

Niewöhner, J. 2011. Epigenetics: embedded bodies and the molecularisation of the milieu. *BioSocieties*, 6(3), 279-298.

Novas, C. and Rose, N. 2000. Genetic risk and the birth of the somatic individual. *Economy and Society*, 29(4), 485-513.

Nutbeam, D. 2008. The evolving concept of health literacy. *Social Science & Medicine*, 67(12), 2072-2078.

Paillet, A. 2000. D'où viennent les interrogations morales ? Les usages rhétoriques des innovations par les pédiatres réanimateurs français. *Sciences Sociales et Santé*, 18(2), 43-66.

Parens, E. and Asch, A. 2000. *Prenatal testing and disability rights.* Washington: Georgetown University Press.

Paul, D.B. 1994. Is human genetics disguised eugenics?, in *Genes and human self-knowledge: historical and philosophical reflections on modern genetics,* edited by F.W. Robert, C.L. Susan and E. Fales. Iowa City: University of Iowa Press, 67-83.

Petersen, A. 2006. The best experts: the narratives of those who have a genetic condition. *Social Science & Medicine*, 63(1), 32-42.

Petryna, A. 2002. *Life exposed: biological citizens after Chernobyl*. Princeton: Princeton University Press.

Pharo, P. 2004. Présentation. *L'Année Sociologique*, 54, 321-325.

Pinell, P. 2004a. Mouvement associatif, in *Dictionnaire de la pensée médicale*, edited by D. Lecourt. Paris: PUF, 762-765.

Pinell, P. 2004b. Pédiatrie. Le processus de spécialisation de la pédiatrie française (XIXᵉ-XXᵉ siècles), in *Dictionnaire de la pensée médicale*, edited by D. Lecourt. Paris: PUF, 853-857.

Popper, K.R. 1963. *Conjectures and refutations: the growth of scientific knowledge*. London: Routledge and Kegan Paul.

Press, N. and Browner, C.H. 1997. Why women say yes to prenatal diagnosis. *Social Science & Medicine*, 45(7), 979-989.

Rabeharisoa, V. 2003. The struggle against neuromuscular diseases in France and the emergence of the 'partnership model' of patient organisation. *Social Science & Medicine*, 57(11), 2127-2136.

Rabeharisoa, V. and Callon, M. 1999. *Le pouvoir des malades. L'Association Française contre les Myopathies et la recherche*. Paris: Editions de l'Ecole des mines.

Rabinow, P. (ed.) 1984. *The Foucault reader: an introduction to Foucault's thought*. New York: Pantheon Books.

Rabinow, P. 1996. *Essays on the anthropology of reason*. Princeton: Princeton University Press.

Rabinow, P. 1999. *French DNA*. Chicago: University of Chicago Press.

Raffle, A.E. 2001. Information about screening. Is it to achieve high uptake or to ensure informed choice? *Health Expectations*, 4(2), 92-98.

Rapp, R. 1999. *Testing the women, testing the foetus: the social impact of amniocentesis in America*. New York: Routledge.

Rapp, R. and Ginsburg, F.D. 2001. Enabling disability: rewriting kinship, reimaging citizenship. *Public Culture*, 13(3), 533-556.

Rapp, R. and Ginsburg, F.D. 2003. Standing at the crossroads of genetic testing: new eugenics, disability consciousness, and women's work. Available at: http://www.gene-watch.org/genewatch/articles/15-1crossroads.html.

Remennick, L. 2006. The quest for the perfect baby: why do Israeli women seek prenatal genetic testing? *Sociology of Health & Illness*, 28(1), 21-53.

Richardson, J.C., Nio Ong, B. and Sim, J. 2007. Experiencing chronic widespread pain in a family context: giving and receiving practical and emotional support. *Sociology of Health & Illness*, 29(3), 347-345.

Rose, G. 1985. Sick individuals and sick populations. *International Journal of Epidemiology*, 14, 32-38.

Rose, N. 1996. The death of the social? Re-figuring the territory of government. *Economy and Society*, 25(3), 327-356.

Rose, N. 2001. The politics of life itself. *Theory, Culture & Society,* 18(6), 1-30.

Rose, N. 2005. Will biomedicine transform society? The Clifford Barclay lecture, February 2nd 2005. Available at: http://www2.lse.ac.uk/PublicEvents/pdf/20050202-WillBiomedicine-NikRose.pdf

Rose, N. 2007. *The politics of life itself. Biomedicine, power and subjectivity in the twenty-first century*. Princeton: Princeton University Press.

Rose, N. 2008. The value of life: somatic ethics and the spirit of biocapital. *Daedalus*, 36-48.

Roth, W.-M. 2005. Making classification (at) work: ordering practices in science. *Social Studies of Science*, 35(4), 581-621.

Scarry, E. 1985. *The body in pain. The making and unmaking of the world*. New York: Oxford University Press.

Scotet, V. et al. 2012. Evidence for decline in the incidence of cystic fibrosis: a 35-year observational study in Brittany, France. *Orphanet Journal of Rare Diseases,* 7, 14.

Singer, M. 1995. Beyond the ivory tower: critical praxis in medical anthropology. *Medical Anthropology Quarterly*, 9(1), 80-106.

Social Studies of Science. 2008. *Special issue: race, genetics, and disease*, 38(5).

Spector, M. and Kitsuse, J.I. 1977. *Constructing social problems*. Menlo Park: Benjamin/Cummings Publishing Company.

Strauss, A. 1961. Professions in process. *American Journal of Sociology*, 66(4), 325-334.

Strauss, A. 1975. *Chronic illness and the quality of life*. St. Louis: C.V. Mosby Company.

Strauss, A. et al. 1985. *Social organization of medical work*. Chicago: University of Chicago Press.

Taussig, K.-S., Rapp, R. and Heath, D. 2005. Flexible eugenics: technologies of the self in the age of genetics, in *Anthropologies of modernity*, edited by J.X. Inda. Malden, Oxford, Victoria: Blackwell Publishing, 194-212.

Thauvin-Robinet, C. et al. 2009. The very low penetrance of cystic fibrosis for the R117H mutation: a reappraisal for genetic counselling and newborn screening. *Journal of Medical Genetics,* 46(11), 752-758.

Timmermans, S. and Angell, A. 2001. Evidence-based medicine, clinical uncertainty, and learning to doctor. *Journal of Health and Social Behavior*, 42, 342-359.

Timmermans, S. and Buchbinder, M. 2010. Patients-in-waiting: living between sickness and health in the genomics era. *Journal of Health and Social Behavior,* 51, 408-423.

Timmermans, S. and Haas, S. 2008. Towards a sociology of disease. *Sociology of Health & Illness*, 30(5), 659-676.

Turner, B.S. 2000. Changing concepts of health and illness, in *The handbook of social studies in health and medicine*, edited by G.L. Albrecht, R. Fitzpatrick and S.C. Scrimshaw. London, Thousand Oaks, New Delhi: SAGE, 9-23.

Van Hoyweghen, I., Horstman, K. and Schepers, R. 2006. Making the normal deviant: the introduction of predictive medicine in life insurance. *Social Science & Medicine*, 63(5), 1225-1235.

Vailly, J. 2004. Une politique de santé 'a priori'. Le dépistage néonatal de la mucoviscidose en Bretagne. *Sciences Sociales et Santé*, 22(4), 35-60.

Vailly, J. 2006. Genetic screening as a technique of government: the case of neonatal screening for cystic fibrosis in France. *Social Science & Medicine*, 63(12), 3092-3101.

Vailly, J. 2007. Dépister les nouveau-nés: évolutions, débats et consensus. *Médecine/Sciences*, 23(3), 323-326.

Vailly, J. 2008. The expansion of abnormality and the biomedical norm: neonatal screening, prenatal diagnosis and cystic fibrosis in France. *Social Science & Medicine*, 66(12), 2532-2543.

Vailly, J. 2011. *Naissance d'une politique de la génétique. Dépistage, biomédecine, enjeux sociaux*. Paris: PUF.

Vailly, J. 2013. Genetics, in *Encyclopaedia of health, illness, behavior, and society*, edited by W.C. Cockerham, R. Dingwall and S. Quah. Malden, Oxford: Wiley-Blackwell, in press.

Vailly, J. and Ensellem, C. 2010. Informing populations, governing subjects: the practices of screening for a genetic disease in France, in *Assessing life: on the organisation of genetic testing*, edited by B. Wieser and W. Berger. München, Wien: Profil, 225-253.

Vailly, J., Niewöhner, J. and Kehr, J. 2011. Introduction. Une question vitale. Connaître, protéger, exposer la vie, in *De la vie biologique à la vie sociale. Approches sociologiques et anthropologiques,* edited by J. Vailly, J. Kehr and J. Niewöhner. Paris: La Découverte, 9-25.

Vassy, C. 2006. From a genetic innovation to mass health programmes: the diffusion of Down's syndrome prenatal screening and diagnostic techniques in France. *Social Science & Medicine*, 63(8), 2041-2051.

Ville, I. 2011. Disability policies and perinatal medicine: the difficult conciliation of two fields of intervention on disability. *ALTER European Journal of Disability Research,* 5, 16-25.

Vinck, D. 1995. *Sociologie des sciences.* Paris: Armand Colin.

Vinck, D. 2010. *The sociology of scientific work.* Cheltenham, Northampton: Edward Elgar Publishing.

Washer, P. and Joffe, H. 2006. The 'hospital superbug': social representations of MRSA. *Social Science & Medicine*, 63(8), 2141-2152.

Waters, D.L. et al. 1999. Clinical outcomes of newborn screening for cystic fibrosis. *Archives of Disease in Childhood Fetal & Neonatal Edition*, 80, F1-F7.

Weber, M. 1968. *Economy and society. An outline of interpretive sociology.* New York: Bedminster Press.

West, S.E.H. et al. 2002. Respiratory infections with *Pseudomonas aeruginosa* in children with cystic fibrosis. Early detection by serology and assessment of risk factors. *Journal of the American Medical Association,* 287(22), 2958-2967.

Wilfond, B.S. et al. 2005. Balancing benefits and risks for cystic fibrosis newborn screening: implications for policy decisions. *The Journal of Paediatrics,* 147(3 Suppl.), S109-113.

Williams, C. 2006. Dilemmas in fetal medicine: premature application of technology or responding to women's choice? *Sociology of Health & Illness,* 28(1), 1-20.

Williams, C. et al. 2005. Women as moral pioneers? Experiences of first trimester antenatal screening. *Social Science & Medicine,* 61(9), 1983-1992.

Wilson, J. and Jungner, G. 1968. Principles and practice of screening for disease. Public Health Papers, World Health Organization.

Wood, M., Ferlie, E. and Fitzgerald, L. 1998. Achieving clinical behaviour change: a case of becoming indeterminate. *Social Science & Medicine,* 47(11), 1729-1738.

Young, B. et al. 2002. Parenting in a crisis: conceptualising mothers of children with cancer. *Social Science & Medicine,* 55(10), 1835-1847.

Documents

AFDPHE. 1999. Proposition d'un programme national de dépistage néonatal de la mucoviscidose. Rapport de l'AFDPHE et des membres du Groupe de travail. Paris.

AFDPHE. 2001a. Dépister pour des enfants en bonne santé. Le dépistage néonatal. Guide pratique pour les professionnels de santé. Paris: AFDPHE et Groupe de travail sur l'information.

AFDPHE. 2001b. 3 jours, l'âge du dépistage. Paris: AFDPHE, Assurance maladie – Sécurité sociale, Ministère de l'emploi et de la solidarité.

AFDPHE. 2004. Le dépistage néonatal de la mucoviscidose en France. Statistiques nationales 2002-2003. *La Dépêche,* 50.

Agence de la biomédecine. 2010. Rapport annuel. Bilan des activités. Saint-Denis.

CCNE. 2004. Avis 83. Le dépistage prénatal généralisé de la mucoviscidose.

Club Mucoviscidose régional. 1989-2002. 35 comptes rendus de réunions.

Gueganton, L., Rault, G. and De Braekeleer, M. 2004. Evaluation des procédures d'annonce du diagnostic de la mucoviscidose, de l'impact psychologique et de l'adaptation parentale. Fondation de France et Fondation Centre-Hélio-marin de Roscoff.

HAS. 2009. Etat des lieux en santé publique. Le dépistage néonatal systématique de la mucoviscidose en France : état des lieux et perspectives après 5 ans de fonctionnement.

Laurent-Seguin, O. 1999. *Un cri d'espoir. Le combat d'une mère contre la mucoviscidose.* Paris: Le Pré aux Clercs.

ONM. 2001. Rapport sur la situation de la mucoviscidose en 1999. Paris: Observatoire national de la mucoviscidose.

ONM. 2004. Rapport sur la situation de la mucoviscidose en 2001. Paris: Observatoire national de la mucoviscidose.

Proposition d'une étude pilote. 2002. Dépistage de la mutation F508del en début de deuxième trimestre de grossesse. Estimation du risque d'attendre un enfant atteint de mucoviscidose. CHU de Poitiers.

Scotet, V. 2001. Epidémiologie moléculaire de la mucoviscidose en Bretagne. Thèse de Doctorat en sciences de la vie et de la santé. Brest: Faculté de Médecine de Brest.

Index

(ab)normal or (ab)normality, 10, 16, 18, 46,
    72, 93, 98, 100, 119-129, 131, 133-
    134, 140-142, 149-150, 153, 157,
    171, 173, 175, 179-181, 189, 202
    See also norm
abortion, 35, 139, 142, 186, 192
announcement, 24, 172-174
anxiety, 5, 101, 105, 109, 111, 113, 116,
    125-127, 134, 141, 178-179, 182,
    191, 201-202
autonomy, bioethical principle, 89
    of clinicians, 104
    of patient organizations, 99
    of patients, 87, 111
    of subjects, 88
    parental, 89
    See also responsibility or responsible

benefits, 10-12, 18, 21, 21n1, 42, 46, 48-
    50, 53, 64, 66-70, 72-73, 75-79,
    83-84, 89, 92, 99-100, 102, 111-
    112, 118, 127, 150, 155, 171, 197,
    200, 204
bias, 49, 59, 76-78, 80-83, 151
bioethics, 3, 31, 34n7, 54, 108
bioidentity, 38, 203
biolegitimacy, 37
biological life, 8, 18, 144, 146, 149-150,
    154-155, 164, 168, 201, 203
    See also social life and life
biomedicalization, 6-7, 19, 201-202
    See also medicalization
biopolitics, 7, 9, 194
    biopolitical practices or figure, 195,
        204
    biopolitization, 38
    See also biopower and life
biopower, 7-9
    See also biopolitics and power
biosociality, 38, 160, 168, 203

blackbox, 68, 70
body, physical or medicalized, 5, 7, 9, 145-
    147, 151, 154, 160, 173, 198
    social, 116
borderline or mild forms, 13-14, 77, 113,
    121-122, 125, 127-130, 131n2,
    132-133, 136, 138, 141-143, 148,
    163, 185, 197, 200, 202
bureaucracy, ethical, 112
    of virtue, 116

carrier, 31, 38, 55, 92, 97,131, 134-135,
    139, 141, 146, 181
    germ, 155
    See also heterozygote
case, 41, 63, 65, 67, 102, 107, 135-136,
    150
    patient cases, 93 100
    case-oriented approach, 101, 131-133,
        138, 140, 142, 199
cautious, attitude, 2, 75, 77, 84, 132, 142,
    180
certainty, attitude of, 66, 70, 85
    concerning the disease, 121, 140
    of genetic tests, 88
    See also uncertainty
choice, 1, 9, 12, 18, 33, 42, 54, 84, 87-89,
    111-112, 115, 129, 144, 150, 169,
    184, 186, 190, 200
chronic, illness or disease, 1, 11, 145-148,
    152, 164-165, 167, 176
    fatigue, 167
    infection, 72, 152, 156-158, 161
    pancreatitis, 135
citizenship, 88-90, 99, 199
classification, 122, 125, 127-128, 130-131,
    135, 184
    of levels of evidence, 79
    of types of language, 78
coalition, 22, 35-36, 42

compassion, 2, 6, 39, 43, 63, 200
  compassionate, 34, 37, 62, 123, 203,
    205
complexity, 2, 83, 116, 122
condition of possibility, 6, 43, 53
configuration, 27, 30, 35, 90, 116, 185,
    200, 205
consent, 9-10, 12, 14, 54-55, 87-89, 103-
    116, 125, 170, 173, 190, 197, 199-
    200, 203, 205
construction or constructed reality, 22, 198
  constructionism or constructionist, 22-
    23, 25, 37, 39-44, 48, 51
  cultural, 120
  of evidence, 61, 168, 199
  of the medicalized body, 151
  of the research object, 16
  social, 22-23, 25, 38, 39, 41-42, 48, 51,
    59, 63, 64, 68, 197-198
conviction, 17, 34, 61, 65-68, 78, 84, 117-
    118, 197, 200
criteria for newborn screening, 10, 69, 195
  public health, 54
critique, 8, 16-17, 74, 85, 169, 189
cross contamination, 73
  See also infection

death, 1, 2, 7, 24, 53, 80-82, 85, 127-128,
    147, 151, 153-154, 160, 167-168,
    203
detachment, 16-17
  See also involvement
determinism, 2, 87
diagnosis, 48, 71-72, 101, 113, 115, 117,
    119, 121, 126-127, 131, 131n2,
    153, 167, 170-173, 175-177, 186,
    189-191, 202
  early, 61-62, 65-67, 115, 141
  misdiagnosis, 65, 170, 176, 201, 204
  over-diagnosis, 5, 101, 141
  pre-diagnosis, 173
  pre-implantation diagnosis, 144
  See also prenatal diagnosis
disparity, 7, 88, 159
  See also inequality
doubt, 44, 50, 66, 70-71, 75, 84, 100, 129,
    179-181, 197-198, 200

emotion, 18, 32-33, 37, 61, 66, 81, 85, 168,
    199
  emotional experience, 161
  emotional involvement, 16
  emotional relations, 12
  emotionally charged, 152
emplotment, 152
epidemiologist, 38, 58, 68, 79, 93, 101
epidemiology, 7, 27, 38, 58
  epidemiological foundation, 22
  epidemiological study or perspective,
    26, 38-39, 47, 51, 62-64, 68, 80,
    114, 131, 161
epigenetics, 2
episteme, 27, 58
epistemic, attitude or framework, 18, 60-
    62, 69, 100
  data, 52
  tension, 84
  turning point, 50
eradication of the disease, 184, 185, 192,
    194-195
ethical government, 145, 157, 185, 189
  ethical practice, 69, 145, 194, 200
  ethical or moral subject, 145, 185, 195,
    200
  ethical substance, 145, 192, 200
  ethical work, 145, 157, 200
ethics, 9, 31, 46, 75, 97, 99, 109, 190, 192,
    200, 205
  morality and, 31
  See also ethos
ethos, 34, 46
  See also ethics
eugenics, 33-34, 55, 63, 69, 87, 99, 184,
    188-190, 192, 194-195, 204-205
evidence, 16, 18-19, 58-61, 64, 66, 68, 70-
    71, 73-75, 78-80, 82-85, 91, 100,
    120, 155, 168, 198-199, 202
  level of, 79, 85, 117-118
evidence-based medicine or EBM, 50, 59-
    61, 59n3, 64, 68, 70-71, 74-76, 79,
    83, 85, 198-199
experience, 16-17, 30, 32, 35, 46, 59-60,
    65-68, 70, 84-85, 87, 89, 94, 100,
    102-103, 115, 119, 129, 136-138,
    144-147, 161, 168-169, 173, 177-

179, 181, 183-184, 189, 193, 195, 199

false negative, 49, 156, 175-176, 192
false positive, 49-50, 100, 170, 177, 192
field of experience, 9, 12, 55, 84, 90, 197
freedom, 8, 33-34, 103, 116, 164, 186, 199-200, 205

genetic counselling, 32-33, 45-46, 69, 88-89, 134, 136-138, 141, 184-185, 188, 193, 200, 205
geneticization, 87
genetic test or testing, 3, 49, 55, 69, 88-89, 94, 109-110, 112, 114, 123-125, 128, 141, 153, 183, 192, 195, 197, 204-205
germ, 72-74, 83, 100, 147-148, 150, 153-157, 159-161
government, 8-9, 12, 21, 57, 64, 90, 93, 99, 101, 103-104, 109, 116-117, 145, 157, 168, 182, 185, 189, 199, 200, 203-204
    governmentality, 16, 18-19
    See also ethical government

heterozygote, 32,69, 124, 141, 143, 180-185, 197
    screening of, 31-35, 55, 69, 190, 200, 205
    See also carrier
hope, 2-4, 11, 26, 63, 87, 90, 153, 205
hygiene, 73-74, 148-150, 161, 163, 167, 174, 198

iatrogenic disease, 74
    iatrogenesis, 74
immuno-reactive trypsin or IRT, 48-50, 109, 122-126, 135, 177
individual perspective, 5-7, 18, 23, 27, 33, 40, 59, 73, 88-90, 99-100, 103-104, 108-109, 111, 115-118, 122, 131-133, 137, 141, 185, 194, 199-200, 202, 205
    action, 15
    individualizing the space, 156
    sum of choices, 184
    See also population

inequality, 6, 8, 19, 119, 146, 155, 161-163, 167-168, 198
    See also disparity
infection, 11, 18, 66-67, 72-74, 81, 83, 146, 150, 152-156, 158-163, 166, 168, 176, 198
    cross infection, 115, 159, 168, 198, 203
    See also cross contamination
interdisciplinary approach, 15, 202
interest, 8, 16, 48, 50, 60, 105, 107, 133
    community or coalition of, 35-36
    corporatist or interest group, 44,90, 97-98
    parents', 10, 106
    professional, 17, 79, 105-106
    public, 42
involvement, 13n8, 16, 44, 92, 164, 171-172
    See also detachment

knot, philosophical or sociological, 12, 116
knowledge, 2-3, 6, 9-10, 12, 15-18, 23, 26-27, 43, 46, 51, 53, 55, 57, 60-61, 64-66, 68, 70, 76, 80-81, 84-88, 94, 100-101, 104, 107, 123, 127, 131, 136, 140, 142, 165, 167, 182, 191, 197, 199, 202, 205
    form of, 9, 26, 53, 123, 168, 197

legitimacy, 55, 108, 194
    of knowledge or scientific, 61, 63, 71, 79, 81, 85, 107
    of screening or prenatal diagnosis, 10, 34, 39, 40-41, 53, 140, 185, 193-195, 200
    legitimate or legitimizing actors or centre, 7, 22, 28, 30, 44-45, 91-92, 94-95, 105, 107, 140, 199
    See also biolegitimacy
life, 2, 4, 6-8, 10, 12, 18-19, 35, 53, 64, 72, 77, 81, 85, 121, 128, 130, 137-138, 140, 143-154, 161, 163, 167, 169, 171-177, 183, 187-189, 191, 194-195, 201, 203
    life expectancy or lifespan, 1, 11-12, 51, 63, 72, 74, 79-85, 96-97, 102, 131, 151, 168, 170, 175, 190-191, 197, 199, 201

life itself, 7
life sciences, 6, 15
lifestyle, 166, 167
life-threatening, 1, 66
mental life, 167-168
politics or policy of, 9
prospect of; real-life, 32
See also biological life, social life,
biopolitics and biopower
living condition, 8, 19, 32, 146, 161-162,
164, 167-168, 198

market, 3, 48, 105, 204
media, 2, 4-5, 8, 26, 36, 38, 40-43, 67-68,
83, 107, 203
medicalization, 5-6, 8-9, 74, 111
medicalized body, 151
See also biomedicalization
molecularization, 2
moral space, 12, 19, 120, 201, 204-205
mutation, R117H, 124, 131, 135, 138, 141
ΔF508, 124, 190

norm, 12, 18, 88, 117, 120-122, 133-134,
138, 142-143, 175, 192
See also (ab)normal or (ab)normality

object, 9, 16, 31, 51, 54, 87-88,133, 157,
172
See also objectivation and subject
objectivation or objectivizing, 63, 109,
147, 199
See also object and subjectivation
origin, 2, 10n6, 11, 16, 38, 54, 54n14, 113,
121, 124, 154, 161-163, 167

patient organization or patient advocacy
group, 2, 4-5, 13, 13n8, 18, 23-24,
27-28, 30, 35-36, 38, 40, 42-
43, 46-47, 80-81, 89-90, 94-99,
106-107, 116-117, 150, 160, 168,
199-200, 203
phenylketonuria, 10n6, 44-45, 71, 91-92,
103, 191, 193
policy, 12-13, 17-18, 21-23, 25, 27, 29, 34-
35, 38-40, 42-44, 50, 52-53, 57, 68,
80n8, 85, 90, 95, 99, 101, 106, 108,
116, 141, 169, 183, 197, 200, 202

health, 5-6, 19, 21-22, 25n4, 30, 35, 41,
43, 50, 59, 72, 93, 107, 108n1
strategies, 8
public, 9, 21, 55, 85
techniques or technology, 100-101, 132
See also political and public action
political, 3-4, 8, 12, 15, 18, 34, 39-40, 42-
44, 47-48, 50, 52-53, 58, 61, 86-90,
93, 96-100, 104, 107, 116-118,
120, 132, 161, 167, 194, 197, 199-
200, 202-205
scientists or science, 26, 34, 47
space, 12, 19, 201, 204-205
strategies, 7-8, 12, 143
structures, 8, 16-17
technique, 18
See also policy and public action
population, 2, 4-7, 10, 10n6, 11, 18, 25-27,
33, 38-39, 43, 48-49, 51, 53-54,
59-61, 75, 77, 82, 89, 91, 97-101,
104, 107, 109, 111-113, 116-119,
121, 123-125, 127, 132, 135, 137,
141, 162, 181-184, 194, 197, 199-
201, 204-205
See also individual perspective
power, 7-9, 18, 37, 42, 58, 61, 65, 86-89,
92-93, 96, 99-101, 104-108, 116-
117, 132, 181, 199-200, 205
effects of, 104-105, 108, 119
microphysics of, 8
over life, 7
relations, 8, 15, 17-18, 47, 90-91, 94,
101, 116, 161, 199
strategies, 107, 199
See also biopower
predisposition, genetic, 1, 3, 5
prenatal diagnosis, 13-14, 18, 27, 31, 35-
36, 62-63, 68-69, 88, 99, 119, 122,
135-136, 138-144, 142n6, 146,
161, 168-169, 181-183, 185, 187-
188, 191-195, 200-201, 205
prenatal screening, 31, 33, 111, 184, 186,
188-194, 197
pressure group, 47, 96-99, 117, 199
prevention or preventing, 5-6, 9, 13, 29,
33, 45, 53, 59, 65, 71, 92, 98, 101,
108, 141, 185, 193-195, 198, 201

problematization or social problem, 2, 5-6, 22-23, 25-26, 34, 36-37, 39, 41-42, 44, 47, 51, 53-54, 63, 97, 183, 197-199

public action, 21-22, 26, 43-44, 53-55, 58, 61, 87, 199
See also policy and political

quality life, 12, 18-19, 143, 146-148, 150-151, 154, 161, 166-167, 169-172, 177, 181-182, 191-192, 194, 201

quality of life, 2, 18, 67, 111, 115, 140, 143-146, 150-151, 154, 161, 170, 191, 201

randomized controlled trial or RCT, 59, 59n2, 71, 75, 83, 84-85, 197

rare disease, illness or condition, 2, 10-11, 39, 44, 53-54, 63-65, 92, 98, 102, 108, 108n1, 110, 111, 119, 131, 200

rare mutation, 134

rationalist or rationality, 51, 57-59, 61, 66, 198

reassure, 3, 93, 126, 132, 148, 165, 177, 180, 186

refutation or refutability, 74, 179

relativism, 58

resistance, 8, 39, 51, 59, 74, 103-104, 157

responsibility or responsible, 5-6, 13, 30, 33, 44-45, 52, 53n13, 54, 74, 75, 80-81, 84, 88-89, 94, 103, 105, 108, 111-112, 118, 160-161, 185
See also autonomy

risk, 3-6, 11, 31, 33, 35, 42, 49, 67, 69, 73-74, 77, 84, 87-89, 98-100, 102, 111-112, 114-116, 119, 132-140, 142-144, 149-150, 154-155, 158-160, 163, 166, 168, 176, 180-181, 183-184, 189-190, 192-194, 198, 203, 205

rumour, 18, 61, 81-82, 85

science or scientific, 3-4, 6-7, 12-13, 13n8, 14-16, 18, 21-23, 26-27, 29-30, 35, 47-48, 51, 53, 55, 57-61, 64, 66, 68-71, 74-75, 77-86, 89-90, 97, 131, 133, 141, 143, 190, 197-198, 202, 204

self-evidence or self-evident, 17, 25, 40, 43, 51, 53, 62, 64-65, 67-68, 113, 116, 198

semantic network, 18, 137, 146-147, 154, 181

sign, 53, 72, 84, 121, 127

social hypochondria, 126

social life, 18, 144-146, 148-150, 152, 154, 167, 201
See also biological life and life

solidarity, 2, 24n4, 40, 43, 160, 200, 203-204

space, 18, 21, 25n4, 29, 73, 78, 90, 99, 102, 106, 120, 146, 154, 156-157, 168, 177, 181-182, 190, 201, 204
public, 49, 67
tertiary spatialization, 160
See also moral and political space

statistics or statistical approach, 9, 27, 34, 39-40, 45, 50, 58, 60, 63-64, 75-76, 80, 85, 99, 123, 125-128, 132-133, 137, 151, 194, 197

stigma or stigmatization, 19, 146, 157, 160-161, 204

structure or structural constraints, 8, 15-16, 22, 26, 88, 108, 115, 155, 167, 194, 202

subject, 8-9, 18, 31, 87-91, 94, 96, 98, 104, 108, 114-117, 173, 197, 199, 205
legal, 54, 109, 113
See also object, ethical or moral subject and subjectivation

subjectivation, 88-89, 111, 113, 116, 199
See also subject and objectivation

suffer or suffering, 6, 13, 16, 22, 32-33, 35, 37, 40-41, 46, 48, 51, 53, 62, 65, 67, 71-72, 76, 80, 82, 94, 96, 98, 106-107, 123, 136, 144, 146-147, 151-152, 155, 161-164, 169-170, 172, 174-175, 177, 182, 184, 185, 195, 200-201, 203, 205

symptom, 51, 61-62, 65, 71-72, 101-102, 115, 121, 124-125, 128-129, 131, 134, 136, 138, 142-144, 146-148, 152-154, 157, 162, 173, 175, 177-178, 181-183, 202, 204
asymptomatic, 132, 135

sweat test or ST, 48, 51, 122, 126-128,
131-132, 134-135, 171, 173, 175,
177-183

technoscientific or technoscience, 6, 12,
48, 73, 141, 201
temporality, 121, 201
the 'other', 8, 155, 160-161, 168, 205
threshold of birth, 194-195, 201
threshold of screening, 123-124, 126, 177,
182, 200
timeframe, 101-102, 126-127, 169-170,
170n1, 172-174, 176-178, 180,
182, 202
treatment, 5, 10-11, 19, 24, 26, 45-46, 53,
59n2, 60-61, 63, 65-67, 71, 75-76,
77n6, 82, 84-85, 87, 89, 92-93, 97,
100, 102-103, 105-107, 112, 115,
122, 126, 143, 146-152, 154-155,
159, 162-167, 169-172, 176-177,

181, 183-184, 187, 191-192, 201-
202
true or truth, 9, 12, 18, 51, 57-60, 61, 64,
72, 75, 78-83, 85, 87, 106, 118,
131, 175, 198

uncertainty, 21n1, 60, 66, 70, 82, 85, 88,
111, 112, 121-122, 125, 128-129,
131, 136-138, 140-142, 144-145,
153, 168, 178-179, 198
attitude of uncertainty, 70, 140
See also certainty

well-being, 5-7, 107, 143-144, 146
window of opportunity, 34
words or wording, 24, 78, 81-82, 111, 125,
129, 131, 147, 178-179, 182
worry or worrying, 3, 49, 81, 111, 126,
130-131, 134, 158, 175, 177-180,
182, 201-202

For Product Safety Concerns and Information please contact our
EU representative GPSR@taylorandfrancis.com Taylor & Francis
Verlag GmbH, Kaufingerstraße 24, 80331 München, Germany